The Gift Nobody Wants

By Dr. Paul Brand and Philip Yancey

Fearfully and Wonderfully Made
In His Image

THE GIFT NOBODY WANTS

Dr. Paul Brand and Philip Yancey

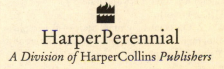

HarperPerennial

A Division of HarperCollins *Publishers*

•

Zondervan

A hardcover edition of this book was published in 1993 by HarperCollins Publishers under the title *Pain: The Gift Nobody Wants*.

First HarperPerennial edition published 1995.

Designed by C. Linda Dingler

The Library of Congress has catalogued the hardcover edition as follows:

Brand, Paul W.
    The gift nobody wants / Dr. Paul Brand and Philip Yancey. — 1st ed.
        p.   cm.
    Includes bibliographical references and index.
    ISBN 0-06-017020-4 (cloth)
1. Brand, Paul W.   2. Physicians—United States—Biography.   3. Physicians—Great Britian—Biography.   4. Physicians—India—Biography.   5. Leprosy—Biography.   6. Pain—Biography.
I. Yancey, Philip.   II. Title.
R154.B779A3   1993
610'.92—dc20
[B}   92-56225

ISBN 0-06-092552-3 (pbk.)
95 96 97 98 99 ❖/HC 10 9 8 7 6 5 4 3 2 1

For my mother,
Granny Brand

Contents

Part Three: Learning to Befriend Pain

Foreword

———◆———

C. Everett Koop, M.D., Sc.D.

Whenever I let my mind wander, and wonder who I would like to have been if I had not been born C. Everett Koop, the person who comes to mind most frequently is Paul Brand. I had known fragments of his life story for years. I had heard him speak on several occasions and was fascinated by his direct approach and gentle manner. Then, after I joined the Public Health Service as Surgeon General in 1981, I found that, in a sense, he worked for me.

Paul Brand was then directing part of the research for the oldest leprosy facility in the United States, the Gillis H. Long Hansen's Disease Center in Carville, Louisiana. There I came in close contact with him, watched him at work in the laboratory, witnessed his interaction with patients, and noted the strong and sincere mentoring relationship that developed between Paul Brand and his students, young and old, able and disabled. During my watch, he justified the enormous expenditure on research in leprosy, a disease that affects few in the United States, by demonstrating the applicability of that research to patients with diabetes, which affects 25 million.

What a joy to see Paul Brand in action! Humble when he could have been proud; kind above and beyond the need of the moment; gentle, to what might seem an unnecessary degree; and, finally, competent, with a capital *C*.

Shortly after I assumed my post as Surgeon General, my wife, Betty, had a joint replaced in her right hand with a marvelous

Teflon substitute. The surgery was excellent, but because of lack of attention to the nonglamorous, very essential bits of postoperative care, she ended up with a seriously disabled hand. She grieved for the loss of her hand for a short time, but since then she has managed well with a functional hand that can flex, although she cannot extend her fingers.

Paul Brand is as good a hand surgeon as there is in the world, so I took Betty to a Public Health Service meeting in Phoenix, Arizona, where I knew Paul would be on the program. I asked whether he would see her in consultation, which he willingly and immediately did. In watching his interaction with my wife and her hand, everything I'd heard and known about Paul Brand came into exquisite focus. His humility was evident from the start. His gentleness was unbelievable. His kindness in the assessment of her condition and in the advice he gave her was enough to make up for the bad news he had to deliver. And of course competence undergirded it all.

I used to teach medical students, "When you examine an abdomen, watch the patient's face, not his belly." What impressed me most was that Paul Brand, knowing what might hurt, kept his eyes trained on Betty's face. He apologized immediately if he hurt her. He never downplayed her discomfort, but imparted a kind of philosophy about pain that put it in a different realm.

I recount that story as a fitting introduction to this book because the book, while it conveys the story of a fascinating life, is mainly about one man's growing understanding of pain—its purpose, origins, and relief. As a surgeon, scholar, investigator, and philosopher gifted with rare insight, Paul Brand has lived and worked among the pain-afflicted. His extraordinary experiences have a strong thematic unity which allows him to present a rather startling perspective on pain. But before you think that might mean dull reading, there are wonderful helps in this book for each of us because Paul Brand opens the window onto new ways of looking at pain, and that translates into something of worth for you and me.

Paul Brand offers an opportunity to look at pain not as your enemy, but as your friend. I know a lot about pain—I have dealt with it all of my professional life—yet I gained a more profound understanding of it from this book. Were I a victim of chronic pain, I would probably call the knowledge gained a godsend.

I once gave Paul Brand the Surgeon General's Medallion, the highest honor a Surgeon General can bestow on a civilian. After finishing this book, I'd do it again, if I could. My esteem for Paul Brand is greater than ever.

Part One

—◆—

My Path into Medicine

1
Nightmares of Painlessness

⬦

He jests at scars who never felt a wound.
Shakespeare, *Romeo and Juliet*

Tanya was a four-year-old patient with dark, flashing eyes, curly hair, and an impish smile. I examined her at the national leprosy hospital in Carville, Louisiana, where her mother had brought her for a diagnosis. A cloud of tension hung in the air between the little girl and her mother, but I noticed that Tanya seemed eerily unafraid. She sat on the edge of the padded table and watched impassively as I began to remove blood-soiled bandages from her feet.

Testing her swollen left ankle, I found that the foot rotated freely, the sign of a fully dislocated ankle. I winced at the unnatural movement, but Tanya did not. I resumed unwrapping the bandages. "Are you sure you want these sores healed, young lady?" I said, trying to lighten the atmosphere in the room. "You might have to start wearing shoes again." Tanya laughed, and I thought it odd that she did not flinch or whimper as I removed the dressings next to her skin. She looked around the room with an expression of faint boredom.

When I unwrapped the last bandage, I found grossly infected ulcers on the soles of both feet. Ever so gently I probed the wounds, glancing at Tanya's face for some reaction. She showed none. The probe pushed easily through soft, necrotic tissue, and I could even see the white gleam of bare bone. Still no reaction from Tanya.

As I puzzled over the girl's injuries, her mother told me Tanya's story. "She seemed fine as an infant. A little high-spirited maybe, but perfectly normal. I'll never forget the first time I realized she had a serious problem. Tanya was seventeen or eighteen months old. Usually I kept her in the same room with me, but that day I left her alone in her playpen while I went to answer the phone. She stayed quiet, and so I decided to begin dinner. For a change she was playing happily by herself. I could hear her laughing and cooing. I smiled to myself, wondering what new mischief she had got into.

"A few minutes later I went into Tanya's room and found her sitting on the floor of the playpen, fingerpainting red swirls on the white plastic sheet. I didn't grasp the situation at first, but when I got closer I screamed. It was horrible. The tip of Tanya's finger was mangled and bleeding, and it was her own blood she was using to make those designs on the sheets.

"I yelled, 'Tanya, what happened!' She grinned at me, and that's when I saw the streaks of blood on her teeth. She had bitten off the tip of her finger and was playing in the blood."

Over the next few months, Tanya's mother told me, she and her husband tried in vain to convince their daughter that fingers must not be bitten. The toddler laughed at spankings and other physical threats, and indeed seemed immune to all punishment. To get her way she merely had to lift a finger to her teeth and pretend to bite, and her parents capitulated at once. The parents' horror turned to despair as wounds mysteriously appeared on one of Tanya's fingers after another.

Tanya's mother recounted this story in a flat, unemotional tone, as if she had resigned herself to the perverse plight of rearing a child with no instincts of self-preservation. To complicate matters, she was now a single mother: after a year of trying to cope with Tanya, her husband had deserted the family. "If you insist on keeping Tanya at home, then I quit," he had announced. "We've begotten a monster."

Tanya certainly didn't look like a monster. Apart from the sores on her feet and her shortened fingers she looked like a healthy four-year-old child. I asked about the foot injuries. "They began as soon as she learned to walk," the mother replied. "She'd step on a nail or thumbtack and not bother to pull it out. Now I check her feet at the end of every day, and often I discover a new wound or open sore. If she twists an ankle, she doesn't limp, and so it twists again and again. An orthopedic specialist told me she's permanently damaged the joint. If we wrap her feet for protection, sometimes in a fit of anger she'll tear off the bandages. Once she ripped open a plaster cast with her bare fingers."

Tanya's mother had come to me on the orthopedist's recommendation. "I've heard your leprosy patients have foot problems like this," she said. "Does my daughter have leprosy? Can you heal her hands and feet?" She wore the helpless, plaintive expression I had often seen on the parents of young patients, the expression that tugs at a doctor's heart. I sat down and gently tried to explain Tanya's condition.

Alas, I could offer little hope or comfort. I would do further tests, but it seemed apparent that Tanya suffered from a rare genetic defect known informally as "congenital indifference to pain." She was healthy in every respect but one: she did not feel pain. Nerves in her hands and feet transmitted messages about changes in pressure and temperature—she felt a kind of tingling when she burned herself or bit a finger—but these carried no hint of unpleasantness. Tanya lacked any mental construct of pain. She rather enjoyed the tingling sensations, especially when they produced such dramatic reactions in others.

"We can get these wounds healed," I said, "but Tanya has no built-in warning system to defend her from further injury. Nothing will improve until Tanya understands the problem and consciously begins to protect herself."

Seven years later I received a telephone call from Tanya's mother in St. Louis. Tanya, now eleven, was living a pathetic existence in an institution. She had lost both legs to amputation: she had refused to wear proper shoes and that, coupled with her failure to limp or to shift weight when standing (because she felt no discomfort), had eventually put intolerable pressure on her joints. Tanya had also lost most of her fingers. Her elbows were constantly dislocated. She suffered the effects of chronic sepsis from ulcers on her hands and amputation stumps. Her tongue was lacerated and badly scarred from her nervous habit of chewing it.

A monster, her father had called her. Tanya was no monster, only an extreme example—a human metaphor, really—of life without pain.

Without Warning

Tanya's particular problem occurs rarely, but such conditions as leprosy, diabetes, alcoholism, multiple sclerosis, nerve disorders, and spinal cord injury can also bring about the strangely hazardous state of insensitivity to pain. Ironically, while most of us seek out pharmacists and doctors in search of relief from pain, these people live in constant peril due to pain's *absence*.

I first learned about painlessness while working with leprosy, a disease that afflicts more than 12 million people worldwide. Leprosy has long provoked a fear bordering on hysteria, mainly because of the horrible disfigurement that may result if it goes untreated. The noses of leprosy patients shrink away, their earlobes swell, and over time they lose fingers and toes, then hands and feet. Many also go blind.

After working for a while with patients in India, I began to question the medical presumption that leprosy caused this disfigurement directly. Did patients' flesh simply rot away? Or might their problems, like Tanya's, trace back to the underlying cause of insensitivity to pain? Perhaps leprosy patients were destroying themselves unwittingly for the simple reason that they too lacked a system to warn them of danger. Still researching this theory, I visited a large leprosy hospital in New Guinea where I observed two grim scenes that have stayed with me ever since.

A woman in a village near the leprosarium was roasting yams over a charcoal brazier. She pierced one yam with a sharp stick and held it over the fire, slowly twirling the stick between her fingers like a barbecue spit. The yam fell off the stick, however, and I watched as she tried unsuccessfully to spear it, each jab driving the yam farther underneath the hot red coals. Finally, she shrugged and looked over to an old man squatting a few feet away. At her gesture, obviously knowing what was expected of him, he shambled over to the fire, reached in, pushed aside the hot coals to retrieve the yam, and then returned to his seat.

As a surgeon specializing in human hands, I was appalled. Everything had happened too fast for me to intervene, but I went immediately to examine the old man's hands. He had no fingers left, only gnarled stubs covered with leaking blisters and the scars of old wounds. Clearly, this was not the first time he had thrust his hand into a fire. I lectured him on the need to care for his hands, but his apathetic response gave me little confidence that he had listened.

A few days later I conducted a group clinic at the neighboring leprosarium. My visit had been announced in advance, and at the scheduled time the administrators rang a loud bell to summon patients. I stood with other staff in an open courtyard, and as soon as the bell rang a crowd of people emerged from the individual huts and barrackslike wards and began to move toward us.

An eager young patient caught my eye as he struggled across the edge of the courtyard on crutches, holding his bandaged left leg clear of the ground. Although he did his awkward best to hurry, the nimbler patients soon overtook him. As I watched, this man tucked his crutches under his arm and began to run on both feet with a very lopsided gait, waving wildly to get our attention. He ended up near the head of the line, where he stood panting, leaning on his crutches, wearing a smile of triumph.

I could tell from the man's gait, though, that something was badly wrong. Walking toward him, I saw that the bandages were wet with blood and his left foot flopped freely from side to side. By running on an already dislocated ankle, he had put far too much force on the end of his leg bone, and the skin had broken under the stress. He was walking on the end of his tibia, and with every step that naked bone dug into the ground. Nurses scolded the man sharply, but he seemed quite proud of himself for having run so fast. I knelt beside him and found that small stones and twigs had jammed through the end of the bone into the marrow cavity. I had no choice but to amputate the leg below the knee.

Those two scenes have long haunted me. Closing my eyes, I can still see the two facial expressions: the weary indifference of the old man who plucked the yam from the fire, the ebullient joy of the young man who ran across the courtyard. One eventually lost his hand, the other his leg; they had in common an utter nonchalance toward self-destruction.

Fearful Glimpse

I always thought of myself as one who cared for patients who lacked pain, not as one doomed to live in that state. Until 1953. At the end of a study program sponsored by the Rockefeller Foundation, I spent a few days in New York City waiting for the ocean liner *Ile de France* to sail back to England. I checked into a cheap student hostel and prepared for a speech I was scheduled to deliver the next day at the American Leprosy Mission. Four months of travel had taken a toll. I was tired, disoriented, and a touch feverish. I slept fitfully that night and arose the next morning feeling little better. By sheer power of will I managed to keep my engagement and struggle through the speech, fighting off waves of nausea and dizziness.

On the subway ride back to the hostel that afternoon, I must have fainted. When I came to consciousness, I found myself sprawled across the floor of the swaying train. Other passengers were studiously looking away, and no one offered any help. They probably assumed I was drunk.

Somehow I got off at the right stop and staggered to the hostel. I dully realized I should call a doctor, but my inexpensive room had no telephone. By now burning with fever, I collapsed on the bed, where I lay through the night and into the next day. Every few hours I would awake, stare at the strange surroundings, make an effort to get up, then sink back onto the bed. Late in the day I rang for the bellman and gave him some money to buy orange juice, milk, and aspirin.

For six days I did not leave that room. The faithful bellman checked on me daily and replenished my supplies, but I saw no other human being. I drifted in and out of sleep and consciousness. In my dreams I rode on the back of a water buffalo in India and walked on stilts in London. Sometimes I dreamed of my wife and children; other times I doubted whether I even had a family. I lacked the presence of mind, and even the physical ability, to go downstairs and phone for help or cancel my appointments. All day long I lay in a room which, its window shades drawn tight, was dark as a tomb.

On the sixth day my door opened and in the blinding light of the doorway I could barely make out a familiar figure: Dr. Eugene Kellersberger of the American Leprosy Mission. He was smiling, and had each arm wrapped around a paper bag full of groceries. At that moment Dr. Kellersberger seemed to me an angel sent from heaven. "How did you find me?" I asked weakly.

Dr. Kellersberger said that I had looked ill the afternoon I spoke at the mission. A few days later he called a surgeon he knew I would be meeting and learned I had missed the appointment. Concerned, he pulled out the Manhattan Yellow Pages and called every hotel listed until he found one that recognized his description. "Brand, yes, we have a Brand here," the hotel operator had told him. "An odd fellow. Stays in his room all day and lives on orange juice, milk, and aspirin."

After determining that I was suffering from nothing more than a bad bout of influenza, Kellersberger forced additional nourishment down me and looked after me during my final few days in the United States. Though still weak and unsteady, I decided to keep my scheduled sailing on the *Ile de France*.

Although I rested on the voyage, when we docked at Southampton seven days later I found I could barely cope with the luggage. I broke out in sweat at the slightest exertion. I paid a porter, boarded the train to London, and hunkered down against the window in a cramped compartment. Nothing on the other side of the glass interested me in the slightest. I just wanted an end to this interminable trip. I arrived at my aunt's house physically and emotionally drained.

Thus began the darkest night of my entire life. I pulled off my shoes to prepare for bed, and as I did so a terrible awareness hit me with the force of a wrecking ball. *I had no feeling in half my foot.* I sank into a chair, my mind whirling. Perhaps it was an illusion. I closed my eyes and pressed against my heel with the tip of a ballpoint pen. Nothing. No sensation of touch whatsoever in the area around the heel.

A dread fear worse than any nausea seized my stomach. Had it finally happened? Every leprosy worker recognizes insensitivity to pain as one of the disease's first symptoms. Had I just made the wretched leap from leprosy doctor to leprosy patient? I stood up stiffly, and shifted weight back and forth on my unfeeling foot. Then I rummaged in my suitcase for a sewing needle and sat down again. I pricked a small patch of skin below my ankle. No pain. I jabbed the needle deeper, probing for a reflex, but there was none. A dark speck of blood oozed out of the hole I had just made. I put my face between my hands and shuddered, longing for pain that would not come.

I suppose I had always feared that moment. In the early days of working with leprosy patients, every time I took a bath I made a visual check for skin patches. Most leprosy workers did, I knew, despite heavy odds against contagion.

A rap on the door broke my reverie and I jumped. "Are you all right in there, Paul?" my aunt asked. "Would you like some hot tea?"

Instinctively I found myself responding just like my early-diagnosis leprosy patients: I covered up. "Oh, I'm fine," I said, in a calculatedly cheerful voice. "I just need rest. It's been a long journey." But rest did not come that night. I lay on the bed fully clothed except for shoes and socks, perspiring and breathing heavily.

From that night on, my world would change. I had crusaded to combat prejudice against leprosy patients. I had scoffed at the possibility of contagion, assuring my staff they were in little danger. Now the story of my infection would spread through the ranks of leprosy workers. What would this do to our work?

What would this do to my life? I had gone to India in the belief that I would serve God by helping to relieve suffering. Should I now stay in England and go underground, so as not to create a stir? I would need to separate myself from my family, of course, since children were unusually susceptible to infection. How glibly I had coaxed patients to defy the stigma and forge a new life for themselves. Welcome to the society of the accursed.

I knew all too well what to expect. My office files were filled with diagrams charting the body's gradual march toward numbness. Ordinary pleasures in life would slip away. Petting a dog, running a hand across fine silk, holding a child—soon all sensations would feel alike: dead.

The rational part of my mind kept cutting in to calm the fears, reminding me that sulfone drugs would likely arrest the disease. But already I had lost the nerve supplying portions of my foot. Perhaps the nerves to my hands would go next. Hands were my stock in trade. I could not possibly use a scalpel if I suffered any loss of the refined sensations from fingertips. My career as a surgeon would soon end. Already I was accepting leprosy as a fact of life, *my* life.

At last dawn came and I arose, unrested and full of despair. I stared in a mirror at my unshaven face, checking my nose and earlobes for signs of the disease. During the night the clinician in me had taken over. I mustn't panic. Since I knew more about the disease than the average doctor in London, it was up to me to determine a course of treatment. First, I must map out the affected area of insensitivity to get some sense of how far the disease had progressed. I sat down, took a deep breath, jabbed the point of the sewing needle into my heel—and yelped.

Never have I felt a sensation as delicious as that live, electric jolt of pain. I laughed aloud at my foolishness. Of course! It all made perfect sense now. As I sat hunched on the train, my body too weak for the usual restless motion that redistributes weight and pressure, I had cut off the blood supply to the main branch of the sciatic nerve in my leg, causing a temporary numbness.

Temporary! Overnight the nerve had renewed itself and was now faithfully spitting out messages of pain and touch and cold and heat. There was no leprosy, only a weary traveler made neurotic by illness and fatigue.

That single sleepless night became for me a defining moment. I had caught only a fleeting glimpse of life without touch and pain, yet that glimpse was enough to make me feel frightened and alone. My numbed foot seemed like a foreign appendage grafted onto my body. When I had put weight on it, my foot felt exactly as if I had not put weight on it. I will never forget the desolation of that sensation like death.

The opposite happened the next morning when I learned with a start that my foot had come back to life. I had crossed a chasm back to normal life. I breathed a prayer, *Thank God for pain!* that I have repeated in some form hundreds of times since. To some people that prayer may seem odd, even oxymoronic or masochistic. It came to me in a reflexive rush of gratitude. For the first time I understood how leprosy victims could look with envy upon those of us who feel pain.

I returned to India with renewed commitment to fight leprosy, and to help my patients compensate for what they had lost. I became, in effect, a career lobbyist for pain.

Discordant Thirds

My professional life has revolved around the theme of pain, and by living in different cultures I have observed at close hand diverse attitudes toward it. My life divides roughly into thirds— twenty-seven years in India, twenty-five years in England, and more than twenty-seven years in the United States—and from each society I have learned something new about pain.

I served my medical internship in London during the most harrowing days and nights of the Blitz, when the Luftwaffe was pounding a proud city into rubble. Physical hardship was a constant companion, the focal point of nearly every conversation and front-page headline. Yet I have never lived among people so buoyant; now I read that 60 percent of Londoners who lived through the Blitz remember it as the happiest period of their lives.

After the war I moved to India, just as Partition was tearing the nation apart. In that land of poverty and omnipresent suffering

I learned that pain can be borne with dignity and calm acceptance. It was there too that I began treating leprosy patients, social pariahs whose tragedy stems from the absence of physical pain.

Later in the United States, a nation whose war for independence was fought in part to guarantee a right to "the pursuit of happiness," I encountered a society that seeks to avoid pain at all costs. Patients lived at a greater comfort level than any I had previously treated, but they seemed far less equipped to handle suffering and far more traumatized by it. Pain relief in the United States is now a $63-billion-a-year industry, and television commercials proclaim better and faster pain remedies. One ad slogan bluntly puts it, "I haven't got time for the pain."

Each of these groups of people—Londoners who suffered gladly for a cause, Indians who expected suffering and learned not to fear it, and Americans who suffered less but feared it more—helped to form my outlook on this mysterious fact of human existence. Most of us will one day face severe pain. I am convinced that the attitude we cultivate in advance may well determine how suffering will affect us when it does strike. Out of that conviction comes this book.

My thoughts about pain developed over many years as I worked with people who suffered from pain and people who suffered from the lack of pain. I have chosen the form of a memoir, with all its loops and detours, for that is how I learned about pain: not systematically, but experientially. Pain does not occur in the abstract—no sensation is more personal, or more importunate. The scenes I will relate from my early life, random, seemingly disconnected like all memories of early life, eventually contributed to a whole new outlook.

I readily admit that my years of working among pain-deprived people have given me a skewed perspective. I now regard pain as one of the most remarkable design features of the human body, and if I could choose one gift for my leprosy patients it would be the gift of pain. (In fact, a team of scientists I directed spent more than a million dollars in an attempt to design an artificial pain system. We abandoned the project when it became abundantly clear we could not possibly duplicate the sophisticated engineering system that protects a healthy human being.)

Few experiences in life are more universal than pain, which flows like lava beneath the crust of daily life. I know well the typical attitude toward pain, especially in Western societies. J. K.

Huysmans calls it "the useless, unjust, incomprehensible, inept abomination that is physical pain." Neurologist Russell Martin adds, "Pain is greedy, boorish, meanly debilitating. It is cruel and calamitous and often constant, and, as its Latin root *poena* implies, it is the corporeal punishment each of us ultimately suffers for being alive."

I have heard similar complaints from patients. My own encounters with pain, though, as well as the specter of painlessness, have produced in me an attitude of wonder and appreciation. I do not desire, and cannot even imagine, a life without pain. For that reason I accept the challenge of trying to restore balance to how we think about pain.

For good and for ill, the human species has among its privileges the preeminence of pain. We have the unique ability to step outside ourselves and self-reflect, by reading a book about pain, for example, or by summoning up the memory of a terrifying ordeal. Some pains—the pain of grief or emotional trauma—have no physical stimulus whatever. They are states of mind, concocted by the alchemy of the brain. These feats of consciousness make it possible for suffering to loiter in the mind long after the body's need for it has passed. Yet they also give us the potential to attain an outlook that will change the very landscape of the pain experience. We can learn to cope, and even to triumph.

2
Mountains of Death

Illness is the doctor to whom we pay most heed: to kindness, to knowledge
we make promises only: pain we obey.
Marcel Proust

Eight years old, returning home with my family after a trip to
Madras, I peered out the train window at scenes of rural India. To
me, village life seemed exotic and full of adventure. Naked children played in the irrigation canals, splashing water at each other.
Their fathers, shirtless men in cotton loincloths, were at work
tending the crops, herding goats, and carrying loads on bamboo
balance poles across their backs. Women in loose-wrapped saris
walked along the paths with large platters of dried dung patties
balanced on their heads.

The train ride lasted all day. I napped in the afternoon, but at
dusk as the sun softened from angry white to tranquil orange I
again took up my post beside the window. It was my favorite time
of day in India. Huge, shiny banana leaves fluttered with the first
puff of evening breeze. Rice paddies gleamed like emeralds. Even
the dust shimmered gold.

My sister and I always made a game of searching for the hills
where we lived, and this time I spotted them first. From then on
our eyes were drawn to the horizon, a pale, curvy line of blue that
only gradually turned solid and purple. As we grew closer I could
see the glint of sun reflecting off white Hindu temples in the
foothills. Just before sundown, I was able to pick out five distinct
ranges of mountains, including the Kolli Malai range, our home.
Our family got off the train at the last stop, transferring first to a
bus and then to a bullock cart before arriving after dark in the
town where we would spend our final night on the plains. I went
to bed early, resting up for the next day's climb.

Modern visitors ascend into the Kolli mountains on a spectacular highway featuring seventy switchback curves (each one neatly labeled: 38/70, 39/70, 40/70), but as a child I either scrambled on foot along a steep, slippery path or rode in a canvas contraption called a *dholi*, slung from porters' shoulders on bamboo poles. Walking at eye level with the porters' glistening legs, I watched their toes dig into the muddy soil and their legs part the ferns and thick lantana shrub. I especially watched the tiny leeches, thin as silk threads, that leaped from the shrub, fastened to those legs, and gradually swelled with blood. The porters seemed not to mind (leeches inject a chemical that controls clotting and pain), but out of sheer disgust my sister and I anxiously checked our own legs every few minutes for signs of unwanted guests.

At last we arrived at a remote settlement on the very top of the Kolli Malai, four thousand feet above the valley floor. The porters deposited our belongings on the porch of a hardwood bungalow, the house I had lived in since my birth in 1914.

Common Language

My parents had come to India as missionaries, settling initially in a station on the plains. Although my father had trained as a builder, he and my mother had taken a brief preparatory course in medicine. When word got out, locals began calling them both "Doctor" and a steady stream of sick people lined up outside the door. Rumors of the foreigners' medical skills spread even into the five nearby mountain ranges, of which the Kolli Malai was the most mysterious and feared: mysterious because few plains people had climbed above the band of clouds that usually shrouded Kolli peaks, feared because that climate zone harbored the *Anopheles* mosquito, carrier of malaria. The very name *Kolli Malai* meant "mountains of death": Spending a single night there, it was said, would expose a visitor to the deadly fever.

Despite these warnings, my parents moved into the hills, where, they had heard, twenty thousand people lived with no access to medical care. We lived in a settlement built mostly by my father's own hands. (Six carpenters had come up from the plains to help him, but five soon fled, afraid of the fever.) Before long my parents had opened a clinic, a school, and a mud-walled church. They also made room for abandoned children—the hill tribes left unwanted children beside the road—and something akin to an orphanage grew up.

To a child, the Kolli hills were paradise. I ran barefoot along the rock cliffs, and climbed trees until my clothes were coated with sap. Local boys taught me to leap like a monkey onto the back of a water buffalo and race the beast around the fields. We stalked lizards and croaking frogs in the rice paddies until Tata, guardian of the terraces, chased us away.

I did my school lessons in a tree house, my mother having fastened assignments to a rope for me to haul them up to my private classroom high in a jackfruit tree. My father tutored me on the mysteries of the natural world: the termites he had foiled by building our house on stilts capped with upside-down frying pans, the sticky-toed geckos that clung to my bedroom walls, the agile tailor bird that stitched together leaves with its beak, using bits of grass stalk as a stitching thread.

Once, Dad took me to a termite colony, its tall mounds standing in rows like organ pipes, and cut out a large window to show me the arched columns and winding passageways within. We lay on our stomachs together, chins propped on our hands, and watched the insects scurry to repair their fine architecture. Ten thousand legs worked together as if commanded by a single brain, all frantic except the queen, big and round as a sausage, who lay oblivious, pumping out eggs.

For entertainment I kept a carnivorous sundew plant, bright green and tinged with red, that snapped shut whenever I dropped a fly inside. During afternoon nap periods I listened for the rats and green snakes poking around in the ceiling beams and behind the stove. Sometimes at night I read by insect-light, my book held open by a jar of glowworms and fireflies.

I cannot imagine a better environment in which to learn about the natural world, and especially to learn about pain. It was as close as our daily meals. Our cook did not buy a chicken precut and shrink-wrapped, but rather selected one from the pen and chopped its squawking head off. I watched it run crazily until the blood stopped spurting, then I brought it to the kitchen for cleaning. When time came to kill a goat, the entire settlement gathered as the butcher slit its throat, peeled back the skin, and divided the meat. I stood on the perimeter, at once repelled and transfixed.

Because of pain I took great care at night when I walked to the outhouse across ground patrolled by scorpions. On hikes I kept alert for a plain-looking beetle that, if surprised, would rear up and with unerring aim squirt a jet of stinging liquid into the intruder's eye. I stayed on guard for snakes too: cobras, vipers, and the "eleven-step-adder" whose potent venom, Dad said, would kill a man before his eleventh step. My father had a kind of victim's admiration for such creatures. He marveled at, and tried to explain to me, the exquisite chemistry of venom, drawing diagrams of the hinged fangs and the erectile tissue that allowed snakes to project their poison through hollow channels in their teeth. I listened raptly and continued to give all snakes a wide berth.

Early on, I recognized a hard justice in the law of nature, where pain served as a common language. Plants used it in the form of thorns to ward off munching cows; snakes and scorpions used it to warn away lumbering humans; and I used it, too, to win wrestling matches against larger opponents. To me such pain seemed fair: the legitimate defense of creatures protecting their turf. I was impressed by David Livingstone's written account of being attacked by a lion and dragged through the grass. While dangling from the lion's jaws, like a field mouse carried by a house cat, he thought to himself, "After all, he is the king of beasts."

Fakirs and Forceps

On our rare trips into a large city like Madras, I saw a different kind of human suffering. Beggars thrust their hands in the windows even before the train shrieked to a stop. Because physical deformity tended to attract more charity, amputees wore brightly decorated caps of leather on their stumps, and beggars with large abdominal tumors arranged them for public display. Sometimes a child was intentionally crippled to increase its earning power, or a mother would rent out her newborn to a beggar who would put drops in the baby's eyes to make them pink and runny. As I walked along the sidewalks, tightly gripping my parents' hands, beggars held out these skinny, rheumy-eyed babies and asked for alms.

I gawked, for our mountain village had nothing to rival these scenes. But in India they formed part of the urban landscape and the philosophy of Karma taught people to accept suffering, like weather, as an unavoidable part of fate.

During a festival local villages often received a visit from one of the very impressive *fakirs*, who seemed to defy all rules of pain. I saw one man push a thin stiletto-type blade through his cheek, tongue, and out the other cheek, then slowly withdraw the blade with no sign of bleeding. Another stuck a knife sideways through the neck of his child, and I broke out in goose bumps as the tip came out the other side. The child held very still and did not flinch.

Walking on coals was a simple trick for a good fakir. I once saw one dangling like a spider, high in the air, suspended from a cable by meat hooks forced through folds of skin on his back. As the crowd gestured and called out, he floated above them, smiling and serene. Another fakir, wearing what looked like a shirt made of small balloons, danced through the crowd on stilts. Coming closer, I saw that his chest was covered with dozens of limes fastened to his skin with tiny skewers. As he jumped up and down on the stilts, laughing, the limes slapped rhythmically against his chest.

Local people credited the fakirs' powers to the Hindu gods. My father refuted them. "It has nothing to do with religion," he said to me in private. "With discipline, these men have learned to control pain as well as bleeding, heart rate, and breathing." I did not understand such things, but I did know that whenever I tried sticking so much as a straight pin in my flesh, my body recoiled. I envied the fakirs' mastery over pain.

With my penchant for tree climbing and buffalo riding, I had some personal knowledge of pain, and to me it was wholly disagreeable. Colic was the worst pain I had felt. I knew it came from roundworms, and I fancied them doing battle inside me as my bowel tried to move them on and out. Gratefully, for a change, I downed spoonfuls of the vile remedy, castor oil.

Malaria, I had simply learned to live with. Every few days, and always at the same time, my fever shifted into an active phase. "Snake time!" I called out to my playmates around four o'clock in the afternoon and dashed for the house. Most of them had malaria, too, and so they understood. Body temperature shoots up and down, and when the chills hit, back muscles go into spasm, causing the body to twist and turn like a snake. Warmth offers some relief, and even on the hottest day I would dive under heavy wool blankets to help calm the bone-rattling chills.

Pain, I learned, had the mysterious power to overrule everything else in life. It took priority over such essentials as sleeping, eating, and afternoon play. I would no longer climb certain trees, for example, in deference to the tiny scorpions that lived in their bark.

My parents' work reinforced this lesson about pain almost daily. In rural India the most common physical complaint was the acute pain of toothache. A man or woman would show up, having walked from a village miles away, with facial features distorted by pain and a rag wrapped tightly around the swollen jaw. My parents, with no dental chair, drill, or local anesthetic to offer, had only one remedy. Dad would sit the patient on a rock or abandoned termite mound, perhaps say a brief prayer aloud, then apply his dental forceps to the tooth. Most cases went without a hitch: a twist of the wrist, a grunt or scream, a little blood, and the ordeal was over. Often the patient's companions, who had never seen a toothache end so abruptly, broke into applause, cheering the forceps which held the offending tooth.

This procedure presented my mother, a small woman, with more difficulty. She used to say, "There are two rules to pulling teeth. One is to slide your forceps down as far as you can, near the roots, so the crown won't break off. The second rule: Never let go!" In some cases it appeared that the patient extracted his own tooth by pulling away as Mother hung on to the forceps at all costs. Yet the patients who yelled the loudest and fought the hardest would come back another time. Pain compelled it.

Compassionate Healers

It was my parents' practice of medicine that endeared them to the Kolli Malai people. My father had studied tropical medicine for one year at Livingstone College, a school to prepare missionaries; my mother relied on what she had learned at the Homeopathic Hospital in London. Despite the limitations of their training, both of them managed to exemplify the original motto of Hippocrates: Good medicine treats an individual, not merely a disease.

My parents were traditional missionaries who responded to whatever human need they saw around them. Together, they founded nine schools and a string of clinics. In agricultural pursuits, Mother had little success growing garden vegetables in the Kollis, but her orchard of citrus trees prospered. My father preferred to work in his area of specialty, the building trade. He taught carpentry to young village boys, and then tile making when it became necessary to replace the settlement's thatch roofs. Traveling on horseback along weedy bridle trails, he also set up half a dozen farms for mulberry trees (to feed silkworms), bananas, oranges, sugar cane, coffee, and tapioca. When tenant farmers received unfair treatment from the landowners on the plains, my father led a delegation of a hundred of them to district headquarters, speaking on their behalf to the British colonial officials.

Despite all this good work, Jesse and Evelyn Brand met with complete failure in their cherished goal of establishing a Christian church among the hill people. A local priest who specialized in spirit worship, sensing his livelihood at risk, had broadcast a warning that any converts to the new religion would incur the wrath of the gods. We feared physical danger, and whenever I saw the priest I would hide. A few poisoned cows underscored his threat, and although my parents conducted church services every Sunday, few attended and no one dared become a Christian.

Then, in 1918–19, an epidemic of Spanish influenza broke out worldwide, reaching even into the Kollis, where it killed with such ferocity that it shattered any sense of community. Rather than nursing a sick member back to health, terrified neighbors and family fled into the woods. My father determined that, thus deserted, many of the influenza victims were dying from malnourishment and dehydration, not the disease itself. He mixed a batch of rice gruel in an enormous black cauldron outside our home and for many days kept the soup replenished. He and Mother went out into the villages on horseback, spooning soup and purified water into the mouths of the forsaken residents.

Eventually, both the hostile priest and his wife fell ill. Everyone deserted them except my parents, who regularly took food and medicine into their home. Nursed by his "enemies," the priest realized he had badly misjudged them. He asked for papers for adoption. "My son was to be priest after me," he told my father, "but no one in my religion has cared enough to help me. I want my children to grow up as Christians." A few days later I stood on the porch of our bungalow and watched as a tearful ten-year-old boy made his way across the fields. He was carrying a feverish nine-month-old baby girl, along with a packet of documents from the priest and his wife. That is how my sister Ruth and her brother Aaron joined our family, and also how the church in the Kolli Malai received its first local members after six years of fierce resistance.

From my parents I learned that pain sends a signal not only to the patient but to the surrounding community as well. Just as individual pain sensors announce to other cells in the body, "Attend to me! I need help!" so do suffering human beings cry out to the community at large. My parents had the courage to respond, even when it involved risk. With little training and few resources my father treated the worst ailments of his day—bubonic plague, typhoid, malaria, polio, cholera, smallpox—and I know without a doubt what would have happened if a mutation like the AIDS virus had appeared in the hills of Kolli Malai. He would have packed his meager bag and headed for the source of the cries of pain. His approach to medicine flowed out of a deep sense of human *compassion*, a word whose Latin roots are *com + pati*, meaning "to suffer with." Any deficit in their training my parents overcame by that instinctive response to human suffering.

I stayed in the Kolli hills until 1923, when I reached the age of nine. Then my sister Connie and I went to England to acquire a more formal education. I felt alien there: plants lost their foliage for half the year; tree-climbing coated my clothes with a layer of coal soot; I was expected to wear shoes all day, and itchy wool sweaters; and instead of a tree house, I had to sit in a classroom to study my lessons. I managed to adjust after a while, but I never felt completely at home. I lived for the long, detailed letters from my parents, delivered in a thick bundle whenever a steamship docked from India.

My father continued his tutorial in nature appreciation via mail, filling his letters with drawings and notes on what he had discovered during walks through the forest. Mother mostly wrote about neighbor families, individual patients, and church members. The missionary work flourished over the next few years. The little church grew to fifty members and my parents treated twelve thousand patients a year in the clinics. Farming, carpentry, and silk industries were thriving, and a store had opened up in the settlement.

In 1929, to my great joy, my parents announced they would return to England the following year for a twelve-month sabbatical. As that time approached, their letters—and mine—began to take on a more urgent and personal tone. Almost six years had passed since I left India. I was fifteen years old now, facing decisions about my future. Where should I live? What career should I choose? What about further schooling? As I wrestled with these choices, I realized how much I relied on my parents for wise counsel. We had much to catch up on, and I could hardly wait to see them.

In June 1929, however, a telegram arrived announcing my father's death. It gave few details, just a report that he had collapsed after a two-day bout with blackwater fever, a virulent complication of malaria. The mountains of death had claimed yet another victim. He was forty-four. "Break news gently to the children," the telegram read; "The Lord reigneth."

I did not feel the pain of grief at first. I felt a sudden thickening of what I had sensed for six years as my father faded from a living person I could hold and smell into a remembered vision of a former life far away. To deepen the sense of unreality, I continued getting his letters for several weeks after the telegram announcing his death, until the sea mail caught up. Dad told of patients he had treated, and described how high the silver oaks had grown on the path behind the bungalow. He wrote of how much he looked forward to seeing us in March, just ten months away. One last letter came, and then no more.

I mainly felt numbness. Over and over I repeated to myself, *No more letters. No more forest hikes. No more Dad.* Then came a long letter from my mother giving the details of his death. His body's resistance had been low because a fall from a horse the year before had limited his physical exercise, she said. His temperature had hit 106°. Mother blamed herself for not immediately setting off for medical help: a local doctor had misdiagnosed the fever. She told of the loud, wailing grief of the villagers, and praised the dedication of thirty-two men who spent three days transporting a granite tombstone across the fields and up the hill to the churchyard.

After that, my mother's letters tended to ramble. She seemed distraught, and the family dispatched a niece to India to persuade her to come home. She finally returned more than a year later, and I saw for the first time the devastating work of grief, the shared pain. Mother lived in my memory, the memory of a nine-year-old, as a tall, beautiful woman overflowing with energy and laughter. But down the gangplank, gripping the railing all the way, came a hunched-over figure with hair prematurely gray and the posture of a woman in her eighties. I had grown, yes, but she had also shrunk. I could hardly force myself to call her Mother.

On the train ride to London she told the story of Dad's death over and over, continually berating herself. She must go back, she said, and carry on the work. But how could she manage in the Kollis alone, without Jesse? The light had gone out of her life.

As it turned out, my mother managed quite well. A year later, ignoring family entreaties for her to stay in England, she returned to the bungalow high in the Kolli Malai. Traveling mountain trails on Dobbin, the horse that had belonged to my father, she resumed the work of medicine, education, agriculture, and teaching the Gospel. She outlasted Dobbin, and broke in a succession of hill ponies. When she grew older and began falling from horseback— "the horses are getting too old for this," she reported—she walked the hills, leaning heavily on tall bamboo poles which she grasped in each hand. The mission officially "retired" her at age sixty-nine, but that mattered not at all. She carried her work from the Kollis to four nearby mountain ranges. "Mother of the Hills," they called her, and those are the words carved on her tombstone now, in a grave beside my father's just down the slope from the bungalow where I grew up. She died in 1975, a few weeks shy of her ninety-sixth birthday.

Family Legacy

My mother became something of a legend in the hills of South India, and whenever I visit there now I am treated like the long-lost son of a beloved queen. The people of the settlement place a floral lei around my neck, serve me a feast on banana leaves, and put on a program of songs and traditional dances in the chapel. Inevitably, some of them stand and reminisce about Granny Brand, as they call her. On my last visit, the main speaker was a professor in a nursing school. She said she was one of the children abandoned by the roadside and "adopted" by my mother, who nursed her to health, gave her a place to live, and arranged for her education all the way through graduate school.

Not as many people remember my father, although an Indian doctor inspired by his life recently moved to the Kollis and opened the Jesse Brand Memorial Clinic. The house where we lived as a family still stands, and out back I can see the site of my tree house high in the jackfruit tree. I always visit the graves with their twin tombstones, and each time, I weep for the memory of my parents, two loving human beings who gave themselves so fully to so many. I had few years with them, far too few. But together they left me a priceless legacy.

I admired my father's even temperament, his scholarship, and his calm self-assurance, all of which my mother lacked. But through an abundance of courage and compassion she found her own way into the hearts of the hill people. The story of the guinea worm, the focal point of many horrible scenes of suffering from my childhood, may serve to capture their differences in style.

The guinea worm parasite infested most of the hill people at one time or another. Ingested in drinking water, the larvae penetrated the intestinal wall, got into the bloodstream, and migrated to soft tissues, usually settling down next to a vein. Though only the width of the lead in a pencil, the worms grew to enormous lengths, as much as a yard. You could sometimes see them rippling under the skin. If a sore developed, for example on the hip of a woman who carried a water pot, a guinea worm's tail might protrude through the boil. Yet if the woman killed the partially exposed worm, the rest of its body would decay inside her, causing an infection.

My father treated hundreds of guinea worm infections. Normally, I loved watching him work, but whenever one of these patients showed up I ran and hid. Buckets of blood and pus would gush out when Dad lanced the swollen arm or thigh. He would stab along the line of abscesses with his knife or scalpel, probing for any residue of the decaying worm. With no anesthetic available, the patient could only grip the arms and hands of relatives, and stifle a scream.

Ever the inquisitive scientist, my father also studied the parasite's life cycle. He learned that the adult form was extremely sensitive to cold water, a fact he took advantage of. He had a patient stand in a pail of cold water for a few minutes until, *prick*, a guinea worm tail popped through the skin and busily started laying eggs in the water through its oviduct. My father deftly seized the tail of the guinea worm and wound it around a small twig or matchstick. He pulled hard enough to get a few inches of the worm around the twig but not so hard as to break it off, then taped the twig to the patient's leg with adhesive. The worm would gradually adjust downward to relieve the tension on its body, and several hours later my father could wind a few more inches around the twig. After many hours (or several days in the event of a long guinea worm), he would pull out the entire length of the guinea worm, and the patient would be rid of the parasite, with no danger of infection.

My father perfected the technique and took great pride in his skill at coaxing out the offenders. My mother never matched him in technique, and despised the messy process of treatment. After his death she concentrated instead on prevention, applying what he had learned about the parasite's life cycle.

The guinea worm problem centered around the water supply. An infested villager who stood in the shallow well to dip a bucket was giving the guinea worm an ideal opportunity to pop out and lay eggs; these hatched into larvae that some other villager would scoop into a bucket and drink, activating the cycle all over again. Mother led an all-out crusade to reform village water practices. She lectured the people, making them promise they would never stand in the wells and ponds, or drink water without first straining it. She badgered the government into stocking the larger ponds with fish to eat the larvae. She taught villagers to build stone walls around their wells in order to keep animals and children out of the drinking water. My mother had boundless energy and unshakable conviction. It took fifteen years, but in the end she eradicated guinea worm infections from the entire range of hills.

Years later, when officials from the Malaria Eradication Unit came to the Kollis with plans to spray DDT and kill the *Anopheles* mosquito, they met suspicious villagers who blocked their path, threw stones, and chased them away with dogs. The officials ended up dealing with a wrinkled old woman named Granny Brand. If she approved, the villagers said, they would go along. She had their trust, the most precious commodity any health worker can earn. She did approve, and the war against the *Anopheles* continued until malaria was effectively abolished from the Kolli Malai. (Unfortunately, the *Anopheles* has now become resistant to most insecticides, and drug-resistant malaria is making a comeback across India.)

My mother tried to bequeath to me the legacy of my father's scientific work. During her year of rest and recuperation in England after his death, she frequently spoke of her dream for me to return to the Kollis as a doctor. The hills of India sounded far more appealing than cold, clammy England, but I cut short all her talk of medicine.

Over time, childhood memories of medicine had distilled into a few scenes of suffering, and I now found these scenes abhorrent. There was the revolting scene of my parents working on a woman tormented by guinea worms, including one whose dragon tail poked out of the corner of her eye. And the memory of my father's most challenging patient: a man who survived a mauling by a bear, his scalp torn from ear to ear. There was one more scene, too, perhaps the most haunting of all.

My father would not even let us watch him work on the three strange men who approached the clinic one afternoon. He confined us to the house, but I sneaked out and peered through the bushes. These men had stiff hands covered with sores. Fingers were missing. Bandages covered their feet, and when Dad removed those bandages I saw that their stumpy feet had no toes.

I watched my father, mystified. Could he actually be afraid? He did not banter with the patients. And he did something I had never before seen: he put on a pair of gloves before dressing their wounds. The men had brought a basket of fruit as a gift, but after they left Mother burned the basket along with my father's gloves, an unheard-of act of waste. We were ordered not to play in that spot. Those men were *lepers*, we were told.

I had no further contact with leprosy in my childhood, but as time passed I viewed medicine with the same mixture of fear and revulsion that I had felt as a child when my father treated such people. Medicine was not for me. Pain and suffering, I wanted to avoid at all costs.

3
Awakenings

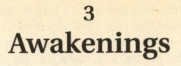

A surgeon does not slip from his mother's womb with compassion smeared
upon him like the drippings of his birth. It is much later that it comes.
No easy shaft of grace this, but the cumulative murmuring of the
numberless wounds he has dressed, the incisions he has made, all the sores
and ulcers and cavities he has touched in order to heal. In the beginning
it is barely audible, a whisper, as from many mouths. Slowly it gathers,
rising from the streaming flesh until, at last, it is a pure calling.

Richard Selzer, *Mortal Lessons*

If someone had suggested to me during school days in England
that my life's work would center on clinical research into pain, I
would have laughed aloud. Pain was to be avoided, not researched.
Nevertheless I did end up in medicine, and I must explain how I
got there.

I was a terrible student. Sometimes when the teacher's back
was turned I crept out a window onto the roof and shinnied down
the drain spout to escape school. While classmates pumped their
heads full of abstract knowledge, I was pining for the natural
world I had known in the Kolli hills. I made urban London more
tolerable by raising songbirds and mice in the basement of our
family estate home and by building a crude telescope observatory
on the roof. The nighttime view gave me a tenuous link to the
Kollis, where I had often gazed into a deep sky unmarred by haze
or ambient light and listened to my father explain the mysteries of
the universe. The nostalgia usually turned into homesickness—in
England even the stars were out of place.

When I was graduated from English public school at age sixteen, I balked at the prospect of spending four to six years in a stifling university classroom. I decided to take up construction, in
order to fulfill my father's original dream of building houses in the

Kolli hills. Over the next five years I learned carpentry, architecture, roofing, bricklaying, plumbing, electricity, and stonemasonry.

Stonework was my favorite. I felt a happiness I had not known since India, where as a child I had sat at the edge of a quarry and watched local stonecutters work magic with tools unchanged in three millennia. I began with Bath sandstone, progressed to granite, and finished my apprenticeship working with marble. Marble gives very little margin for error: one errant stroke of the hammer creates a "stun," a ganglion of tiny cracks that run deep into the block and destroy its lovely translucency. On vacations I would visit the great cathedrals of Britain and run my hands over the rippled texture of stone pillars and arches, awed by the realization that each tiny ridge marked the rise and fall of a medieval mason's wooden mallet.

In my final assignment after five years, I helped supervise the construction of an office building for Ford Motor Company, just then venturing into England. Clearly, I had moved beyond what would be useful in the Kolli hills. It was time to get on with overseas plans. For no other reason than to follow in my father's footsteps, I suppressed my feelings against medicine and signed up for the one-year course he had taken at Livingstone College Medical School.

Coming to Life

The Livingstone course brought together thirty-five international students, all committed to careers overseas. "You will learn to recognize symptoms, prescribe medicines, dress wounds, and even perform minor surgeries," the leaders told us during orientation. "You'll get hands-on experience, because local charity hospitals have agreed to let you students assist with incoming patients." I blanched, remembering those awful childhood scenes of blood, pus, leprosy, and guinea worms.

Before long, though, I discovered that the science of medicine could tap into the sense of wonder I already felt toward nature. I can still recall my first glimpse of a living cell under a microscope. We were studying parasites, my old adversaries from India, where dozens of times I had suffered from dysentery. Early one morning I decided to examine a living amoeba.

I crossed the dewy lawn to the garden pond, scooped water in a teacup, and let myself into the laboratory while other students were still at breakfast. Bits of decomposing leaves floated in the water, and it reeked of decay and death. Yet when I touched one drop of that pond to the microscope slide, a universe sprang to life: scores of delicate organisms, excited by the warmth of my microscope lamp, flitted this way and that. They looked like miniature jellyfish. Edging the slide sideways I saw a limpid blue blob plumping itself forward. Ah, there it was—an amoeba. This creature's distant relatives in India had cost me many hours of lost playtime. It looked innocent, primordial. Why did it so vex my intestines? How could it be disarmed? I began coming back to the laboratory after hours for further exploration.

Even more surprisingly, I found I also enjoyed the clinical work. On assignment in a dental clinic I learned that the procedure of pulling teeth with the proper tools and anesthetics bore little resemblance to those gruesome scenes in the Kollis. Tooth extractions drew on the manual skills I had developed as a carpenter and mason, and had the excellent advantage of ending someone's toothache. I fleetingly wondered whether I had made a mistake choosing against medical school. Had I wasted the last five years in the building trade? Yet surely I dare not discard all that training and start over in a new profession. Putting my doubts aside, I finished the term at Livingstone and enrolled in a preparatory course at the Missionary Training Colony, my final step before returning to India as a missionary builder.

A quintessentially British institution, the Colony combined the rigors of Sparta, the ideals of Queen Victoria, and the jolly teamwork of the Boy Scouts. The founder, who had lived in rural Ethiopia, determined that his charges would emerge from the Colony equipped to survive in any corner of the Empire. We slept in long wooden huts with single-thickness walls that stood no chance against English weather. Every morning before daybreak, in rain, sleet, or snow, we jogged in formation to a park, underwent a regimen of calisthenics, then returned to take a cold bath (the Colony disdained such luxuries as warm water). We repaired our own shoes, cut each other's hair, prepared our own meals. Summers, we went on six-hundred-mile treks through the Welsh and Scottish countryside, pulling supplies behind us in a wagon-wheel cart.

The two-year Colony course also included a stint at a charity hospital, and it was here that my interest in medicine finally drove me to action. One night as I was working in the emergency room, ambulance attendants wheeled in a beautiful young woman, unconscious. The hospital staff lurched into their controlled-panic response to a trauma patient: a nurse dashed down a corridor for a bottle of blood while a doctor fumbled with the transfusion apparatus. Glancing at my white dresser's coat, he thrust a blood pressure cuff in my direction.

I could not get a reading, nor could I detect the faintest flicker of a pulse on the woman's wrist. Her skin had an unearthly paleness, a sign of internal hemorrhaging, and her brownish hair seemed jet-black in contrast to her thin-lipped, parchment face. In the glare of hospital lights she looked like an alabaster saint from a cathedral. As the doctor searched her chest with his stethoscope, I noticed that even her nipples had whitened. Only a few freckles stood out against the pallor. She did not seem to be breathing, and I felt certain she was dead.

Just then the nurse arrived with a bottle of blood. The doctor punctured the woman's vein with a large needle and fastened the bottle high on a metal stand so that the increased pressure from elevation would force the blood faster into her body. The staff told me to keep watch over the emptying bottle while they scurried off to cross-match her blood type and get more blood.

Nothing in my memory can compare to the excitement of what happened next. Alone in the room, nervous and frightened in the presence of death, I held the woman's cold, damp wrist. Suddenly I felt the slight press of a pulse. Or did I? Was it my own pulse that I felt? I searched again. It was definitely there, a faint, rhythmic tremor against my middle finger.

The next bottle of blood arrived. A spot of pink appeared like a drop of watercolor on her cheek and began to spread into a full flush. Her lips darkened pink, then red, and her body quivered with a kind of sighing breath. A third bottle was connected. My own heart pounding, I watched a drama unfold. Her eyelids fluttered and began to part. She took a deep breath, then another. She squinted at first, then blinked a few times, her pupils constricting in reaction to the bright lights. At last she looked straight at me and, to my amazement, she spoke. "Water. Water, please," she said in a soft, raspy voice. "I'm thirsty." I ran to get some water.

That young woman entered my life for only an hour or so, but the experience transformed me. No one had told me medicine could do this! I had seen a corpse resurrected. By the end of my first year at Missionary Training Colony, I was incurably in love with medicine. I swallowed my pride, resigned from the Colony, and in 1937 enrolled in medical school at University College Hospital, London.

Parting the Veil

I will never forget my first anatomy class under H. H. Woolard, nicknamed "the monkey man" because of his theories linking humans and apes. A short man with an oversized head, glisteningly bald, strode into the classroom and all chatter ceased. With a rather haughty demeanor, he stood before us and slowly surveyed the room, allowing his eyes to rest on each individual student. For a full sixty seconds there was silence. Then he let out a huge, breathy sigh. "Just as I expected," he said with disgust. "They've given me the usual lot of pasty-faced, sallow, sunken-chested specimens."

He paused for the words to have their full effect before continuing. "I was like you once. I studied all day and smoked all night to stay awake. I now attribute my miserable stature to bad habits in my student days. I expect to die of a heart attack soon. My advice to you is simple: Get outdoors and run!" He then launched into a fierce lecture on the deleterious effects of smoking: it destroys your heart, stunts growth, and ruins your lungs, he said.* Afterward, as if to seal his warning with a suitable object lesson, Woolard divided us into teams of eight and led us to the dissection lab to meet our cadavers.

---

*Woolard's fears proved prophetic: before I left medical school he died of a heart attack while walking along one of the school corridors. This was decades before any Surgeon General's reports on smoking, and the dangers of tobacco had not been firmly established. At University College I participated in an experiment to test a possible link between hypersensitivity to tobacco and Buerger's disease, a condition of thrombosis of the veins. First I had to get the tobacco smoke in a usable form. I persuaded our senior resident, a pipe smoker, to cooperate by attaching his bowl and stem to a deep U-tube: smoke curling from the pipe passed through a bubbling solvent that extracted the tobacco gases. We ended up with a thick liquid resembling a runny brown oyster, which we used in skin patches on various people, some smokers and some not. We found no solid evidence of tobacco hypersensitivity on the skin, but the experiments did have the side effect of curing our resident of smoking. When we saw the vile, mucous substance collecting in our glass tubes—impurities that normally would be inhaled—all of us swore off smoking forever.

My dissection team was assigned a cadaver with a name, and a very respectable one at that. "You are awarded the great honor of dissecting Sir Reginald Hemp, a high court judge," Professor Woolard told us gravely. Students usually practiced on nameless indigents, and Woolard made sure we appreciated the privilege we had been granted. "Sir Reginald was a magnificent human being," he continued, as we stared at the wrinkled, bluish corpse. "He has given you the honor of exploring his body, which he generously donated for medical research. From him you will learn the wonder and dignity of the human being. In this laboratory I expect the same atmosphere of respect that I might find at a nobleman's funeral."

For weeks we carved away in a fog of formalin as fans whirred overhead, straining to drive out the pervasive odor. Day after day my colleagues and I snipped through the layers of tissue and bone that had been Sir Reginald Hemp. We learned some of his eating habits, and devised elaborate theories to explain the scars and abnormalities we found within. Indeed, in Hemp's lungs we came across the kind of cellular damage Woolard had warned us about in our first class; evidently, the judge had died of lung cancer.

Sometimes Professor Woolard himself visited the room, taking up a scalpel to demonstrate the finer points of dissection. Once he happened to wander in while two male students were playing a game of catch with their cadaver's kidney. Woolard's domelike head turned red as an aorta, and I feared for a moment that his heart would give way on the spot. He composed himself enough to pillory the offenders, and then gave us all a withering extemporaneous speech on the sacred honor of each and every human body. That speech, delivered with both passion and eloquence by this renowned man, made a huge impression on us students, cowering like schoolchildren caught in a prank.

I had not yet decided on a career in surgery when I encountered H. H. Woolard, but the spirit he imparted would stay with me forever. It was one thing for Sir Reginald Hemp to let medical students rummage through his body after death; it is quite another for living human beings to invite a surgeon to part the veil of skin, enter, and then explore portions of their bodies they themselves have never seen. I am reminded of that privilege, learned from a corpse, every time I draw a scalpel across the skin of a living patient.

My decision to enter surgery, made a few years later, was influenced by another instructor, a man who held the exalted position of surgeon to England's royal family and who bore a grand name befitting his role: Sir Launcelot Barrington-Ward.

Sir Launcelot trained his students like a drill sergeant, trying to instill in us the proper reflexes needed in medical emergencies. "What is your most useful instrument in the event of massive bleeding?" he asked each newcomer assisting him in surgery. "The hemostat [artery forceps]," the assistant would usually respond, proud of himself for coming up with such a quick answer. "No, no, that is for small blood vessels," Sir Launcelot growled through his mask. "In an emergency, a hemostat applied too abruptly may do more harm than good. It may crush nerves, tear vessels, destroy the wrong tissue, and complicate the healing process. You have a perfect instrument with a broad, soft pad rounding off the end of your thumb. Use your thumb!" A few days later he would ask the same assistant the same question, just to test reaction time.

I can still see Sir Launcelot across the operating table, utterly serene, with his thumb resting on a tear in a patient's vena cava. He winks at me and says, "What do you think, Mr. Brand—shall we clamp it or shall we sew it up?" By example he was communicating one of the most important lessons for a young surgeon: Don't panic. "You make mistakes when you panic," he would say, "and fast bleeding breeds panic, so don't rush in with instruments. Use your thumb until you're certain what to do, then do it carefully and deliberately. Unless you can overcome the panic instinct, you'll never make a surgeon."

I listened to Sir Launcelot's advice, but not until a real emergency presented itself did I know whether I had the temperament for surgery. That moment came sooner than I expected. I was working in the large outpatient department, dealing with everyday problems: dressings that needed changing, a child who had pushed a pea too far into his ear canal. Just to the side was a small operating room reserved for minor outpatient surgery, and suddenly a nurse in a blood-spattered uniform shot out of that room. She had an awful, stricken look on her face. "Come quickly!" she called to me. Rushing next door, I saw a surgical intern holding a wad of dressings over the neck of a young woman. Dark red blood had formed a pool under the dressings and was now spilling from the woman's neck onto the floor.

The intern, white as a corpse, gave me a rushed explanation,

"It was just a lymphatic gland in her neck. My chief wanted it taken out for a biopsy specimen. But now I can't see anything for the blood."

The patient herself had a look of terror. Having come in for a minor outpatient procedure under local anesthetic, she now found herself apparently bleeding to death. She was thrashing about and making gurgling noises.

I had pulled on a pair of gloves while the intern was talking. When I lifted off the pack of dressings I saw a small incision, less than two inches, with a virtual forest of forceps protruding from the wound. Most of them must have been applied blindly through the dark blood welling up from below.

"Use your thumb!" I could hear the advice Sir Launcelot had drummed into us. I hastily removed all the forceps and simply pressed down with my gloved thumb, letting its surface fill the breach. Bleeding stopped. My own pulse was racing, but I did nothing but hold my thumb there for several minutes until the panic in the room, in me, and in the patient subsided.

Then, speaking in low tones, I said, "Now then, let's clean up a bit—and nurse, could you please send for an anesthetist? Why don't you go down the hall and see who's on duty." Gradually I could sense the patient relax under my thumb. I explained that we would finish the job and close the wound for her, and that she'd be far more comfortable if we had her sleep through the repair.

When she was finally asleep, and with my thumb pressing on the bleeding site, I had the intern extend the skin incision a little, and I probed until I found the source of all the blood. At once I saw what had happened. The intern had been following a routine procedure for a biopsy: inject novocaine into the neck area, make a small incision, grasp the nodule with forceps, pull, dissect around it, and snip the nodule at the base. One problem he had not anticipated, however: the roots of the nodule had extended downward and wrapped themselves around the surface of the jugular vein. His snipping had inadvertently cut out a segment of the wall of that huge vein. The woman had indeed been in danger of bleeding to death. But now we had relaxed time to repair the defect and close the wound.

An encounter with blood transfusion had convinced me I should go into medicine, and this encounter with the opposite, severe blood loss, helped convinced me I should pursue surgery. I had always liked the mechanical process of surgery, even from dissection days. But until it was tested, I had not known my instinctive response to a medical emergency. Now I believed I could handle the pressures of an operating room.

Verge of Revolution

I chose surgery because it seemed the most concrete way to offer help. War with Germany had broken out and hospitals were filling up with bomb casualties who needed surgical repair. Besides, at that time much of medicine *was* surgery; otherwise, a doctor's task was mostly diagnosis.

Physicians distinguished themselves primarily by their ability to predict the course of the disease. How long will the fever last? Any lingering aftereffects? Will the patient die? Patients recovered from diseases, but credit was due mainly to their own immune systems, reinforced by a little outside assistance. The concept of radical cure by specific medication lay beyond the bounds of medicine. Once we had identified and classified the bacterium or virus causing an illness, we were as helpless as doctors from a previous century. The word *antibiotic* had not yet come into use.

The influenza epidemic of 1918–19, the same one that had established my father's reputation on the Kolli Malai, clearly demonstrated that impotence. Deaths from the epidemic totaled 20 million worldwide, surpassing even the carnage of World War I. The greatest medical specialists of the day could do nothing more than my father had done: stand beside dying patients, bathe them, and offer soup or other nourishment. The aura of fear and mystery that surrounds AIDS as I write this in the early 1990s—a disease we can isolate, identify, and accumulate knowledge about, but without a clue as to how to cure—applied to a wide array of diseases half a century ago.

Any slight infection represented a mortal danger, for we simply had no way to slow it. Streptococcus originating from a needle prick could travel up a nurse's arm—you could watch the progress of a fine red line under her skin—and kill her. A septic boil at the base of the nose had dire consequences, for it could travel along a vein right to a sinus and then into the brain. Never, ever, squeeze a boil on the nose, we would warn patients. In treating eye injuries, at the earliest sign of infection the eye was usually removed rather than risk a sympathetic reaction in the other eye. Wartime added new hazards, for the wounds of battle made a fine breeding ground for the sporing bacteria that caused gas gangrene. To complicate matters, the hospital environment introduced its own dangers. If, while working on a soldier's grenade wound, we accidentally admitted staphylococcus into an area of bone, we triggered a whole sequence of chronic disease. We could operate again and carve out the site of infection, but the sepsis almost certainly would appear somewhere else, in an ankle or a hip joint.*

Into this stifling atmosphere of helplessness blew the first breezes of change and hope. First we heard promising reports about syphilis. Everyone in a cosmopolitan city like London knew the jerky, pavement-slapping walk that marked the assault of syphilis on the central nervous system, a probable prelude to blindness, dementia, and, ultimately, death. Doctors sometimes resorted to a drastic treatment for the worst cases: they would deliberately infect patients with malaria, hoping the fevers would cook away the syphilis, and then treat the malaria with quinine. In the 1930s, though, came word of successful treatment of syphilis with derivatives of arsenic. There were dangers, to be sure, especially to the liver. But I can still remember how novel, almost miraculous, it seemed to be able to stop a disease in its tracks.

In 1935 German scientists made the exciting discovery that certain synthetic chemicals actually killed bacteria without harming tissue, especially a red chemical called Prontosil (which had the startling side effect of turning patients bright pink). British scientists, who smuggled in some Prontosil at the onset of the war, analyzed the dye and identified the active ingredient, sulfanilamide, which became the first of a whole new generation of sulfa drugs. When the story circulated across England that a sulfa drug

---

*It had taken the heroic efforts of Ignaz Semmelweis and Joseph Lister to convince the medical establishment that hospitals themselves were incubators of lethal germs. Deaths from childbirth dropped 90 percent in one year when Semmelweis persuaded Viennese hospitals to start scrubbing their hands and using chlorine water. As late as 1870, one in four surgery patients died of infections introduced by the surgery (commonly called "hospital gangrene" or "mortification of the wound"). England's Joseph Lister countered with a disinfectant spray, filling his operating theater with a fine mist of carbolic acid, and taught all surgeons the laborious task of preparatory scrubbing. Even in my student days, surgery in a hospital still sometimes resulted in infection. Operations were occasionally performed at home to avoid hospital bacteria.

had saved Winston Churchill from a deadly bacterial infection in North Africa, the term "miracle drug" entered the vocabulary.

We students, interns, and residents in the early 1940s had the vague sense of living in a breakthrough era in the history of medicine. Sometimes older professors would say wistfully, "Oh, to be starting out now!" It soon became apparent that I had happened to enter medical school at the very threshold of a revolution.

I sensed the change in medicine most dramatically in two separate research projects during my tenure at University College. The first project, conducted just before the chemical breakthroughs, was spearheaded by an upperclassman named Ilingworth Law, an engineer who had entered school at age forty-five to begin a second career in medicine. Law puzzled over the infections that tended to radiate through a hand from an injury site on a finger. Dissecting the hands of cadavers, he studied the hydraulics of fluids in the fingers. He would inject a suspension of water and carbon black (specks of black dust about the size of pus molecules) into the fingers, then repeatedly bend and straighten them, tracing the route of the carbon black.

I remember Ilingworth's enthusiasm when he discovered that the simple motion of flexion was the main agent for distributing infection throughout the hand. "We can stop the infection from spreading!" he said triumphantly. "All we have to do is immobilize the finger to keep it from bending. We can contain the infection in a local area and then drain it." His techniques caught on quickly at our hospital, and before long his professor was publishing papers on them, giving little or no credit to Law himself.

The ability to contain the spread of infection stood at the frontier of medicine in 1939. Yet four years later we residents were experimenting with a new medication that promised what no drug before had dared to promise: penicillin, possibly the greatest single advance in medical history, had come into use.

The details of Alexander Fleming's discovery of penicillin in 1928 have rightfully become the stuff of legend. He worked in a cluttered, mildly chaotic laboratory, and his research often showed a touch of whimsy. (He liked to swab selected germs in a pattern on a culture dish so that the chromogenic bacteria emerging twenty-four hours later would form a picture or a word. Bacteria would in effect sign their own names: "egg" or "tears," for example, on an agar surface coated with egg white or human tears.)

The first penicillin spores entered Fleming's laboratory

entirely by chance, probably blown in through an open window. In a museum in England I have seen the original culture dish on which Fleming first noticed penicillin's unusual properties. He was trying to grow staphylococci bacteria, not mold, and on the edges of the dish, colonies of staph glow brightly, like galaxies at the edge of the universe. Closer to the center, though, they turn pale, mere ghost-images. And around the patch of mold itself the agar plate is dark; no bacteria are visible. The black hole of *Penicillium notatum* has swallowed them all.

For twelve years, off and on, Fleming worked with penicillin. Despite its remarkable ability to kill harmful bacteria, penicillin showed little potential as a drug: it was toxic and unstable and broke down quickly inside the human body. Still, Fleming kept enough of the mold (a rare one, as it turned out) growing to supply himself and others.

In 1939, more than a decade after Fleming's discovery, Howard Walter Florey, a young Australian pathologist at Oxford, took an interest in penicillin. He could not have picked a worse time to launch an expensive research project: his application for a government grant arrived three days after Britain declared war on Germany. On the very day Hitler's panzers drove the British Army toward Dunkirk, Florey performed his first clinical tests on mice, injecting them first with streptococci, then with penicillin. The experiment showed so much promise that Florey, after learning of the defeat at Dunkirk, smeared penicillin spores into the lining of his coat so that in event of a German conquest he could smuggle the mold out of the country. Later that year he conducted clinical tests on human patients, with dramatic success.*

Florey's lab became a penicillin factory. He grew the mold in milk churns, pottery, gasoline cans, biscuit tins, any container he

---

*Florey learned why Fleming's clinical trials had failed: the penicillin obtained even after elaborate purification procedures was 99.9 percent impure. Once Florey had learned to purify the drug and increase its potency, it took only a small amount of penicillin to kill bacteria. The tiny amounts we prescribed then would astound a modern doctor. In 1945 I conducted tests on behalf of the Medical Research Council to determine the right dosage to cure babies of staphylococcus infections in the bloodstream. We found that a daily dose of 1,000 units penicillin per kilogram of body weight would suffice to kill all traces of the infection. Today, because of resistant strains, a doctor would need to prescribe a hundred times that amount.

could find. Allied governments, quick to recognize the drug's potential for use against infections in wounded servicemen—and also against gonorrhea, which in some places was causing more casualties than the enemy—offered full-scale backing. An old cheese factory was sequestered to grow penicillin. The Distiller's Company agreed to convert some of their huge vats from the brewing of alcohol to the brewing of mold. This enormous effort produced a grand total of twenty-nine pounds of purified penicillin in 1943. Americans hoarded their quantities in anticipation of D-Day. British authorities restricted the drug to use by servicemen and carefully meted out supplies to approved hospitals.

I was doing rotations at London suburban hospitals when I had my first direct contact with penicillin. At Leavesdon, an evacuation hospital, I treated some of the victims of the British retreats at Boulogne and Dunkirk. Word of the miracle drug had spread like a prairie fire among the troops. "No matter how bad your wound, this stuff will keep you alive," the rumor went. At that time no drug, not even morphine, was more precious or more craved. Soldiers selected for treatment believed they would gain an invincibility against all disease; they would gain new life.

Yet there were a few problems with the miracle drug. Distillers had not perfected the purification process and the thick, yellowish solution was highly irritable to living tissue. Inject it in a vein and the vein would thrombose, or close tight in self-defense. Inject it into the dermis and the skin would become necrotic. We could only give it intramuscularly, preferably in the buttocks, where the needle could sink deep. It burned like acid, and the soldiers' buttocks became so sore they had to sleep on their stomachs. Worst of all, the drug had to be administered every three hours.

It was in the Leavesdon evacuation hospital in those early days of the penicillin program that I learned an indelible lesson about the powerful, even overwhelming role the mind plays in pain perception. "We feel one cut from the scalpel more than ten blows of the sword in the heat of battle," said Montaigne. One of my patients, a man named Jake, bore out the literal truth of that statement.

The Frightened Hero

Jake had been evacuated from the beaches of Boulogne. His friends loved to recount the tale of his heroism. During an attempt to advance and destroy an enemy position, Jake got pinned down in the no-man's-land between trenches. A blast from an artillery shell shattered his legs. He managed to wriggle over to the relative safety of a foxhole, where he looked down and saw that his legs were a mess. A few minutes later one of Jake's buddies fell to the ground nearby. From his foxhole, Jake saw him lying in an open field, unconscious and exposed to enemy fire. Jake somehow pulled himself out of his foxhole, crawled over to his friend, and, his own shattered legs trailing behind him, dragged himself and his friend back to safety.

Jake had been selected for the new penicillin therapy to combat severe secondary infections in his legs. According to his friends, no one deserved it more. Jake himself, however, failed to appreciate this honor. He could handle the daytime injections when his buddies were awake and he had much else to concentrate on, but the wake-up calls at 2:00 and 5:00 A.M. were more than he could stand. The night nurse complained to me that Jake cried like a baby when she approached his bed at night. "Please, no! Go away!" he would yell. He fought her and grabbed her wrist when she moved the needle toward him.

"He's hopeless, Dr. Brand," said the nurse. "I don't think I can give him the treatment. Besides, he's disrupting the ward."

It fell to me as house surgeon to reason with Jake. I decided on a blunt, man-to-man approach. "Jake, all the guys tell me you are a hero. Not even the pain from two broken legs could stop you from saving your buddy in no-man's-land. Now tell me, why are you giving us so much trouble over a needle prick in your backside?"

His face became that of a petulant child, "It's not just a needle prick, Doc. That penicillin may be good stuff, but it burns and it stings! There isn't a place on my backside that's not sore."

"Yes, I know it stings, Jake, but you're a hero. You've proved you know how to handle pain."

"Oh, on the battlefield, yes. There's a lot more going on out there—the noise, the flashes, my buddies around me. But here in the ward, I have only one thing to think about all night in bed: that needle. It's huge, and when the nurse comes down the row with her tray full of syringes, it gets bigger and bigger. I just can't take it, Dr. Brand!"

* * *

Sometimes a single scene can help crystallize ideas and hunches that have been floating in suspension for years, and my bedside conversation with Jake did that for me. Having heard his story from other soldiers, I had a vivid mental picture of the battlefield hero defying all protective instincts, including pain, for the sake of his friend. But the night nurse gave me an equally vivid picture of Jake the coward, his face contorted in fear, awaiting the nighttime needle. Those two images, brought together by our conversation, underscored an important fact about pain: pain takes place in the mind, nowhere else.

As I would soon learn, the human brain in essence advises the pain system what it wants to be told. Having changed Jake's bandages and studied his X rays, I had some idea of the millions of pain signals that had reported in from his shattered legs. But much else was occupying Jake's brain at the time of the injury, and those screaming messages of pain simply did not register. Later, in the total absence of any competing activity or thought, an oversize penicillin needle made a far more compelling and urgent case for attention.

While dealing with Jake, I also grasped the wisdom that lay behind the approach to medicine we learned in those days. We practiced a more general treatment of the whole person because we had so little specific help to offer. But Jake showed why all good medicine must take into account the "whole" person. Somehow I had to convince Jake that the battle he now fought in a recovery ward was as meaningful as the battle he had fought so gallantly on a beach at Boulogne.

4
Pain's Lair

———◆———

*Common sense, though all very well for everyday purposes, is easily
confused, even by such simple questions as "Where is the rainbow? When
you hear a voice on a gramophone record, are you hearing the man who
spoke, or a reproduction? When you feel a pain in the leg that has been
amputated, where is the pain?" If you say it is in your head, would it be
in your head if the leg had not been amputated? If you say yes, then what
reason have you ever for thinking you have a leg?*

Bertrand Russell

My interest in pain had actually been kindled a few years before I
decided on surgery, during a detour in my medical training. I had
begun my second year of studies in September 1939, just as Nazis
marched into Poland, and England responded with a declaration
of war. The authorities decided that London, a prime target for
German bombers, was no place for juniors to study medicine.
They shipped most of my class off to Cardiff, Wales, and it was in
that sleepy coastal city that I first delved into the mysteries of pain
and sensation.

I do not know the name of my most memorable acquaintance
in Cardiff, a middle-aged Welshman with a shock of dark hair and
bushy eyebrows. I never saw the rest of his body, for it had been
severed from his head. I had proposed an ambitious project for my
required dissection: to expose the twelve cranial nerves of the head
and follow them to their site of origin in the brain.

Normally our cadavers came with empty skulls, their brains
removed for the benefit of neurosurgery students. "Don't worry,"
my gentle old adviser Professor West said, "I think I can locate a
head for you." Before long the Welshman's head appeared, brain
intact.

The lab schedule called for dissection three mornings a week, but I found myself coming back every free hour, often late into the night. The smell of formaldehyde never left me, lingering on my skin to affect the taste of food, toothpaste, and even water. Looking back, the scene seems a bit macabre. The Medical College in Cardiff occupied a stone Edwardian building complete with gables, parapets, and angular hallways—a perfect setting for a Gothic horror story. In a large room sealed with blackout cloth I sat alone by a hooded laboratory lamp, hunched over a cadaver head. Leonardo da Vinci wrote of his "fear of passing the night hours in the company of these [dissected] corpses, quartered and flayed and horrible to behold." Yet even da Vinci, under orders from Rome, averted his gaze from the human brain.

Journey Inward

To a surgeon, nothing quite compares to the sensation of cutting through living skin. Trace a thin line with your scalpel and skin springs open to reveal moist, colorful layers underneath. The tissue talks to you through the knife, informing the delicate pressure sensors on your fingertips of your precise location.

In contrast, pickled skin is mute. Make a cut, and nothing springs open. Every layer has the same cheesy consistency, giving you no idea how deep the knife has plunged. For this reason medical students tend to make a mess of dissections and wonder whether clumsiness will disqualify them from surgery. Fortunately, cadavers do not sue for malpractice, and the students eventually learn that a living body, though less forgiving of mistakes in dissection, is far less prone to cause them.

I had not yet operated on living bodies when I made the dissection in Cardiff, but thanks to my experience in carpentry I felt comfortable working with tools on a variety of materials. (It frightens me to realize that some surgeons hold their first saw when they cut a human bone and turn their first screwdriver when they screw a steel plate to it!) Starting at a point between the eyebrows, I made a midline cut along the ridge of the nose, through the lips, and over the chin down to the neck. Next I cut in the other direction, bisecting the scalp. I peeled back the skin on one side of the face and stripped away fat, connective tissue, and even the glistening facial muscles, for I was on a hunt for thin white nerves.

Of the many nerves in the human body, only the twelve cranial nerves bypass the spinal cord with a hotline to the brain. Flick a finger at my eye and I blink. Chew gum while talking and your tongue darts perilously in and out of chomping molars to steer the gum and suck its juices, all the while snaking from teeth to roof of mouth to lips to teeth again, forming syllables of sound. These speedy movements, guided by sensory input, are made possible by the cranial nerves' short, direct path to the brain.

The first cranial nerve, the olfactory, was easy to track. Chipping away bone from the upper nasal cavity near the eyebrows, I exposed the cribriform plate, a penny-size patch of bone and spongy tissue supporting millions of tiny hairs. The advance guard of smell, these cilia wave in the breeze like stalks of rice, trapping odorous molecules in a bed of mucus for the olfactory bulbs to analyze. They seemed very fragile, and I knew that a severe blow to the head could shear off those receptors, leaving the victim in a permanent state of smell-lessness. Since anatomically the two olfactory bulbs are pieces of the brain itself extended outward, I did not have to trace the nerve far. The roof of the nose is the floor of the brain.

After laying open the olfactory nerve I shifted my focus a few inches to the four cranial nerves concerned with vision. Three of these nerves control eyeball movements (the largest, the optical nerve, carries digitized images from the retina to the brain). Coordinating six tiny muscles, they furnish an advanced tracking system that allows us to lock in, say, on a goldfinch and follow its erratic, dipping flight across the horizon. The same nerves govern the minuscule jerks and glides required by the act of reading.

Saccade is the name anatomists give to the eyeball's tiniest movements, borrowing the French word for the motion a horseman makes when he jerks abruptly on the reins. The metaphor fits: if the six opposing eye muscles did not remain taut, like reins on a spirited horse, our eyes would drift up or down, or out to the edges, or toward the nose. I cleaned the nerve pathways to those six muscles with a sense of wonder. They get the greatest workout of any muscle, moving about 100,000 times each day (equivalent to leg muscles walking fifty miles). They even participate in our dreams: the brain shuts down other motor pathways, but for some reason condones rapid eye movements (REM) during sleep.

I will not linger over details of the other cranial nerves, which had made it possible for the Welshman to taste, hear, swallow, speak, move his head and neck, and also feel the sensations of lips, scalp, and teeth. As the dissection deadline neared I became more and more obsessed with my project, skipping classes to spend time with my cadaver head. The bombings (German planes were soon targeting Cardiff) and the war outside seemed remote as I moved farther and farther inward, into the brain itself tracking my prey into a region of absolute mystery.

When working on the bony surface of the skull, I would pound with a mallet and chisel, as in my stonecutter days. Other times, as I pricked away thin layers of fat and fibrous muscle, I breathed shallowly and took care to keep the blunt edge of the scalpel toward the nerve. I remember a slight slip of the knife as I tried to follow the nerve that carries taste sensations along its shortcut route through the ear canal. *Oops!* It was the type of mistake that gives a surgeon nightmares: if operating on a patient, I would have put an abrupt end to the pleasures of eating and drinking. I artfully pieced the nerve together with glue, breathing a prayer of thanks that I was working on a cadaver, not a living person.

After a month of tedious dissection, I added a few cosmetic details to my cadaver head. I painted the cranial nerves with a yellow pigment, the color of fresh butter, so they would stand out against the background of bone and white matter. The purplish tint of veins made a nice complement, and I added some color to the pale arteries. I felt proud of the final result: twelve distinct yellow lines meandered through bone and muscle on their way to the wrinkled brain, at which point they fanned out magnificently.

Professor West beamed his approval and put the specimen on display, and for a few days I entertained schoolboy fantasies of a career in brain surgery. As it happened, I did not become a neurosurgeon, but those weeks spent with a cadaver head helped to form my understanding of the odd alliance that exists between the brain and the rest of the human body.

The Ivory Box

Above all, the dissection project taught me to appreciate the splendid isolation of the human brain. To remove the thick mantle of skull I had drilled a line of evenly spaced holes, threaded a fine Gigli saw between them, worked the saw back and forth, and lifted off the squares like trap doors. A cloud of fine bone dust drifted through the room that day and I, exhausted, came away impressed with the body's means of protecting its most valued member.

Ironically, the organ the body trusts to interpret the world lives in a state of solitary confinement, shut off from that world. The organ that gives us consciousness lies beyond our conscious awareness: unlike the stomach, it makes no noises; unlike the heart, it is not felt as it toils; unlike the skin, it cannot be pinched. The skull—so thick that to cut through it I had to lean at an angle and put all my weight behind the saw—seals the brain from every direct encounter with reality. Ensconced in an opaque skull, the brain never "sees" anything. Its temperature varies only a few degrees, and any fever exceeding that would kill it. It hears nothing. It feels no pain: a neurosurgeon, once inside the skull, can explore at will with no need for further anesthetic. All sights, sounds, smells, and other sensations that define life come to the brain indirectly: detected in the extremities, escorted along the nerve pathways, and announced in the common language of nerve transmission. To a secluded brain, it does not matter where the data originate. Butterflies and blowflies, equipped with organs of taste on their feet, can sample a spilled soft drink by wading in it. Cats scout the world with whiskers.

The year I was in Cardiff, laboratories in Plymouth, England, and Woods Hole, Massachusetts, made the first recordings of actual electrical signals from the nervous system. By inserting electrodes into the oversized axons of a squid, the scientists could eavesdrop on individual nerve cells. They heard a series of clicks and pauses closely resembling the pattern of Morse code. The entire animal kingdom uses the same simple "on/off" pattern of reporting information to the brain. A neuron in the human ear, for example, detects vibration at a certain frequency and sends a signal, pauses a thousandth of a second, and if the stimulus persists sends another signal. The brain itself never feels the vibration; it simply receives a report, in a form not unlike the digital code used on modern compact discs.

Nerve transmission relies on an elegant combination of chemistry and electricity. Along the "wire," or axon, of an excited nerve, sodium and potassium ions dance in and out of a permeable membrane, changing the electrical charge from positive to negative as the charge travels up the axon in a wave pattern. All perceived sensations—the smell of garlic, a view of the Grand Canyon, the pain of heart attack, the sound of an orchestra—

reduce to this process of nerve cells spitting charged ions at each other.* The brain has the task of interpreting all these electrical codes and presenting them to consciousness as a visual image or sound, a smell or a jolt of pain, depending on their nature and origin.

At the cellular level the pain network crackles ceaselessly with information, most of which never achieves the rank of conscious pain because our bodies handle the signals appropriately. Sensors in my bladder continually report on distension, and sensors on the surface of my eye report on lubrication. If I respond by going to the bathroom and by blinking regularly, these will not become pain; but if I deliberately ignore their gentle reminders for a few hours, I'll feel excruciating pain. The health of the body depends largely on its attentiveness to the pain network.

Neurons are the largest cells in the human body—in the leg, they can reach a yard in length—and the only cells not replaced every few years. As I dissected the Welshman's brain in Cardiff, I began to visualize the design of nerve cells as something like a great tree uprooted in a winter storm: a tangled network of roots in the extremities joined to a tangled network of branches in the brain by a long, straight trunk (the axon). In an extremity like a finger or toe, a neuron depends on "root hair" dendrites to discuss with surrounding neurons what sort of signal to send the brain. A large neuron may share information with other neurons along the way, crossing as many as ten thousand synapses. But a sensation like pain, whether originating in the fingertip or in the foot, does not really register until it completes the circuit and reaches the brain.

Santiago Ramón y Cajal, the father of modern brain science, described brain neurons as "the mysterious butterflies of the soul,

---

*Nerve transmission was a hot topic during my years in medical school. Scientists had known for many years that muscle contraction involved an electrical signal, but did not understand the mechanism involved. In 1936 the German pharmacologist Otto Loewi was awarded the Nobel Prize in Medicine for his discoveries in the field. Loewi had been stymied in his attempt to understand the exact process of nerve transmission until one night it came to him in a dream. He awoke, scribbled a few words on a scrap of paper, and contentedly went back to sleep. But the next morning his scribble proved illegible, and details of the dream eluded him all day. Amazingly, that night the dream repeated. This time Loewi jumped from bed and rushed to his laboratory. By dawn he had discovered the basic nature of nerve transmission in frog muscles: an electrical charge conveyed through a chain of chemical reactions.

the beating of whose wings may some day—who knows?—clarify the secret of mental life." Exploration of the nervous system tends to bring out comments like that. Nowhere are the Creator's fingerprints more visible than in the brain, where mind and body come together.

Looking at the Welshman's brain through magnifying loops, I could see the upper end of the nerve "tree," with its branches crisscrossing each other in a tangle of soft white threads. Each neuron has a thousand or so junctions with other neurons, and some cells in the cerebral cortex have as many as sixty thousand. A gram of brain tissue may contain as many as 400 billion synaptic junctions, and the total quantity of connections in one brain rivals the number of stars in the universe. Every bit of data carried along nerve threads sets off an electrical storm among other cells, and in the utter isolation of its ivory box the brain must rely on these connections to make sense of the buzzing chaos of the world outside. Sir Charles Sherrington, a Nobel Laureate and well-known neurophysiologist at my school in London, likened brain activity to an "enchanted loom" composed of patterns of tiny lights flickering on and off. From all this rapid-fire activity—five trillion chemical processes a second—we form patterns of meaning about the world.

Many times, as I worked late at night in a room dark but for the oval cast by the lab lamp, I wondered about the Welshman and the electrical storms within his brain. What messages had his auditory nerve relayed: Mozart or the big band sound? Had he worked in a noisy factory that gradually dulled his hearing? Had he a family? If so, the first babbles of his children and the love-whispers of his wife had followed the route of the nerve I was dissecting at that moment.

The mandibular branch of the very large fifth cranial nerve had presented a dissection challenge, for the nerve tunneled through the jawbone, emerging in numerous places to supply sensation for the lips and teeth. When I chiseled through bone and enamel to expose the slender axons in the teeth, I came across untreated dental cavities. I thought back to childhood memories of blinding toothache pain; the Welshman's nerve must have carried similar messages of torment. Yet that same nerve also carried subtle sensations from the lips—every pleasure from every kiss had traveled the identical pathway to the brain.

Whatever its source in the head—tooth decay, scratched

cornea, pierced eardrum, canker sore—pain travels along one of the twelve cranial nerves and presents itself to the brain in a code identical to that used for conveying hearing, smell, vision, taste, and touch. How could the brain sort out such mixed messages? I came away from my dissection project awed by the economy and elegance of the system that transcribes the vast phenomena of the material world.

The brain dissection in Cardiff set me thinking about sensation and taught me a fundamental truth about the nature of pain, the truth I would later see played out in patients like Jake the soldier. As I stared at the Welshman's dissected head I realized that sensations of pain, like all others, enter the brain in the neutral, dot-dash language of nerve transmission. Anything more—an emotional response or even the perception "It hurts!"—is an interpretation supplied by the brain.

Master Conjurer

While my classmates and I were studying medicine in Cardiff, Winston Churchill was establishing a war command center underneath Whitehall Palace in London. Often Churchill spent the night there, sleeping on a cot in a makeshift bedroom sheltered from German bombs by a thick slab of reinforced concrete. Since he rarely toured the fronts in person, Churchill had to make crucial military decisions in that command center on the basis of reports that came in from all over the world via telegraph and telephone lines. Colored markers on huge wall maps displayed the daily progress of Allied forces. If Montgomery needed reinforcements in North Africa, he wired for help. If ship captains of Atlantic convoys desired more naval support, they sent in a request.

That underground command center served as the brain for the British war machine, the one place where the needs and requirements of the entire army could be weighed. Yet its very isolation made Churchill vulnerable to mistakes: what if an important message never got through, or a German agent managed to sneak in disinformation? From the thousands of communications that came in, each one subject to human error, headquarters personnel had to devise a "best guess" policy to serve the good of the whole.

The human brain, too, must rely on incomplete and sometimes erroneous information. After sifting through millions of bits of data, the brain provides an interpretation based on its "best guess," in which memory plays a large role. From the moment of birth onward, the brain actively constructs an internal model of the external world, a picture of how the world works.

Each day after dissecting and attending classes in medical school I would go home, open the door, and warmly greet my Cardiff landlady, Granny Morgan. At least that was the version of reality presented by my brain after it had evaluated a series of coded messages. Touch corpuscles in my fingers sent in reports of a pressure of 124 grams per square centimeter while nearby temperature sensors reported an input of two calories per second. My brain, receiving these signals from thousands of nerve fibers in my right hand, assembled a composite impression of a warm object imposing upward and downward thrusts on that hand, and, comparing these sensations with its data bank of past experiences, it then diagnosed a handshake.

Meanwhile, millions of rods and cones in my eye identified zones of shading and color which the brain sifted through and recognized as a pattern matching the face of Granny Morgan. (Only engineers who have tried to program computers for facial recognition can fully appreciate the complexity of this chore.) And tiny hairs in my inner ear sent in reports of molecular vibrations at specific tonal frequencies; the brain related these thousands of bits of code to the past record of my landlady's voice.

When I reduce mental activity to its constituent parts, I marvel that I can ever know what goes on in the world outside. Yet the process occurs instantaneously, below the level of consciousness, as soon as I hear the voice and look into the face of a friend. Over time, I have learned to trust the image of reality presented to me by my brain.

(Naturally, the brain sometimes guesses wrong.* Close your eyes and press on the skin in the corners by your nose. You will see

---

*Psychology textbooks give examples of simple *illusions*—from a Latin word meaning "to mock, or ridicule"—that demonstrate how easily our brains can be fooled. Lifting two cans of equal weight, we'll judge the smaller can lighter, even if it has 20 percent more weight in it, simply because we expect it to feel lighter. (Blindfolded, we would judge both equal.) We are duped into thinking two parallel lines uneven if a third line intersects them at an angle. We'll think one line longer than another if it ends with arrow vectors pointing inward instead of outward. Hollywood has built an entire industry on illusion. The brain cannot dwell on twenty-four patches of false light because the sudden pressure provokes the optic nerve to fire off signals that the brain, using its "best guess," interprets and renders as light. Similarly, a blow to the head may cause a person to "see stars." Neurological disorders may further confuse the brain. I knew a man in my student days who suffered from Ménière's syndrome. The balancing mechanisms in his inner ear, gone awry, would suddenly send false messages that he was tilting to the right. Receiving these misguided signals, the brain ordered a series of corrective moves, and he would throw himself violently to the left. We learned to place a cushion on his left side to protect him from injury.)

This basic awareness of how the brain works—isolated, it constructs a "best guess" inner picture to interpret the outer world—clarified my thinking about pain. As a child I had instinctively viewed pain as an enemy "out there" attacking me at the site of injury: when a scorpion stung my finger, I squeezed the finger and ran into the house crying to show it to my mother. Now I learned from the Welshman's brain that pain is not out there, but rather "in here," inside the ivory box of skull. Paradoxically, pain seems like something done to us, though in reality we have done it to ourselves, manufacturing the sensation. Whatever we might conceive of as "pain" occurs in the mind.

The sounds of traffic outside, the smell of cut lilacs on the table, the itchiness of my wool pants—all these, like pain, arrive in the same neutral Morse code of nerve transmission to await the mind's interpretation. A vibrating eardrum does not constitute hearing (my eardrums vibrate when I'm asleep), and a stubbed toe does not constitute pain. Pain is always a mental or psychological event, a magician's trick the mind knowingly plays on itself. It per-

---

individual frames of still pictures in a second, so it allows them to merge together in the illusion of movement.

An internal picture of reality, of course, depends entirely on what messages reach the isolated brain. Kittens raised in boxes painted with horizontal stripes do not even notice vertical stripes at first: their brain cells have not yet developed a category of "verticalness." For people born with color blindness, the world seems no less "real" than it does to me, and yet our internal pictures are very different. Blind people have auditory dreams: their brains must fashion a sense of reality apart from visual images. Quite probably, the artists Van Gogh, El Greco, and Edgar Degas "saw" their surroundings in such an uncommon way because eye disorders affected their perception. After a cataract operation, Monet was surprised to find so much blueness in the world; he retouched his recent work so it would conform to his new vision.

forms this conjuring feat with such powerful suspension of disbelief that I stop whatever I'm doing and tend to the toe. I cannot avoid the impression that the pain itself is in my toe, not my brain.

Sufferers from migraine, whiplash, or bad back sometimes hear the catty comment, "Your pain is in your head." In a most literal sense, all pain is in the head: it originates there, and dwells there. Pain does not exist until you feel it, and you feel it in your mind. Bertrand Russell got it right when he went to the dentist with a toothache. "Where does it hurt?" the dentist asked. Russell replied, "In my brain, of course."

Baptism by Fire

I learned about pain in the abstract in my Cardiff laboratory. Just as I moved back to London in September 1940, the Luftwaffe began attacking that city in full fury and I found myself immersed in human suffering.

Graham Greene, who lived through the Blitz, remembers it like this: "Looking back, it is the squalor of the night, the purgatorial throng of men and women in dirty torn pyjamas with little blood splashes standing in doorways, which remains. These were disquieting because they supplied images for what one day would probably happen to oneself." I mainly recall a state of relentless exhaustion. We students took turns spending evenings and nights fire watching on the hospital roof. It was eerie to look out over a city under total blackout. First we heard the growling sound made by bomber engines. Soon flares floated down slowly, like large yellow flowers siphoned out of the night. Then came the whistle of bombs and bright orange bursts of explosion. The brick buildings in our neighborhood collapsed easily, kicking up huge clouds of smoke and dust, and flames licked through the windows of the ghostly superstructures that remained.

During one period, fifteen hundred planes attacked London on fifty-seven consecutive nights, and antiaircraft guns clattered all night without pause. I remember two especially somber nights. The first was captured in a famous wartime photo: incendiary bombs had ignited a firestorm around St. Paul's Cathedral, and the photo shows the grand dome designed by Sir Christopher Wren backlit by a sky of flame. When I went off shift I told my roommates that St. Paul's would surely fall. The loss felt heavy, a symbol of our civilization being pummeled into ruin. But the next morning as smoke cleared away and the gray sky lightened I saw that somehow, miraculously, St. Paul's had survived and stood alone, defiant, amid several blocks of rubble.

Another night, bombs hit University College. Bomb fragments heavily damaged the quarters for resident doctors, which few lamented: the bricked-up windows made the rooms intolerably stuffy and we were happy to move. What grieved us was that the university library, third best in all England, burned to the ground.

In addition to fire-watching duties, medical students were pressed into service to treat the bombing victims. During heavy bombardment, residents were on call every single night. The real surgeons handled the complex fractures and third-degree burns, while we juniors did such tasks as picking fragments of glass out of people who had been standing near a window when a bomb fell. I remember the janitor of a church who had received a full blast of stained glass window fragments in his face, chest, and abdomen. He joked with us: "Can you tell whether it's Jesus or the Virgin Mary by the pattern of the glass you're pulling out?"

After casualty duty we would grab a few hours of sleep before breakfast—sometimes in a "mattress sandwich" to muffle the noise of the bombing—and then, after downing countless cups of coffee, begin the daytime regimen of studies and clinical work in the wards. I followed this routine for several months until I approached the point of physical breakdown.

One morning while reading a patient's chart I asked the nurse, "Who prescribed this sedative?" "You did," she replied. Horror-stricken, I listened to her account of the previous night: she had awakened me from sleep, described the patient's symptoms, and then taken down my mumbled prescription order. I had no thread of memory of the incident. I must have been functioning at some subconscious level and talking in my sleep. Fortunately, I had made a reasonable decision and the dosage was acceptable, but I knew I dare not put my patients in jeopardy. I asked for, and received, a two-week leave.

Catching a train to Cardiff, I showed up at the familiar house that belonged to my old landlady Granny Morgan. She was a true eccentric—very charming, very Welsh, very deaf, and very Baptist. She carried around a brass ear trumpet about eighteen inches long, which extended up from her head like a ram's horn. Terrified of being caught in her nightclothes during an air raid, she wore all her clothes to bed. And instead of changing skirts, which would risk immodesty (a bomb might hit while she dressed), she wore them in layers, underskirts and black overskirts all pulled up over each other. Despite her oddity, or perhaps because of it, Granny Morgan had become a dear friend, serving as a kind of surrogate parent for us students during our interlude in Cardiff.

Granny Morgan certainly knew how to handle an exhausted medical student. She fed me, pampered me, and let me sleep undisturbed sixteen to twenty hours a day. She did one more thing during that visit: she convinced me I needed a wife. "You won't do better than Margaret Berry," Granny said. "She'll look after you."

Margaret was a charming classmate who had helped tutor me through my first, difficult year of transition from construction work to medical school. She had been evacuated to Cardiff the year after me, and I had put her in touch with Granny Morgan. Granny asked my opinion about marrying Margaret and thrust her ear trumpet in my direction. I shouted that I'd have to think it over. Actually, I had often entertained the idea of marrying Margaret Berry, and the more I contemplated it the more I liked the idea. After two weeks' rest, I traveled back to London and made a point of looking her up. We fell in love, and a year later we were married.

We enjoyed an eight-day honeymoon in the Wye Valley, then settled into separate hectic schedules. Margaret took an assignment across town and I became surgical officer at the Hospital for Sick Children on Great Ormond Street. Since many of England's best doctors had been shipped to the front, I had nearly unlimited opportunity to practice surgical technique. In the daytime I worked on pediatric procedures and at night I supervised the casualty station where mangled victims of bombings were taken. For a budding surgeon, the experience was invaluable; for a newlywed husband, very trying. Margaret and I could only spend alternate weekends together, and the setting for these rendezvous was usually a bomb shelter in the basement with the rest of her family.

About that time, a horrible new weapon appeared in the skies of London: the V-1 rocket, or buzz bomb, as we called it. It flew in a straight line with a tail of flame stretching out behind, and chattered with a noise like a machine gun until the fuel ran out. Twenty seconds of dread silence followed, then the rocket would wobble a bit and fall to the earth with a thunderous crash. I remember one night of fire watching when I calculated that an incoming V-1 rocket would hit Great Ormond Street Hospital dead-on. I sounded the alarm. The buzz bomb whooshed just above the roof I was crouching on, missing by twenty feet, but made a solid hit on Royal Free Hospital a few streets away. I scrambled down from the roof and ran to a scene straight out of Dante.

Walls in the obstetric ward had collapsed and volunteers were already digging in the smoldering ruins for newborns, most of them less than a week old. Out of the rubble they pulled babies speckled with plaster, blood, grime, and glass. The babies' thin, pathetic cries went unheard in the clamor. To the side, mothers in bathrobes gray with debris dust watched with fear and despair flickering across their faces. Volunteers, forming a line like a fire brigade, passed the babies to ambulances that began pulling up outside on a street shiny with broken glass. I dashed back to Ormond Street to prepare to receive these new casualties.

A few months later, I caught a firsthand glimpse of what those mothers must have been feeling. I had fire-watching assignment on the roof of Great Ormond Street Hospital the evening Margaret went into labor with our first child. I dropped her off at a nearby hospital and sped to my watch two miles away. The bombing had never seemed so heavy as that night. I scanned the northern skyline with a feeling of helplessness and gloom, certain that the high-explosive bombs falling there were landing on Royal Northern Hospital where Margaret lay. She came through fine, thank God, and after Ormond's last casualty victim had been treated I rushed to her side to meet my son, Christopher.

Compensations

Although I saw the terrible effects of war every day in the casualty clearing station, I also saw the very best of the human spirit. According to modern-day polls, a majority of Londoners who lived through the Blitz now remember those days with fondness and nostalgia. I would have to agree.

Britain stood very much alone after the fall of France and the Western European nations. Retreating soldiers told horror stories of the lightning panzer brigades, and we expected a German invasion at any moment. Each night, more bombs fell on London. Yet somehow, in that atmosphere of fear and menace, a new sense of community grew up.

One evening I went down the escalator to the London subway, or "tube," where I discovered an entire city of people living on underground platforms and passageways. Some were tucking babies away for the night, some were eating dinner, some were gathered in little clusters telling jokes and even singing. I had to step over dozens of bodies, stretched out on mats and blankets, to catch the train. I learned that these people came each night to escape the bombs and noisy sirens. Authorities at first tried to evict them, but soon reversed policy and outfitted the platform with three-tiered wire mesh bunks.

Whenever I visited the underground city, I came away buoyed by the sense of camaraderie I found there. The scene shattered any stereotype of the British as a standoffish people. Londoners rich and poor assembled nightly, sharing food and goodwill. They swapped stories of narrow escapes from bombs, and made jokes about the impending invasion. Even the pain of bereavement was eased: one person would tell of family members who had been killed, and total strangers would gather around and weep together. The royal family paid a few visits, supposedly to bolster spirits but secretly, I think, to catch some of the infectious spirit for themselves. Above ground many of these people had lost homes, possessions, and loved ones, but below ground they relaxed among friends.

The medical profession also benefited from the new community spirit, for the elite of London signed up as hospital volunteers. Agatha Christie joined the staff of University College. A pharmacist before taking up detective stories (good fodder for her poison plots), she volunteered in the pharmacy as her contribution to the war effort. My wife will never forget a chance encounter with another famous volunteer. One morning while doing a postoperative dressing Margaret noticed a darkly beautiful woman standing near the patient's cubicle. She was wearing a volunteer's uniform, and Margaret offered her the job of taking the soiled, stinking dressings to the refuse bin. Later she learned the woman's identity: Princess Marina of Greece, the recently widowed Duchess of York.

As a doctor in training, I profited especially from the superb doctors who came out of retirement to fill vacancies created by the war. In the midst of the chaos of war, these selfless professors taught me something more important than facts about physiology and pharmaceuticals. University College had challenged us to treat patients, not merely diseases, but now by watching wise, experienced doctors in action we saw the human side of medicine fleshed out. Only later did I recognize how profoundly this approach to treatment can affect the perception of pain.

A surgeon named Gwynne Williams, a war volunteer, typified this "old-fashioned" approach to medicine. From him I learned that in medicine there is no substitute for human touch. "Don't just stand by the bed," Williams told us, "or you'll tend to feel only with the tips of your fingers. Kneel by your patient's side. That way, your full hand rests flat against the abdomen. Take your time. Just let your hand rest there for a while. As your patient's muscle tension relaxes, you will feel the small movements."

Before visiting a patient in our poorly heated hospital, Gwynne Williams would place his hand on a radiator, or immerse it in hot water. Sometimes he walked the wards with his right arm tucked Napoleonically inside a large coat, concealing the hot water bottle that made his hand a good listener. A cold hand would cause a reflex tightening of the patient's abdominal muscles, but a warm, comforting hand coaxed them to relax. Williams trusted his fingers above a stethoscope or even the patient's own descriptions. "How do patients know what's really going on in their intestines?" he would ask with a scowl. "Listen to their intestines directly. And as for a stethoscope—how can you learn anything by shoving a cold piece of metal onto a frightened patient's flesh?"

Williams was right: a trained hand on the abdomen can detect tautness, inflammation, and the shape of tumors that more complicated procedures merely confirm. For fifty years touch has served as my most precious diagnostic tool. And as it informs me about my patient's symptoms, touch simultaneously conveys to my patients a sense of personal concern that may help calm their fear and anxiety—and thus help reduce their pain.

Gwynne Williams constantly sought ways to lower the barriers that tend to create distance between doctors and their patients. "Humility is the one quality a surgeon needs to cultivate," he would say. "Climb down off your pedestal."

I once presented to Dr. Williams my recommendation against surgery for an eighty-year-old woman who had fallen and broken her hip. "She seems frail to me," I said, "and has symptoms of diabetes as well. We could operate on her and reinforce her bones with a metal plate, but that procedure would involve trauma and also a long casting period. It might be too much for her. I suggest letting her lie in traction so that the bone heals on its own, shortened. She'll never regain her mobility, of course, but if someone looks after her, she'll do fine. Surgery is risky."

Williams exploded. "How dare you talk about not taking risks for an old person! Old age is the time to take risks! I'm an old man, and if I break my leg you'd better do everything you can to restore it. Being old is bad enough, but to allow her to become helpless and require others to wait on her is unconscionable." He then discussed the options with the patient, determined her suitability, and scheduled the surgery.

Once again, Williams was right. The woman survived and walked again. From encounters like that I learned that medicine does not merely consist in taking care of body parts. Treating a disease and treating a person are very different concerns, because recovery depends in large part on the mind and spirit of the patient. Suffering, a state of mind, involves the entire person.

5
Mentors in Pain

Here comes the nurse with the red hot poultice,
Slaps it on and takes no notice.
T. S. Eliot

With the treatment of pain now made a national priority by war, some of the best minds at University College took up the subject. One colorful lecturer was a whiz kid named J. H. Kellgrin, a slight, unimposing man with fair skin, hair, and eyebrows. Something of a showman, he conducted dramatic demonstrations of pain and anesthesia in a lecture hall built on a steep slant so that all students would have an unobstructed view.

During one class Kellgrin wheeled in a soldier who had been wounded in battle. "This soldier is feeling intractable pain in his neck and shoulder area," Kellgrin said. The soldier, unable to move his neck, held his head crookedly to one side and stared out at us sideways, looking very apprehensive. Kellgrin announced that he was going to try to locate the source of the man's pain. "Please tell us when you feel the same pain that you recognize as your present neck pain," he instructed the soldier. Kellgrin inserted a long needle in the nape of the soldier's neck.

At once the soldier let out a loud cry, "No! That hurts!"

"Does that feel like the pain that has been bothering you?" asked Kellgrin, impassive.

"No, that's a new pain, in my arm," said the soldier, cowering before him.

Another probe of the needle—"*Ohhh!*"—another scream of agony. Was that the pain? "No! That pain comes from where the needle is, and it's bloody awful!" Kellgrin smiled and moved the needle farther in, probing this way and that.

I could hardly contain my outrage. This was medicine at its

most callous, exploiting a pitiful soldier just to make a classroom point about pain. I waved my hand in the air, ready to protest, but at that moment Kellgrin's needle hit the right spot. "There, that's the pain!" the soldier cried. "You've got what you wanted."

Kellgrin asked in his unruffled way, "Are you quite sure this pain is the same as you've been feeling when you try to move your neck?"

"Yes, I'm bloody sure! Now will you stop all this!" the soldier demanded.

At last Kellgrin emptied the syringe of novocaine, slowly and deliberately, and as he did so an expression of blissful relief spread across the soldier's face. Kellgrin waited for a moment, and then cautiously moved the man's head just a little. Sensing no reaction of pain, he slowly withdrew the needle. He moved the man's neck in a wide circle. The soldier's face first registered fear, then surprise, then amazement. Testing his own shoulder, the soldier found he could now rotate his arm without discomfort. Finally he gave Kellgrin a thumbs-up sign and reached over to thank him. "Let me shake your hand while this still feels good," he said.

Kellgrin brought the lecture to a triumphant close. "Pain is part of a complex system. We have made major progress by identifying the trigger point of this man's pain. It's possible this single injection may provide permanent relief, by calming hypersensitive nerve endings and giving his muscles a chance to relax. If not, we'll continue treatment."

Anesthetists in that day were just beginning to recognize the potential of epidural anesthesia, a way of controlling pain at the level of the nerve roots just before they enter the spinal cord. For me as a student, the expression of relief on the soldier's face became a vivid symbol of a new insight into pain. Until then I had conceived of it as a two-stage process: first, an alarm signal from the periphery (a cut finger, a toothache), then a recognition by the brain. I now had striking proof of a pathway in between. A nerve trunk receives pain messages en route to the spinal cord which the brain may interpret as if they had come from nerve endings farther down the limb. The soldier had "felt" acute pain in his arm and shoulder, even though Kellgrin's needle was sticking in his neck, probing nerve branches near the spinal cord.

A few days later I saw this principle reinforced as Kellgrin treated another wounded soldier. Though his injury seemed minor compared to others in the ward, I had never seen a more pathetic patient. A bullet had entered his thigh, passing near and probably grazing the sciatic nerve, which had brought about a state of extreme tenderness known as causalgia. This tough, superbly conditioned young soldier was now hypersensitive to any sensation. He could not tolerate a sheet resting on his leg. He complained about light shining in his eyes. All day he lay curled in a fetal position, crying for his mother. Messages of pain were flooding in from all over his leg and elsewhere, and ordinary pain medications had very little effect.

As we students held the soldier down, Kellgrin inserted a needle into his lumbar spine and injected an anesthetic into the nerve ganglia controlling the sympathetic nervous system. When we left the room, the soldier was writhing in pain. The next day we found him sitting up in bed, laughing and joking. Kellgrin had once again abolished a pain, this time by knocking out a whole segment of the sympathetic nervous system in order to silence its frantic signals.

Kellgrin was a protégé of Sir Thomas Lewis, known to us as Tommy Lewis, the leading physiologist at University College, a man whose spirit filled the medical school. Sometimes called the "king of cardiology," Lewis had gained fame for his pioneer work identifying the effects of psychological stress on the heart. He was a small, slender man in his sixties, distinguished by a trim beard and a posture permanently bowed from lab work.

Tommy Lewis had a rather gruff manner which he used to maximum effect in intimidating the newer medical students. He had strict notions about which patients we should see. "University College is a teaching hospital," he insisted. "We should not be admitting patients with easy diagnoses." I accompanied him once when he came across one of these obvious cases, and he walked away with an offended air, mumbling "Rubbish, rubbish. Anyone could treat this patient. We want someone more challenging, someone with problems you can sink your teeth into."

At a time when the world was falling apart, we students sometimes questioned the relevance of obscure academic inquiry, but Tommy Lewis did not alter the college's research program one iota. To him, war had little significance except for its side benefit of opening up fascinating new areas for medical research. He had studied the heart during World War I; now he was investigating pain. The book that resulted, *Pain*, first published in 1942, is still read in medical schools today.

Lewis inspired in me a fondness for research. As we studied pain I was pulled into an orbit from which I would never escape, even though much of what I learned would not come into play for many years. Doctors and patients alike tend to regard pain as the symptom of a problem, and their attention quickly shifts to the root cause, the diagnosis. Lewis's scientific detachment allowed him to consider pain as a sensation in itself. Studying under him, for the first time I began to glimpse the possibility of an answer to certain underlying questions. Previously I had thought of pain as a blemish in creation, God's one great mistake. Tommy Lewis taught me otherwise. Seen from his point of view, pain stands out as an extraordinary feat of engineering valuable beyond measure.

During my student days, Lewis was trying to categorize varieties of physical pain. He hoped to quantify the actual experience of pain so that patients could describe their pain as "number eight" or "number nine," rather than relying on vague words like "agonizing" or "excruciating." He was working on three main groupings—ischemic pain, skin pain, and visceral pain—and I volunteered as an experimental subject in ischemic pain.

Laboratory Masochism

Ischemic pain occurs when blood supply is cut off or restricted. In a muscle, for example, ischemic pain results when there is too little blood to supply oxygen and the circulation does not carry away toxic impurities fast enough. The pain comes on slowly in a passive muscle, but in an active muscle ischemia causes muscle spasm. As anyone knows who has been jolted awake by a muscle cramp, ischemic pain can be sudden and severe. A common blood pressure cuff will easily produce it: pump up the cuff until it cuts off all circulation in your arm, and then make a fist a few times. Very soon you will feel a pain so excruciating that you must stop and loosen the cuff.

The ordinary blood pressure cuff did not satisfy Tommy Lewis's thirst for precision, though. After all, it takes a few seconds to pump up the cuff, during which time the greater arterial pressure will sneak in more blood even after venous return is cut off, causing the arm to swell slightly. To correct this problem Lewis devised an instant cuff inflater, a huge spherical glass container, wrapped in rope, that looked like a marine marker. He would pump air into the glass cask until it reached a specified pressure, then connect it to the blood pressure cuff on my arm. When he turned a tap the cuff inflated instantly, halting blood flow in both directions at once.

With my blood supply cut off, I would squeeze a rubber ball once, twice, three times, keeping time to the beat of a metronome and continuing until it began hurting. At the first onset of pain I made a sign, and Lewis noted how many seconds had passed. I continued squeezing until the pain became unbearable and I had to let go. Again Lewis noted the lapsed time. My classmates and I underwent this procedure week after week as Lewis sat beside us with infinite patience. He was looking for two results: the threshold level of when we first felt pain and the tolerance level of how much we could withstand.

Lewis tested subjects from various ethnic backgrounds, uncovering major differences in the way Northern and Southern Europeans perceive pain. Other volunteers participated in experiments to test the power of distraction: for example, those who listened to racy novels being read aloud showed a far higher tolerance for pain. Researchers after Lewis would further refine his pain tests, using new techniques such as high-frequency sound waves, ultraviolet lights, supercooled copper wires, and repetitive spark generators, but all essentially confirmed the findings Lewis arrived at during those war days. I must admit, however, that it seemed slightly bizarre to be sitting in a laboratory inflicting pain on ourselves as other citizens were receiving it in a most involuntary fashion from German bombers.

Just for variety we ischemic volunteers also sampled skin pain and visceral pain. To test skin pain Lewis used the web of skin between thumb and forefinger, since the anatomy there, skin folded back on skin, would guarantee skin pain of a very pure quality. He pinched the thumb web with a calibrated, miniature vise, and with each turn of the screw we responded with a number from one to ten, quantifying the pain. Such pressure-induced pain caused a distinct "burning" sensation, whereas tests with pins and boar bristles produced a "pricking" pain. Lewis found that blindfolded subjects could not distinguish between pains caused by sharp points, hair-pulling, heat, electrical currents, or irritant poisons: all pricking pains felt alike.

Of Lewis's three categories of pain, I found visceral pain the most fascinating. This slower, less localized kind of pain warns of problems deep inside the body. I learned that internal organs, such as the stomach and intestines, have a sparse supply of pain sensors. (This shortage is what makes stomach ulcers dangerous: acid may eat well into the stomach lining before the patient notices any secondary effects.) A surgeon uses anesthetics mainly to get past the barrier of skin. Cut the intestine with a knife, burn it with a cautery, or squeeze it with forceps, and the patient will feel nothing. I have since treated a man in India who had been gored by a bull: he sat calmly in the waiting room holding his intestines in a cloth, like a package from a store, with no signs of visceral pain.

Yet stomach and intestines have exquisite sensitivity to one particular type of pain, the pain of distension. Tommy Lewis's volunteers would gamely swallow a tube rigged with a balloon on the end. Once the tube had moved down through the stomach into the intestine, Lewis would begin blowing up the balloon. Within a few seconds, the volunteers grunted and motioned wild-eyed for him to stop. They were experiencing one of the most acute pains the human body knows: the pain of colic, which results when something tries to pass through a too-small opening, whether in the kidney, gallbladder, or intestine. Internal organs possess nerve cells that respond to the primary dangers they will likely confront; the economical body deems it redundant to have them warn, say, of cutting when skin sensors handle that chore perfectly well.

While learning about pain firsthand in Tommy Lewis's experiments, I also began formally researching the subject in libraries. The dazzling complexity of the pain network astounded me. I began studying pain out of simple curiosity, having no idea I was accumulating a foundation for my life's work. I came away from that early research with an enduring sense of awe and gratitude for the very sensation most people view with resentment.

The body has millions of nerve sensors, distributed not randomly, but in exact accordance with each part's need. A light tap on the foot goes unnoticed, on the groin is felt as painful, and on the eye causes anguish. The German scientist Max von Frey's statistics on skin pain show the difference clearly: it takes 0.2 gram of pressure per square millimeter for the cornea of the eye to feel pain, as opposed to 20 grams on the forearm, 200 on the sole of the foot, and 300 on the fingertips.

The eye is a thousand times more sensitive to pain than the sole of the foot because it faces peculiar hazards. Vision requires that the eye be transparent, thus limiting the number of (opaque) blood vessels immediately available. Any intruder, even a speck of dirt or thread of fiberglass, poses a threat, because with its limited blood supply the eye cannot easily repair itself. For protection the eye has such a hair-trigger response that virtually anything touching it causes pain and trips the blink reflex.

On the other hand, the foot is designed to bear the body's weight: it has tougher supporting structures, a plentiful blood supply, and a thousand times less sensitivity to pain. Fingertips can likewise withstand much duress: carpenters would be rare indeed if the gripping fingers fired off pain signals to the brain at every stroke of a hammer. In each case, a body part's function determines its surrounding structure, and the pain network loyally adapts.

Adding to the system's complexity, pain sensors report in at different speeds. Signals from the skin surface travel at a rate of three hundred feet per second, prompting an immediate response. Touch a hot stove and your finger jerks back even before the pain registers in your conscious brain.* In contrast, pain from the dermis or internal organs creeps along at two feet per second, so that several seconds may pass before it registers. The ache or throb of slow pain is deeper, and tends to persist. Tommy Lewis, ever-observant, wondered why technicians in the new field of radiology never ate soft-boiled eggs. Examining them, he discovered that X-ray beams (early machines were poorly shielded) had destroyed the

---

*The reflex response provides a good illustration of the pain network's sophisticated design. When a danger—touching a hot stove, stepping on a thorn, blinking in a dust storm—requires a quick response, the body delegates it to a reflex loop that functions below the level of consciousness. There's no advantage to thinking about the stove, so why bother the higher brain with an action that can be handled at the reflex level? Yet—and I marvel at the in-built wisdom of the body—the higher brain reserves the right to overrule this reflex loop under unusual circumstances. An expert rock climber clinging to a precipice will not straighten his leg when a falling stone hits the patellar tendon; a society matron will not drop a too-hot cup of tea served in Wedgwood china; the survivor of a plane crash will repress reflexes and walk shoeless across shards of glass and hot metal.

nerve sensors on their outer layers of skin, thus silencing the early warning system of fast pain. The technicians had learned to avoid handling hot eggshells because the delayed slow pain was far worse, and would not easily go away.

Hairbrush Doctor

Tommy Lewis used to puzzle over what prompts a pain sensor to send its signal. When people attending a concert clap their hands together, they feel no pain at first. Each time the hands come together, the soft onion shapes of pacinian corpuscle cells compress, firing off notice of a pressure sensation. If members of the audience continue clapping for ten minutes in hopes of an encore, though, their hands start to feel tender, and if they go on much longer they will experience real discomfort. Why? The last few claps are no stronger than the earlier ones, so the pressure has not increased. Somehow as the palms of the hands become red and swollen, indicating tissue damage, nerve cells perceive this danger and send signals of pain in addition to pressure.

Similarly, if a splash of hot cooking oil lands on the back of my hand, I hold it under cold water until it feels better. The burn leaves a small red mark, which I forget about—until I take a bath at night. Suddenly the water which feels fine to one hand feels hot and uncomfortable to the other. Temperature sensors in both hands are recording the same heat flow, but the slightly damaged skin has become hypersensitive and its pain detectors adjust their thresholds accordingly.

Before researching the subject in any depth I had imagined the pain network as a series of "wires" that run directly from the extremities to the brain, like individual fire alarms linked to a central fire station. I soon learned how naive that conception was. Pain is a sophisticated interpretation drawn from many sources.

Graham Weddell, another protégé of Tommy Lewis and a junior lecturer at University College, approached scientific mysteries with the enthusiasm of a martyr. Aided by an Indian assistant, he cut tiny windows in the flesh of his own arm and isolated out individual nerve fibers, which he wired to an oscilloscope. Weddell then applied various stimuli—heat, cold, pinprick, acid— to his hand and noted the results displayed on the oscilloscope screen. He ended up with a forearm that looked like a practice field for a bad tattooist, but along the way he gained a new under-

standing of pain: it works more as a perception than a sensation.*
To become pain signals, the firings of individual neurons must
summate in time, through repeated signals, or in space, by involving nearby neurons. The self-mutilating procedures convinced
Weddell that pain signals from isolated neurons have little meaning; what matters are their interactions with surrounding cells and
the interpretation supplied by the brain.

Weddell noticed early on that the laboratory setting had a
powerful effect on the pain experience. Pain was never "objective."
Consistently, first-time volunteers for our experiments reported
feeling pain much sooner than the regulars. Even after being
assured they could turn off the painful stimuli by hitting a switch,
they did not fully trust the testing process, and that anxiety altered
their perception of pain. They simply hurt more easily and
quickly. Similarly, in experiments with the skin pain vise, most students reported lower levels of pain from the same pressure when
they were allowed to turn the screw themselves. The fear they felt
when somebody else turned the screw made the perception of pain
much higher. (This fact points to one of the main limitations of
laboratory experiments. What I allow a trusted colleague to inflict
on me in a controlled environment is a wholly different experience
from pain I might encounter in the outside world where I am subject to fear, anger, anxiety, and helplessness. On the other hand,
pain that I report as significant in a laboratory, such as a pinprick, I
may not even notice if I am involved in a carpentry project—or on
a battlefield.)

Graham Weddell was a great favorite among students, perhaps because he seemed like an overgrown student himself: he
never brushed his hair, he preferred the unorthodox point of view
on almost any subject, and he roared approval at off-color jokes.
As a counterpoint to his work on pain, Weddell began investigating pleasure. First he studied the anatomy of the erogenous zones
by dissecting the genitalia of female monkeys. Then, somewhat
characteristically, he recruited volunteers among the female stu-

---

*Weddell went on to become a respected researcher in the field of
pain. He traveled the globe, testing his theories on subjects in Africa and
Asia. Once, he was having trouble explaining to some Nigerian tribesmen
why he wanted them to undergo certain tests. His translator interjected,
"He's like a chicken scratching around in the sand until he finds something."
Weddell loved telling that story. He said it was the finest definition of scientific research he had ever heard.

dents who agreed to let him stimulate the nerves of the clitoris electrically. To his surprise, he found no nerve ending that could be designated a "pleasure nerve." In fact, the main feature of the erogenous landscape was an abundance of the free nerve endings normally associated with pain.

Weddell concluded that sexual pleasure, too, is more perception than sensation. Sensors of touch, temperature, and pain dutifully record the mechanical aspects of one body coming into contact with another. But pleasure involves an interpretation of those reports, a process heavily dependent on subjective factors such as anticipation, fear, memory, guilt, and love. Physiologically, sexual intercourse between two lovers and the ordeal of rape involve the same nerve endings—but one registers as beauty, the other as horror. Pleasure, even more than pain, emerges as a by-product of cooperation among many cells, mediated and interpreted by the higher brain.

Any ticklish child knows the thin line that separates pleasure from pain. I used to enjoy being tickled, and in India my sister, Connie, would sometimes oblige me. A feather lightly pulled across my forearm produced a delicious sensation. And yet the pattern made by a scorpion crawling across my forearm, exerting similar force on the same nerve endings, produced exactly the opposite result: it crossed the divide between pleasure and pain, a divide controlled by the perceiving brain.

The more I investigated pain, the more my thinking about it changed. My early "fire-alarm" conception of pain had closely followed the theory described by René Descartes in the seventeenth century. Descartes developed the first real cause-and-effect theory of sensations after visiting a trick sculpture garden in France operated by hydraulics. When he stepped on a tile, water squirted out of a statue into his eye. Sensations have a similar cause-and-effect relationship, he reasoned: stimulate a nerve ending and it sends a message directly to the brain. He likened pain signals to a sexton ringing a church bell: a pinprick on a finger, like a yank on the rope, causes an alarm to sound in the brain. This sensible theory, explained in his *Treatise of Man*, served science well for nearly three centuries, but as medicine advanced certain exceptions came to light.

In the pain network, for example, an alarm sometimes sounds even when no rope is pulled. When I began to see patients, I encountered the phenomenon of referred pain. I have already mentioned that the economical body assigns pain sensors only to guard against the most common dangers (the intestine warns of distension but not cutting or burning). If a part of the body faces an *uncommon* danger, the body gets around this emergency by "borrowing" pain sensations from other regions. An injured spleen may seek the help of faraway pain receptors in the tip of the left shoulder, and a kidney stone may be "felt" anywhere along a band from the groin to the lower back.

Referred pain makes proper diagnosis of a heart attack a tricky problem for a young doctor. "It's a burning sensation here in my neck," one patient reports. "No, it feels like my arm is being squeezed," says another. Various patients may describe a burning or constriction in the neck, chest, jaw, or left arm. In a sense, the spinal cord is playing a trick on the brain. A warning system located in the spinal cord or lower brain detects a cardiac problem, but, aware that the conscious brain has no felt image of the heart because of its few pain sensors, it instructs skin and muscle cells to act as if they are in serious jeopardy as a favor to their wordless neighbor. Remarkably, the "borrowed" area, say, the left arm, may remain tender to the touch even between attacks of pain. The tissue of the left arm is, of course, as healthy as that in the right arm; reports of damage are mental constructs (we dare not say *mere* mental constructs). The left arm puts on a performance worthy of an Academy Award for the purpose of seizing the attention of a victim who would otherwise not attend to his endangered heart.

Sometimes the body invents pain, and sometimes it squelches legitimate pain signals. For example, when an athlete spreads a liniment on her sore calf muscle, the deep muscle pain magically disappears. In reality, the sensors in her calf muscle are still emitting signals of distress, but new transmissions overwhelm those signals so that they never reach the brain. Irritants in the liniment attract an increased blood supply, creating heat sensations which combine with her hand's rubbing motion to drown out the pain signals from the calf muscle. Sensations of touch, heat, or cold can overpower the message of pain: we rub an itchy mosquito bite, blow on a burn, apply an ice pack to an aching head, squeeze a stubbed toe, lie on a hot water bottle. The action is as instinctive as a dog's licking a wound.

As soon as I understood some of the basic principles behind pain perception, I began to adapt them clinically. Once, a painful boil developed from a rash near my ankle. I knew I must not scratch it, but the temptation was nearly irresistible. I discovered I could get relief from both the pain and the itch if I scratched nearby, just beyond the edge of the rash. Next, I tried brushing my leg up and down with a boar-bristle hairbrush. The leg tingled, and I felt relief even when I brushed my thigh, far from the source of pain. Inundated by new sensations from the stiff bristles, the spinal cord put pain signals on hold and did not relay them to the brain.

I tested the treatment on my patients and it worked like a charm, especially at night. (I remembered that Jake the soldier had the roughest time after dark, when there were fewer things to occupy his mind.) Chronic pain sensations tend to get louder as other sensations die down, and I found that the hairbrush could counteract this pain by stimulating thousands of nerve endings on the skin surface of the same limb. My patients soon dubbed me "the hairbrush doctor."

Today, of course, a doctor can prescribe high-tech Transcutaneous Electrical Nerve Stimulator (TENS) machines to accomplish the same result as my hairbrush, at considerably greater expense. These machines, controlled by the patient, excite nerves to fire a barrage of conflicting sensory messages. (Lest we idealize modern medicine unduly, I should point out that in A.D. 46 a Roman physician practiced electroanalgesia by holding an electric fish against a patient's head.)

Gate-Control Theory

University College continued as a center of pain research long after my student days. Three decades later, in the 1970s, Professor Patrick Wall would collaborate with Ronald Melzack on a theory to explain many of the mysteries of pain that had so puzzled us during war years. Their "spinal gate-control theory" offers a simple and cohesive way of looking at pain.

According to the theory, in a very simplified version, thousands of nerve fibers, some descending from the higher brain and some ascending from the extremities of the body, all come together in a switching station, "the gate" (actually a series of gates), located where the spinal cord joins the brain. So many nerve cells converging in one place creates something of a bottleneck, like a toll booth on an expressway, profoundly affecting the perception of pain. Some messages have to wait to get through, while others may not get through at all.

The gate-control theory caught hold among clinicians because it seemed to account for so many enigmas in the old Cartesian model of pain. Certainly it offers an explanation for my hairbrush routine: the many new touch and pressure sensations crowd out the signals of chronic pain. The gate-control theory also helps explain how a plane crash survivor can walk across hot metal without pain: urgent impulses descending from the higher brain block out all signals of pain from the ascending fibers. Melzack and Wall have used the gate-control theory to shed light on such phenomena as acupuncture and the feats of Indian fakirs (in the first case, stimuli from the needles crowd out other signals; in the second, masters of self-control utilize their cerebral powers to overrule pain signals from below).

Despite many advances in understanding the pain network, even today scientists can barely fathom the complexity of the system that first astounded me in student days. The simple sentence "My finger hurts" encompasses a firestorm of neuronal activity at three separate levels. At the cellular level, reports of minor scratches and skin irritations on my finger vie for attention, most of them never achieving the intensity required to transmit a pain *signal*. If they do get transmitted, my finger's pain signals must compete in the spinal cord with those from other nerve fibers—if I stub my toe, my finger may stop hurting entirely—before being forwarded to the brain as a pain *message*. And as it passes the spinal gate, the pain message may be squelched on orders from the higher brain. Unless the pain message goes on to provoke a *response* in the brain, I'll never know about it—my finger will not "hurt."

6
Medicine India Style

The patience of poverty.
In rice fields, backs bent forever.
Amazing, man outoxens the oxen and still smiles.
The mystery of India, say the Indologists.
Günter Grass

I finished my surgical residency in 1946, a year after World War II ended, and I fully expected to be shipped overseas with British occupation troops for a few years, after which I could return to a quiet career in a research laboratory. But the Central Medical War Committee, overseer of such assignments, proved no match for an irrepressible Scotsman named Dr. Robert Cochrane. The supervisor of leprosy work in southern India, Cochrane had come to London to recruit a surgeon for a new medical college in the town of Vellore. My mother, eager to get me back to India, had told him I might be available.

Although the notion of returning to India held a certain magical appeal for me, several barriers stood in the way. Cochrane waved aside the first objection. "Don't worry, I'll handle the War Committee!" he said, and somehow he persuaded them to accept service in India in lieu of my mandatory army stint. Cochrane had a way of presenting the destiny of the Vellore hospital as a watershed for India and the British Empire.

Family posed a more immediate problem for me. I had missed the birth of our first child, thanks to casualty duty during the Blitz. Now Christopher was two years old and Margaret was approaching the due date of her second pregnancy. I could not bear the thought of leaving at such a time. Margaret herself quashed that objection: "The army would likely send you to the Far East anyway. And I'll have the baby all the same whether you're in Europe, the Far East, or India." She promised to join me in a few months, after the delivery and a little time for recuperation.

Our daughter, Jean, arrived while I was in the very act of packing bags. Two weeks later I hugged my wife, toddler son, and infant daughter and boarded a steamship for India. Heading east on a route through the Suez Canal, I relived the pain I had felt on the reverse journey, when as a nine-year-old I had traveled to England from my boyhood home in the Kollis. My family back in London, my future uncertain, my childhood memories resurrected—I felt very alone on that voyage.

Until the ship docked in Bombay, I had no idea what a grip the land of my childhood had on me. "Smells are surer than sounds or sights to make your heartstrings crack," said Kipling. He should know: he too had inhaled India, a land of limitless redolence. Memories came flooding back as soon as I breathed in the unmistakable atmosphere, a rich bouquet of sandalwood, jasmine, hot charcoal, ripe fruit, cow dung, human sweat, incense, and tropical flower blossoms. My pain vanished, displaced by nostalgia.

Six thousand years of tradition walked around Bombay in various guises: nearly naked Hindu ascetics; Jainists breathing through handkerchiefs to avoid killing insects; Sikhs wearing their trademark beards, handlebar moustaches, and turbans; bald Buddhist monks in saffron robes. Human-powered rickshaws jockeyed for position in the streets with buses, camels, and even an occasional elephant. A farmer was using his bicycle to transport pigs—legs tied together, hanging upside-down from the handlebars, squealing like unoiled machinery.

I drank in the sights like one who has just had patches removed from his eyes. Beauty abounded: the vendor stalls of flowers and bright powdered dyes, the women in flowing silk saris the color of tropical birds, even the horns of bullocks decorated with silver and turquoise. I found myself gawking, once more the nine-year-old child who had gripped his father's hand so tightly in the streets of Indian cities.

Settling In

Other memories surged in during the long train ride from Bombay to Madras. Outside, the steam locomotive puffed out thick clouds of dark smoke. Inside, I shared space with burlap bags of coconuts, baskets of bananas, bundles of rags, and cages full of squawking chickens. A goat in the next compartment kept up a constant bleating. Indian families stretched out on the wooden floor—shiny with the red slime of betel juice—and clambered onto baggage racks to lie atop their goods.

The train climbed through the forested hills east of Bombay, descended into dry, dusty plains, and chugged toward the fertile land of the east. Every few miles a tiny hummock of thatch appeared in the distance, marking one of India's million villages. As we approached the fertile region, irrigation ditches stitched the landscape into squares of lush green. From the train window I watched scenes unchanged in centuries as peasant families threshed and winnowed in the fields. Two men were practicing the ancient method of irrigation. One stood barefoot on a high wooden contraption resembling a playground seesaw. Balancing himself with arms outstretched like a trapeze artist, he walked toward one end of the beam, and as he did so, his shifting weight caused a leather bucket to dip into the irrigation ditch. Then he walked toward the center to level the beam, waited for his companion to swing it around in a semicircle to another ditch, and walked back toward the bucket of water, which now sloshed its contents into the new ditch. The two would repeat that procedure a thousand times, all day, every day. The mystery of India.

From Madras I went by car to Vellore, a city of about 100,000, and moved into the crowded quarters allocated to hospital employees. Within a few days I was feeling Indian again. I stored my shoes in a closet and went around barefoot or in sandals. I wore loose-fitting cotton clothes. I bathed Indian style, dipping a metal ladle into a bucket of water heated over an open fire and then pouring it over my head. I went to sleep beneath a slowly turning ceiling fan, soothed by the clear metallic "Hoo . . . hoo" of the coppersmith birds, and awoke to the raucous sound of crows.

I arrived in Vellore during the cool season, and as summer approached I encountered heat such as I had never known as a child in the mountains. Afternoons, the temperature sometimes climbed past 110°. We treated barefoot Indians who had blistered the soles of their feet just by walking on the hot asphalt streets. The simple act of breathing brought on perspiration. Some offices hung reed curtains at the door and hired boys to spray water on them all day, but on really hot days the curtains dried instantly.

Palm-leaf fans simply shifted hot air from one place to another. Clothes were hot compresses. At night the thin mosquito net I crawled under smothered like a wool blanket.

Nothing in Vellore was air-conditioned, not even the operating room. I became very unpopular among surgical nurses and assistants because I refused to use the ceiling fan, fearing (with some justification) that it would stir up germ-laden dust which might fall into the wound. Sometimes we operated for twelve straight hours, pausing between each long operation to change our sopping scrub suits and gowns.

In that climate an adult requires six quarts of liquid a day, but I found that when I drank so much I broke out in a severe case of "prickly heat," a hideous skin rash that results from constant sweating. I had a nearly irresistible urge to scratch, but I could not possibly do so while wearing my sterile surgical gown and gloves, and, besides, I knew that scratching would bring on boils and infections. Another doctor warned me not to scrimp on the liquids, though. "I know the temptation," he said. "When I first came to India I cut back on fluids to reduce the sweating and clear up the prickly heat. It worked. But when I stopped drinking so much, I wasn't taking enough water to keep the urea dissolved and it crystallized into stones. Frankly, Paul, you have a choice. Prickly heat or kidney stones. Having had both, I strongly recommend the prickly heat." I heeded his advice and kept drinking my daily quota.

Adjusting to India took its toll on my body. Any resistance to local diseases I had developed in childhood had long since faded away, and I fought successive bouts with dysentery, hepatitis, influenza, and dengue. Dengue, the worst of the ailments, was commonly called "break-bone fever" because for about a week it feels as if all the bones in your back and legs are broken.

After I had six months to adjust to Vellore, Margaret and our two small children set sail from England, and in June of 1947 our family was reunited at last. I had been working nonstop, and Margaret's arrival forced me to settle into a more normal routine. We moved into the top floor of a stone bungalow near the medical college and most days Margaret joined me at the hospital, where she had taken a position in pediatrics.

The Vellore hospital had been founded in 1900 by an American missionary, Dr. Ida Scudder. It began as a medical college for young women, based initially in a small dispensary that measured no more than ten feet by twelve feet. The school flourished, and eventually opened its doors to male students. By the time we arrived, the hospital had grown into a sprawling four-hundred-bed complex of buildings. Somehow, despite the hospital's size, the staff had retained the strong sense of Christian community that Dr. Scudder had first inspired. We felt we were among family.

Margaret and I both had to adapt to the Indian style of medicine, however. I learned, for example, that many Indian patients viewed a doctor almost as a priest. One busy morning a woman followed me all through my rounds, lurking in the shadows as I went from room to room. "What is it?" I asked her. "Didn't I just treat your husband?" She nodded yes. "And did you get the prescription from the pharmacy?" Again, a nod. "Have you given it to him?" This time, a no. "Doctor, can you come and give the medicine to him with your good hands?" she asked. At first I was somewhat irritated by the Indians' insistence on touch and on family interaction in all decisions. Soon I came to see its wisdom, a wisdom I now wish we in the West recognized more.

Following Ida Scudder's vision, the Vellore hospital sought to blend modern medicine into an Indian context and not simply replicate Western methods. It was the first Asian hospital to offer thoracic surgery, kidney dialysis, open heart surgery, electron microscopy, and neurosurgery. Its reputation was such that Arabian princes would sometimes fly to India and make the journey to the backwater town of Vellore for treatment of a health problem. And yet the hospital maintained a distinctly Indian flavor. Hallways sometimes resembled a boisterous marketplace. Patients lay in open wards of forty or fifty beds, and in most cases their families, not the cafeteria, provided food. (The staff kept an eye out for women who would light a charcoal brazier in the wards, creating a fire hazard.) If a patient died, the ever-present family would break into howls, chest beating, and high-pitched keening right in the ward or hallway. This was India, where illness and death were accepted parts of the cycle of life and no one saw the need to shelter other patients from the bad news.

Lacking air-conditioning, the hospital kept its windows open most of the time, and street noise—the clatter of bullock carts, the buzz of motorbikes, the cries of food vendors—filtered in. For a time the hospital had a problem with crows that conspired to steal patients' food. One of the canny birds would lead the assault, flying in an open door to tug at the tray cloth with its beak, and when all the food had spilled onto the floor coconspirators swooped in for the feast. Once, a crow brazenly flew into the autopsy lab and plucked from the countertop a human eye that our pathologist was readying for dissection. The hospital soon crow-proofed its corridors with fine steel mesh; it is still working on ways to keep the monkeys out.

Improvisation

More than anything else, practicing medicine in India called for creativity. Because limited resources prevented us from automatically ordering the newest labor-saving devices, we were forced to improvise. In addition, something was always going wrong that no textbook had prepared us for: a power blackout in the middle of surgery, a report of rabies in the hospital, a water shortage, an unknown pyrogen in the blood bank. We had to scratch our heads and come up with a new approach.

If a new technology, such as image-intensifier X rays, offered an immediate diagnostic benefit, we tried to obtain the best equipment available. One of our Indian radiologists mastered the art of cineradiography and made outstanding moving pictures of the inner workings of the human body. (He also gained some notoriety thanks to a bizarre film. This radiologist persuaded an Indian snake-swallower to let him feed barium meals to his liveliest snakes. Then in front of an X-ray camera the obliging street entertainer swallowed each of the snakes, one by one, let them frolic a while in his stomach, and regurgitated them. The resulting film—viewers see snakes, outlined in white by the barium, squirm down the esophagus, wriggle and knot in the man's stomach, then thrust upward above a heaving diaphragm—made quite a hit at international radiology conferences.)

Our anesthesia department, in contrast, was sparsely supplied. At first we used a simple wire mask with twelve layers of gauze clamped onto it. The anesthetist would soak the gauze in ether, position it over the patient's mouth for the proper duration, and check under the eyelid periodically to gauge the ether's effect. We had no monitors providing readouts of blood gases, blood pressure, or heartbeat rate, but in India the plentiful labor supply could often substitute for technology: an assistant stood by with the sole duty of checking blood pressure and listening through a stethoscope for any irregularities. In retrospect I can see that we operated in rather basic conditions, but I console myself with the memory that very few people died on operating tables at Vellore.

It took years for us to master the subtleties of blood transfusion, a relatively new science. When I began at Vellore, the hospital had no blood bank. For orthopedic surgeries we relied on a jerry-rigged device that suctioned out and recirculated a patient's own blood. In an emergency we used the arm-to-arm method of transfusion, which was quite dramatic. After being tested for compatibility the donor, usually a relative, would lie on a high table above the endangered patient. The doctor would put a needle into the vein of the healthy person, then run a tube down, and insert the other end into the vein of the one in need. Life flowed directly from one person into the other.

Eventually we got a blood bank functioning. Most Indians were reluctant to donate blood, but the free market system overcame their resistance. Rickshaw drivers discovered they could get as much money for donating a pint of blood as they earned pulling a rickshaw for a day. Before long we had to devise a skin tattoo system to monitor the frequency of their donations, for by using false aliases and traveling to other hospitals some of them were donating up to a pint of blood a week!

Sometimes we performed surgeries in a village setting rather than in the hospital. At first I feared terrible complications from such outdoor procedures, but we learned the village environment presented no real danger if we strictly followed an aseptic method. An agar plate set under a tree in the open air might grow more bacteria than a plate set in a hospital corridor, but those bacteria would certainly be less harmful and surely less immune to antibiotics. In the average Indian hospital, germs from the worst communicable diseases, some of them in resistant strains, float freely through the hallways. Not so in the rural setting, where the most common germs are those to which the ordinary villager already has developed natural resistance. I have performed numerous operations during surgery camps—including one in which I had to borrow a set of chisels from a local carpenter and boil them—and I cannot remember a serious sepsis resulting.

Anton Chekhov sometimes performed his surgeries—and autopsies—outdoors under a tree. His descriptions of the fears and superstitions of Russian peasants remind me of what I occasionally encountered in rural India, where we had to contend with traditional remedies. For example, since superstitious families thought it important for their child to be born under a good sign of the horoscope, midwives employed a variety of techniques to alter the time of birth. With the mother in a sitting position the midwife would have a strong man sit on her shoulders in order to put pressure on the birth canal and delay labor. Alternatively, to speed up delivery the midwife might pound on the poor woman's abdomen.

The single most difficult obstacle we faced in health work was impure water. Without doubt, more Third World children have died from dehydration due to diarrhea than from any other cause. We could control the water quality at the hospital, but in the villages the water supply was usually the source of the illness. In the cure lay the disease: the more a child drank to combat dehydration, the more infected he or she became. Oddly enough, the plentifulness of coconut trees in southern India offered one way around this dilemma.

Back in London I had worked with Dick Dawson, a surgeon who had been captured by the Japanese during the war and assigned to the work crews constructing the infamous Burma-Siam railroad. Conditions were appalling. The crews worked in swamps, and since their captors provided no latrines, soon all the water was contaminated by sewage. Dysentery set in and the malnourished British prisoners fell by the score. As medical officer of the regiment, Dawson grew more and more distraught, helpless to prevent the soldiers' deaths.

Suddenly one day, while sitting in a tent in the midst of that hellish scene, Dick Dawson had a revelation. Looking out over the putrid, steaming swamp, he noticed tall and graceful trees growing in the midst of a bog. From the tops of the trees hung shiny green coconuts. There it was—a bountiful supply of sterile fluid full of nutrients! Dawson ordered the healthiest soldiers to shinny up the trees and pull down the greenest coconuts (only the green ones would do, before their juice thickened into white coconut milk). From then on Dawson managed to rehydrate most cases of dysentery by transfusions of coconut water. He whittled the slim, hollow twigs of bamboo to use as needles, and fastened them to rubber tubes. One needle went into the coconut, one into the soldiers' veins.

Dick Dawson's technique came in handy in parts of India, where sterile fluids could not be obtained. Usually we fed the coconut water to patients through the mouth, but village hospitals sometimes used coconuts as a temporary source of intravenous

(IV) fluids. To visitors from England or the United States, it was jarring to see a metal IV stand rigged with a rubber tube snaking up from the patient's arm to a fresh coconut. Yet the fructose mixture in the sealed coconut was as sterile as any product from a medical supply house. Countless cholera and dysentery victims have been saved through such a village-based treatment.

The heat, the sometimes-primitive conditions, the oddities of Indian medicine, the regular bouts with dysentery and tropical fevers—all these required some getting used to, but the difficulties were more than offset by the sheer thrill of practicing medicine. Indians did not visit a doctor to complain about a runny nose or sore throat; they came to the hospital only when they needed urgent medical attention. I felt like a forensic detective. In England if a patient showed up with an ulcer we treated the ulcer; in India we would treat the ulcer and also check for hookworm, malaria, malnutrition, and a dozen other ailments.

I was amazed by the fortitude of Indian patients and their calm attitude toward suffering. Even after sitting in a crowded waiting room for hours, they did not complain. To them, pain was part of the landscape of life, and could by no means be avoided. Karma philosophy dulled any sense of unfairness about pain; it simply had to be borne.

At times I thought wistfully of the climate-controlled, state-of-the-art operating rooms and laboratories of University College Hospital in London. But my involvement with individual patients, and the freedom I felt to practice my calling, easily made up for any sense of loss. Never had I felt so challenged and fulfilled. Some people look upon expatriate doctors in Third World countries as self-sacrificing heroes. I know better. Most are having the time of their lives. I know too many physicians in the West who spend half their hours filling out insurance forms, wrangling with government health programs, choosing computerized record-keeping systems, shopping for malpractice insurance, listening to pharmacy sales reps. Give me India any day.

A Slower, Wiser Way

The first year in Vellore I served as general surgeon, treating whoever came in the door. I was young, eager, and drunk with the adventure of real medicine. Beginning with my second year I began to specialize in orthopedics, still with no idea of what would constitute my life's work. At first, like any new surgeon, I merely implemented what I had learned in training. In time, though, I found that India was teaching me new approaches to treatment. My favorite memory of those days relates to the treatment of club-foot, or talipes equinovarus. The condition, a genetic deformity, causes the foot to rotate and turn inward.

At the Great Ormond Street Hospital in London I had seen many clubfoot cases because my chief, Denis Browne, was an internationally known expert in this field. (A clubfoot splint still bears Denis Browne's name.) I remember watching with eager student eyes as he, a big man, massaged tiny infant feet with hands so large that his thumb covered the sole of a newborn's foot. With great skill he would surgically manipulate those feet, forcing them into proper position and fixing them with adhesive tape onto the foot-piece of a rigid splint. He insisted on complete correction at the first manipulation, and he got it. I sometimes heard the breaking of ligaments as he worked a foot into its new position.

I was assigned to the follow-up clinic where splints were changed, and in that clinic I began to see the patients who came back years later with problems requiring special shoes and corrective surgery. I never lost my admiration for Denis Browne, an authentic medical genius, but nonetheless I am afraid he did not fully appreciate the harm done to a limb by the scarring that results from coercive pressure. The feet he corrected came out with a beautiful shape, but with no flexibility and much stiffness due to the many torn tissues.

Soon after arriving in India I opened a foot clinic at the Vellore hospital and was nearly trampled by feet. Word of our project spread, and before we had adequate staff we found ourselves facing more patients than we could handle. Looking out over the courtyard, I saw people of all ages leaning on crutches and dragging themselves pitifully across the ground. As I stared out at that crowd, I felt dazed and helpless.

I looked for familiar symptoms and soon found them in the form of clubfoot. Scores of distressed mothers had brought babies afflicted by the disorder. We established a talipes clinic just for these babies, and I trained the Vellore staff in the familiar routine of surgery and forced splinting that I had learned from Denis Browne. We bought a large fragment of a downed World War II airplane, and a local blacksmith cut the metal skin and hammered out little splints for us to use.

Meanwhile, I also began to treat the older patients. Among them, I noticed some who walked in a jerky, bowlegged style I had never before seen. They were actually walking on the outer surfaces of their feet, their ankles almost touching the ground. The soles of their feet, turned inward and upward, faced each other. It was unnerving to see someone walk toward me with the pink soles of both feet fully visible throughout each step. I realized with a start that for the first time I was looking at clubfoot victims in adult life who had never been treated in infancy. Thick calluses covered the "tops" of their feet; many had become infected and ulcerated because the skin on the top of the foot was not designed to be walked on.

I selected a nineteen-year-old patient for treatment, anticipating a long process of splinting followed by an operation of the most radical kind to turn the foot over and fix it sole-downward. As I examined him, I could hardly believe my hands. Massaging and rotating his feet, I found them to be supple and responsive to gentle manipulation, in great contrast to the stiffness I had encountered in my older patients in England. No scar tissue had formed because no doctor had ever forced his feet into a new shape or surgically corrected them. It came to me that I must not introduce scar into this virgin tissue through the use of coercive force. So I simply pressed his feet back in the direction of their correct position until he felt a twinge of pain, and then casted them in place. After a week, on changing the splint, I found the tissues had loosened. Week by week I pressed them a little more, with progressive splinting, until nearly half the deformity was corrected without surgery.

When I finally saw that teenager walk away, for the first time in his life using the soles of his feet, I knew for certain that we had to apply the principle of slow correction to the babies' clubfeet. I announced to the baby clinic that we were to try a new approach. No more forceful manipulation. No more scar-producing surgeries. From now on we would stimulate the tissues to correct themselves. There was one problem: somehow we had to calculate an amount of force strong enough to stimulate the shortened side of the foot to grow, yet not so strong that it would damage tissues and cause scarring.

I will not mention all the methods we tried in arriving at this calculation, only our final and most successful method. The talipes clinic treated babies, and in India mothers breast-feed their babies for at least a year. In this, we found a key. We instructed mothers to bring very hungry babies to the clinic; no one was to feed before the morning treatment.

The clinic already had a well-deserved reputation as the noisiest room in the hospital, and now the waiting room became a cacophony of squalling babies. As soon as a baby's name was called, the mother entered and sat opposite me. She laid her baby across her knees and opened her sari at last, exposing a breast swollen with milk. While the baby sucked greedily at the breast, I removed the old splint and washed the foot, then began to move it around to test the range of movement. Sometimes the baby would turn its eyes toward me and frown, but milk was the overwhelming priority. After assessing the problem, I would get a roll of fine plaster of paris, wet it, and begin to work with the foot.

Now came the critical moment. I stared intently into the baby's eyes. At that point, the baby still had only one interest: food. I moved her foot gently but steadily toward a more correct position. At the first discomfort her eyes shifted and began looking at the foot and at me, the source of the trouble. That was the signal! We quickly wrapped wet plaster of paris bandage around the foot and leg, bending the foot to the farthest position we could achieve that would keep the baby looking and frowning.

If she ever let go of her mother's nipple in order to yell, we had lost the game. We had gone too far, forcing the foot into a position that would put tissue under too much stress. At that first cry of protest we would have to relax, unwrap the plaster, and start over with a new bandage while the baby went back to the breast. We learned that if we crossed this pain barrier, even though we could see no obvious injury, swelling and stiffness would later appear.

Using this technique, we obtained dramatic results of total correction without resorting to surgery. One child might require as many as twenty splint treatments, with each successive plaster cast remaining on for about five days, enough time to allow skin, ligaments, and finally bone cells to adapt to the gentle stresses being imposed on them. After the final treatment, we kept the feet in Denis Browne splints until the child was walking. The correcting influence had to be both gentle and persistent; if we left the foot uncasted for a few weeks, the deformity came right back. If the treatment proved successful, the child ended up with supple limbs and feet in the correct position for walking, with no sign of swelling or scarring. Those few cases requiring surgery at a later stage were a joy to operate on because of the absence of scar tissue.

Through my experience with talipes, I learned a fundamental principle of cell physiology: gentle persuasion works far better than violent correction. We hung a motto over the door of the clubfoot clinic: "The Inevitability of Gradualness." Although I had trained as a surgeon, a specialist in radical correction, I came to prefer the greater thrill of assisting the body in the wondrous process of adapting to stress and healing itself. No matter how skillfully I might operate, I will always leave a wound and spilled blood and torn tissue—the very factors that lead to scarring such as I had found in Denis Browne's patients. If I can persuade the body to correct itself without surgery, then every local cell can devote itself to work toward solving the original problem, not any new ones I might introduce. The body's slower, wiser changes will leave no scar.

Along the way, I learned another lesson as well, a lesson about pain that would become a guiding principle of my career. At the clubfoot clinic I began listening, almost by instinct, to the body's pain signals.

Our ritual with the nursing mothers worked for one reason: it helped us attune ourselves to the baby's tolerance for pain. I knew that if my movement of that little girl's foot merely caused irritation, the body could handle that stress without any damage. Many things can irritate a baby: a stranger's face, wet diapers, a loud noise. The advanced state of hunger, though, ruled out all interruptions except pain. If I rotated her foot so hard that it caused real pain—enough so that she would release the nipple—then I had crossed the barrier pain was designed to protect. Pain protects from damage without discrimination, whether the damage is caused by patients themselves or by their physician.

Very soon I would use similar principles to correct stiff hands in leprosy. But these patients posed a whole new set of problems, problems that would baffle me for a decade. I could not listen to their pain—they had none.

Part Two

———◆·◆———

A Career in Pain

7
Chingleput Detour

———◆———

I was recognizably human; I had at least the usual complement of legs and arms; but I might have been some shameful piece of garbage. There was something indecent about the way in which I was being furtively shuffled out of life.

Peter Greaves, leprosy patient

I was happily settling into the daily routine of teaching surgery until Dr. Robert Cochrane, the indomitable Scotsman who had summoned me to India in the first place, upended that routine by inviting me to his leprosarium.

I knew little about the disease in which Cochrane had achieved world renown. I remembered well the scary scene from my childhood, when my father had confined my sister and me to the house while he treated the men with leprosy. And in Vellore I had often seen forlorn beggars with the deformities characteristic of leprosy. "Why don't you come to my clinic?" I asked these beggars. "At least we could examine you and dress your sores."

"No, *daktar*, we could never come," they responded. "No hospital would let us in. We are lepers." I checked with the hospital, and the beggars were right. Vellore, like every other general hospital in India, had a strict policy against admitting leprosy patients, believing that "lepers" would scare away the other patients. I put the matter out of my mind—until Bob Cochrane insisted I visit his leprosy sanatorium in Chingleput.

Bob had a classic Scottish appearance: ruddy skin, a head full of graying hair, and bristly eyebrows that he used to maximum effect. I had never met anyone so dynamic, confident, and hardworking. Besides overseeing daily operations at the thousand-patient leprosy sanatorium in Chingleput, Cochrane also served as temporary director of the Vellore medical college and headed up government leprosy programs for the entire state. Rising at 5:00 A.M. each day, he worked nonstop—even on the hottest summer days—until 10:00 P.M., when he retired for an hour or two of Bible study.

Cochrane's war against leprosy was at its core a religious crusade. "I'm not interested in Christianity. I'm interested in Christ, which is an entirely different matter," he would say. Citing the example of Jesus, who had broken cultural taboos by reaching out to victims of leprosy, Cochrane led a campaign against the prevailing social stigma. He sent shock waves through the medical community by hiring leprosy patients ("burnt-out" cases he considered noninfectious) to work in his home, one as his personal cook and the other as his gardener.

Most significantly, Cochrane pioneered the use in India of a new sulfone drug from America that stopped leprosy from progressing. For the first time, he could offer leprosy patients genuine hope of arrest of the disease, possibly even a cure.

A Sudden Jolt

Everyone looked upon the sanatorium run by the Church of Scotland as a model facility. Leprosy patients tended to live apart from society, forming their own communities beside a garbage dump or some such remote place. Even leprosy institutions housed their patients in squalid compounds away from population centers. In contrast, Chingleput was a lovely, sprawling campus of neat yellow buildings with red tile roofs. Years before, missionaries had planted long rows of mango and tamarind trees, and as a result Chingleput now stood out like an oasis in the rocky, red-clay terrain south of Madras.

It was a mild, sunny day in 1947 when I finally visited Bob Cochrane at Chingleput. As we strolled down a shady pathway, he filled my ear with more facts about leprosy than I cared to know. "It's hardly contagious at all," he said. "Only one in twenty adults is even susceptible—the rest couldn't contract it if they tried. Leprosy used to be terrible but now, thanks to sulfone drugs, we can arrest the disease at an early stage. If we could just get society to catch up with advances on the medical front, we could shut this place down. Our patients could return to their communities and resume their lives."

In between these minilectures, Cochrane proudly showed me

the cottage industries he had established: weaving, bookbinding, and cobbler shops; vegetable gardens; carpentry sheds. He seemed oblivious to the gargoylish appearance of the advanced leprosy patients, but I had to fight the temptation to avert my eyes from the more disfigured faces. Some had the so-called leonine characteristics of leprosy: a flattened nose, no eyebrows, and greatly thickened forehead and cheekbone areas. A few had so little control over facial muscles that I found it hard to tell a smile from a grimace. I noticed a red-stained, milky film on many eyes, and Cochrane informed me that leprosy often blinds its victims.

After a few minutes I stopped looking at faces, however, for the leprosy patients' hands had captured my attention. As we passed by, the patients greeted us in the traditional Indian way, hands held up and palms pressed together before a slightly bowed head. Never in my life had I seen so many stumps and claw-hands. Shortened fingers jutted out at unnatural angles, their joints frozen into position. I saw other fingers bent downward against the palm in a fixed claw position, with the fingernails actually indenting the flesh of the palm. Some hands lacked thumbs and fingers altogether.

In the weaving shop I noticed one young boy working vigorously at a loom, shooting the shuttle through the weft with his right hand and then reaching out with his left hand to ram a wooden bar against the threads, forcing them together. He picked up speed, probably showing off for the director and his guest, and bits of cotton floated through the air like dust. Cochrane shouted over the clatter of the loom, "You see, Paul, these workers would have to resort to begging outside the leprosarium. Despite their skills, no one would dare hire them." I made a gesture to interrupt Bob and pointed to a trail of dark spots on the cotton cloth. Blood?

"May I see your hand," I yelled to the weaver. He released the pedals and set down the shuttle, and instantly the noise level in the room dropped several decibels. He held out a deformed, twisted hand with shortened fingers. The index finger had lost maybe a third of an inch in length, and as I looked closer I saw naked bone protruding from a nasty, septic wound. This boy was working with a finger cut to the bone!

"How did you cut yourself?" I asked. He gave a nonchalant reply: "Oh, it's nothing. I had a pimple on my finger, and earlier it bled a little. I guess it's opened up again." I took a few photos of his hand to add to my orthopedics files, and we dispatched him to the clinic for bandaging.

"That's a real problem here," Bob explained as the boy left. "These patients go anesthetic. They lose all sense of touch and pain, so we have to watch them carefully. They hurt themselves without knowing it." *How could anyone not notice a cut like that?* I thought to myself. From Tommy Lewis's research, I knew that up to twenty-one thousand sensors of heat, pressure, and pain crowd together in a square inch of the fingertip. How could he feel no pain from such an injury? Yet the boy had indeed shown no sign of discomfort.

We continued the tour and Cochrane, a dermatologist, began describing subtle variations in the color and texture of the dry skin patches symptomatic of leprosy. "Note the different reactions in a macule and a papule, a nodule and a plaque," he said, pointing to patients whose skin had been infiltrated by the disease. I was still thinking of the young weaver with the bloody finger, and the nonstop lecture was beginning to annoy me.

"Bob, I've heard enough about skin," I said at last. "Tell me about bones. Look at the hands of that woman. She has no fingers left, just a stump. What happened to her fingers? Did they fall off?"

"Sorry, Paul, I don't know," he replied brusquely, and resumed his lecture on skin.

I broke in again. "Don't know! But Bob, these patients will need their hands for any kind of livelihood. Something's destroying the tissue. You can't just let those hands waste away."

Cochrane's eyebrows arched upward in a sign I recognized as the final warning before a storm burst. He jabbed a finger in my stomach. "And who is the orthopedist around here, Paul!" he demanded. "I'm a dermatologist, and I've studied this disease for twenty-five years. I know most of what there is to know about how leprosy affects skin. But you go back to that medical library in Vellore and look up the research on leprosy and bones. I can tell you what you'll find—nothing! No orthopedist has ever paid attention to this disease, even though it's crippled more people than polio or any other disease."

Could it be true that not one of the thousands of orthopedic surgeons had taken interest in a disease that produced such terrible deformities? A look of incredulity must have crossed my face because Cochrane responded as if he had read my mind. "You're thinking of leprosy like other diseases, Paul," he said. "But doctors, like most people, put it in a separate category altogether. They view leprosy as a curse of the gods. It still has the aura of supernatural judgment about it. You'll find priests, missionaries, and a few crackpots working in leprosy settlements, but rarely a good physician and never a specialist in orthopedics."

I stayed silent, mulling over what Cochrane had said. We were walking under the main arched colonnade of trees toward the dining hall. Cochrane nodded and spoke to the patients we passed. He seemed to know them all by name.

One man motioned for us to stop, and asked whether we would look at a sore on his foot. He squatted on the ground and tried to unbuckle his sandal, but he couldn't manage it with his hand pulled into a claw position. Every time he tried to slide the sandal strap between his thumb and palm in order to tug it free of the buckle, the strap slipped away. "Paralysis from nerve damage," Cochrane remarked. "That's what this disease does. Paralysis, plus complete anesthesia. This fellow can't feel his sandal strap any more than the boy at the loom could feel his cut finger."

I asked the sandal-wearer if I could see his hands. He rose from the ground, the sandal still strapped to his foot, and presented his right hand. The fingers were full-length and intact, but virtually useless. The thumb and four fingers curved in and pressed against each other in the position I recognized as "leprosy claw-hand." As I examined the man's hand, though, to my surprise the fingers felt soft and supple, very unlike fingers made stiff through arthritis or other crippling diseases. I pried the fingers open and slipped my own hand between his bent thumb and fingers. "Squeeze," I said. "As hard as you can."

Anticipating a weak twitch from nearly paralyzed muscles, I was startled to feel a jolt of pain shoot through my hand. This man had the grip of a bodybuilder! The nails of his bent fingers dug into my flesh like talons. "Stop!" I cried. I looked up to see a puzzled expression on the man's face. What a strange visitor, he must have thought. He asks me to squeeze hard, then yells when I do.

I felt more than pain in that moment. I felt a sudden awakening, a tiny electric prod signaling the beginning of a long, boundless search. I had the intuitive sense of stumbling across a path that would send my life in a new direction. I had just spent a very depressing morning, seeing hundreds of hands that cried out for treatment. As a surgeon who loved hands, I had shaken my head in sadness at the waste, for until this moment I had thought them permanently ruined. Now, in this one man's grip I had first-hand proof that a "useless" hand concealed live, powerful muscles. Paralysis? My own hand still ached from his grip.

The man's puzzled look only added to the mystery. Until I cried out, he had no idea he had hurt me. He had lost sensory contact with his own hand.

Creeping Death

Accepting Bob Cochrane's challenge, when I returned to Vellore I checked the literature on orthopedic aspects of leprosy. I learned that 10 to 15 million people worldwide were estimated to suffer from the disease. Since a third of them sustained significant damage to the hands and feet, leprosy probably represented the single greatest cause of orthopedic crippling. One source suggested that leprosy caused more hand paralysis than all other diseases combined. Yet I could find only one article describing any surgical procedures other than amputation, an article that bore the byline "Robert Cochrane."

The afternoon in Chingleput had kindled an interest I could not ignore, and I felt compelled to study this cruel disease further. The pattern of paralysis baffled me because it blatantly contradicted my previous experience with paralysis. The man with the sandal could flex his fingers in, but not extend them out: he could grip my hand like a vise, but could not separate his fingers enough to pick up a pencil. Why had only one part of his hand become paralyzed? As a starting point, I needed to determine which of the three major nerves in the hand was responsible for the partial paralysis.

I set up a weekly visit to Chingleput. Each Thursday after hospital rounds I caught the evening train from Vellore, then hired a horse-drawn cart to transport me the last few miles to the sanatorium. The Cochranes kept a guest room available for me, and after a good night's sleep I would arise to begin a full day of surveying patients. Following dinner with the Cochranes on Friday evening, I would retire early, setting my alarm for 4:30 A.M. Bob taught a morning class at the Vellore medical college on Saturdays, and I could ride back in his car.

I organized an assembly-line team of technicians, and one by one we examined the thousand patients at Chingleput. Testing with a feather and a straight pin, we mapped the sensitivity to touch and pain in the various regions of the hand. Then we measured the range of movement of thumb, fingers, and wrist, and repeated the procedure for toes and feet. We recorded the precise length of fingers and toes, noting which digits had shortened and which muscles seemed to be paralyzed. If facial paralysis was present, we noted that, too. The most interesting cases, we X-rayed.

Since I spent only one day a week in Chingleput, the survey dragged on for several months. Early on, though, I noticed a clear pattern among the patients (80 percent, as it turned out) who had experienced some degree of paralysis of the hand. Almost all of them had lost movement in the muscles controlled by the ulnar nerve. Forty percent also showed evidence of paralysis in areas supplied by the lower part of the median nerve. Oddly, I found no paralysis in the forearm muscles supplied by the upper part of the median nerve. Very few muscles controlled by the radial nerve were affected and we also found no paralysis above the elbow. This was the anomaly I had first noticed in the sandal-wearer, who could bend his fingers but not extend them.

I had never seen such a peculiar pattern. In some diseases paralysis inches relentlessly toward the trunk, affecting all nerves in its path. In others, like polio, paralysis is completely haphazard. Leprosy seemed to attack specific nerves very selectively, with a strange consistency. What could account for the unusual progression?

By now my scientific instincts were fully aroused. Even severely afflicted leprosy patients retained some good nerves and muscles, as the man with the claw-hand had demonstrated on me so powerfully, a fact which opened up the tantalizing possibility of surgical correction. A claw-hand patient could still bend his fingers inward; if I could figure out how to free them to straighten in an outward direction, he would regain a functioning hand.

Before proceeding, though, I had to learn much more. I read everything available about leprosy. I soon discovered why Bob Cochrane had become such a crusader. No disease in history has been so marked by stigma, much of it the result of ignorance and false stereotypes.

Hysteria over leprosy sprang partly from a great fear of contagion. In Old Testament times a person with leprosy or infectious skin diseases had to "wear torn clothes, let his hair be unkempt, cover the lower part of his face and cry out, 'Unclean! Unclean!'" (Lev. 13:45). People with leprosy lived in isolation outside the town walls. In most societies in history, in fact, a similar fear of contagion led to government policies of quarantine.

Yet, as Bob Cochrane had assured me, such fear was largely unfounded. Leprosy may only be spread to susceptible people, a small minority. In 1873 the Norwegian scientist Armauer Hansen identified the agent responsible for leprosy—*Mycobacterium leprae*, a bacillus that closely resembles the tuberculosis bacillus—and since then leprosy had proved to be one of the least communicable of all communicable diseases. Hansen's compatriot Daniel Cornelius Danielssen, "the father of leprology," tried for years to contract the disease for experimental purposes, injecting the bacillus by hypodermic needle into himself and four laboratory workers. These efforts demonstrated incredible courage but little else: all five colleagues were immune.*

(The riddle of transmission remains unsolved to this day. The most vulnerable group seems to be children who have prolonged contact with infected persons, and for this reason in many countries children are separated from their infected parents. Most clinicians favor the theory that leprosy is spread through the upper respiratory system, via nasal droplets communicated through a cough or sneeze. High standards of hygiene tend to reduce the chance of contagion: leprosy workers have a very low infection rate despite their regular contact with patients. Some theorize that the leprosy bacillus breeds in colonies in the soil, which may explain why it stubbornly perseveres in low-income countries where people go barefoot and live in houses with dirt floors. The disease lost its grip on Western Europe, once a primary breeding ground, as the standard of living rose, and the same trend holds true in developing countries today.)

However it spreads, leprosy rarely affects more than 1 percent of the population of a given region. There are a few exceptions to that rule, I learned, and the area around Vellore, India, happened to be one of them; in the 1940s more than 3 percent of the surrounding population had tested positive for leprosy.

Most infected patients stand a good chance of healing the dis-

---

*Hanson met similar failure in his attempts to transmit the bacillus. When he had no success with rabbits, he experimented on a human being by injecting leprosy germs into the cornea of a patient's eye. The woman did not contract the disease, but she suffered pain from the injection and reported him to the authorities. For this breach of ethics Hansen was banned from practicing in Norwegian hospitals for the rest of his life.

ease on their own. These "tuberculoid" cases may suffer patches of
dead skin, the loss of sensation, and a little nerve damage, but no
extensive disfigurement. Many of the symptoms result from the
body's own furious autoimmune response to the foreign bacilli.

One in every five patients, however, lacks any natural immunities. These unprotected patients, classified "lepromatous," are
usually the ones who end up in facilities like Chingleput. Their
bodies seem to put out a welcome mat for the foreign invaders and
trillions of bacilli lay siege in a massive infiltration that, were it by
any other strain of bacteria, would mean certain death. But leprosy
rarely proves fatal. It wrecks the body in slow, debilitating ways.
My patients sometimes used a local word for leprosy which literally means "creeping death."

Sores appear on the face, hands, and feet, and if they go
untreated, infection may set in. Fingers and toes mysteriously
shorten in length. Beggars I saw in the streets of India usually had
raw, suppurating sores and deformed hands and feet. Lacking a
sensation of pain, these beggars had little regard for the dangers of
infection and instead exploited their wounds for their profit
potential. The more aggressive beggars would sometimes threaten
to touch a passerby unless he or she gave alms.

Blindness, a further manifestation of the disease, greatly
complicates the life of a person with leprosy: having lost touch and
pain sensations, he cannot use his fingers to "scout" the world and
test for danger.

As I studied the history of leprosy, I came to have the utmost
respect for the saintly few who, defying society's stigma, looked
past the unsightly symptoms of leprosy and ministered to its victims. For centuries such people had nothing to offer but simple
human compassion. As the disease ravaged Europe during the
Middle Ages, religious orders devoted to Lazarus, the patron saint
of leprosy, established homes for patients. These courageous
women could do little but bind wounds and change dressings, but
the homes themselves, called *lazarettos*, may have helped break the
hold of the disease in Europe, by isolating leprosy patients and
improving their living conditions. In the nineteenth and twentieth
centuries, Christian missionaries who spread across the globe
established many colonies for leprosy patients, such as the one at
Chingleput, and as a result many of the major scientific advances
in understanding and treating leprosy came from missionaries—
Bob Cochrane being the latest in a long line.

At Chingleput, the introduction of sulfone drugs represented a breakthrough every bit as exciting as what I had experienced in medical school with penicillin. The previous treatment, injecting oil distilled from the chaulmoogra tree directly into the patients' skin patches, had side effects almost as bad as the disease. Some doctors preferred many small injections, as many as 320 per week, which left the skin pulpy and inflamed. Desperate, patients sought out such treatment regardless, and some reported improvement. The new sulfone drug had the distinct advantage of being an oral medication. By the time I visited Chingleput, after five years of testing with sulfone, patients were actually showing negative reports of active bacteria. Leprosy had virtually disappeared from their bodies.

Old-time leprosy workers like Cochrane were ecstatic. No longer contagious, their disease now inactive, patients could theoretically be released back to their villages. Hopes dimmed, however, as it became clear that villages had no interest in welcoming home anyone with a history of leprosy. In almost every case, patients had to stay on at Chingleput even after they had been cured.

I was not sure what contribution I could offer leprosy patients, but the more time I spent among them, the more confirmed I felt in my calling. While conducting the research tests I had listened to hundreds of stories of rejection and despair. Banished from home and village, the patients went to Chingleput because they literally had nowhere else to go. They had become social outcasts simply because of their misfortune in contracting a feared and misunderstood disease. For the first time I grasped the human tragedy of leprosy. With Cochrane's encouragement, I also caught a whiff of hope that progress could be made in reversing that tragedy.

Revelation at Dawn

After surveying Chingleput and other leprosy sanatoriums near Vellore, I reviewed the data collected from two thousand patients. Each file folder on a damaged hand included diagrams of the insensitivity and range of movement, as well as photos of bone and skin damage. The pattern I had first noticed at Chingleput, which defied every conventional sequence of paralysis, held true: frequent paralysis in areas controlled by the ulnar nerve, moderate paralysis in the median nerve, and very little in the radial nerve. I could think of no logical reason why the ulnar nerve at the elbow would cause paralysis while the median nerve, one inch away, stayed healthy; or why the median nerve went dead at the wrist while none of the radial nerve muscles was paralyzed.

To add to my confusion, I had sent tissue samples from short-ened fingers to Vellore's professor of pathology, Ted Gault. "What's wrong with these tissues, Ted?" I asked. Again and again he reported, "Nothing, Paul. They're perfectly normal except for the loss of nerve endings."

Normal? I had taken some of the biopsies from fingers that had shortened several inches in length, mere stumps of fingers. How could they be normal? I could hardly believe the reports until Ted let me look through the microscope and see for myself. The tissue showed scars from previous infection, of course, but the bones, tendons, and muscles looked fine, as did the skin and fat. What was causing damage to the hands? The facts did not add up.

I longed to try some corrective hand surgery on patients with motor paralysis, most of whom had not suffered much damage to their hands because their hands were too weak to get into trouble. This group represented the best hope for restoring any leprosy patients to a productive life, and yet I dared not plunge in before learning why certain muscles stayed healthy while others became paralyzed. I needed to know whether some muscles would remain "good," unaffected by the disease, and to do so I would need to examine the full arm's length of affected nerves. Of course, I could not ethically operate on a living patient for the sole purpose of retrieving nerves. Autopsies were the only solution.

Alas, in India autopsies were more problem than solution. Moslem mullahs forbade bodily mutilation after death, even for the purpose of donating organs to science. The Hindu faith required that the entire body be burned to ashes in a purifying fire, and so very strict Hindus resisted amputation for any reason, even if gangrene threatened death; better to die now, they rea-soned, than to be deprived of a limb through all future incarna-tions. To meet its needs for organ transplants and laboratory work, the Vellore hospital worked hard to persuade families to allow autopsies. They also used the bodies of dead prisoners and dere-licts who had no families. (My wife, who had broadcast her need for eyes to use in corneal grafts, vividly remembers a knock on the

door late one evening. She opened it to find a rather spectral figure shrouded in a cloth. He thrust before her a handwritten note
from the local judge which she read by the light of his hurricane
lantern: "Judicial hanging at dawn. Be there to remove the eyes.")

Because leprosy is not a terminal disease, its patients tended
to live long. To get our autopsy, we would have to wait for the natural death in the hospital of a lepromatous patient whose relatives
had no religious objections. I sent an urgent message to every leprosy clinic within traveling distance, up to hundreds of miles away,
asking for immediate notification if any such prospect came along.
"Telephone or telegraph at any time of day or night," I said. My
Portuguese-Ceylonese assistant, Dr. Gusta Buultgens, prepared
boxes of surgical instruments, formalin jars, and anything else we
might need for an autopsy. And we waited.

For more than a month we waited, until one evening the
phone rang at the very end of a full day of surgery. A patient had
died at Chingleput, a mere seventy-five miles away. The Chingleput
hospital had no refrigeration, and had scheduled a cremation for the
next day, but they would grant us access to the body overnight.
Three of us, Dr. Buultgens, an Indian pathology technician, and I,
gulped down dinner, loaded the box of supplies into a Land Rover,
and hit the road.

I felt especially tense and anxious as we headed across the
pitch-black countryside toward Chingleput. Driving is always an
adventure in India, where trucks and cars must share the tarmac
with pedestrians, bullock carts, bicycles, and sacred cows (there are
200 million of these and they have an inviolable right-of-way).
Nightfall adds to the adventure because many bullock carts have
no lights. In addition, some Indian drivers practice a peculiar
courtesy when they see an oncoming vehicle: they turn off their
headlights for a while so as not to blind the other driver, then suddenly switch their headlights on high beam and flash them furi-
ously a few times before switching them off again. You see utter
darkness, a brief hypnotic eruption of light, and darkness again.
Because drivers compensate for the absence of light by liberal use
of the horn, sounds echo menacingly in the darkness.

About halfway to Chingleput, I felt a sensation of intense
heat. Looking down, I saw flames shooting up through the open-
ings for the pedals and licking around my sandaled feet! I jerked
my feet away from the floorboard and steered the Land Rover off
the road into a clump of shrubbery. We all piled out of the vehicle,

nearly falling into an open well. No one was hurt, and a few hand-fuls of sand put out the fire right away. But when I raised the hood, my flashlight revealed a melted snarl of wires and blackened metal. Evidently a thief had loosened a union nut in order to siphon gas out of the fuel line; later, vibrations worked the loose nut off, causing the fuel pump to spray gasoline over the hot engine.

The three of us walked on the road in the moonlight, balanc-ing the autopsy boxes on our shoulders. By now it was past mid-night and we encountered not a single motorized vehicle for two miles. Finally we reached a mission school, where I was able to rouse a teacher and hire a reluctant driver to transport us the rest of the way to Chingleput. We arrived about 2:30 in the morning to find the leprosy compound completely dark. More time passed as we tried to persuade the night watchman to let us begin our dubious task. With some misgivings he guided us along a narrow, rocky trail toward the foothills behind the sanatorium. There, after a long walk, we found a tiny stucco hut, the death place. The watchman lent us a hurricane lantern—the hut had no electric-ity—and quickly retreated. Stretched out on a wooden table before us was the dead man.

The body, an elderly man's, showed evidence of severe defor-mity: claw-hands, shortened fingers and toes, facial deformities. He was a classic "burnt-out case": the leprosy bacilli had done all the damage they could do, and then died out. For our purposes, his body was ideal.

We knew we had to hurry. We had promised the Chingleput superintendent we would complete our task by dawn, now only four hours away, so that normal religious rituals could proceed. We hung the lantern from the roof beam, switched on a pocket flashlight for closeup work, and donned rubber aprons and gloves. Within seconds we were covered with perspiration. The body had lain in this unventilated hut all day under a broiling sun, and, to put it delicately, was fast moving toward a state of overripeness. The setting—a silent moonlit night, the heat, the isolation, a corpse full of germs—was worthy of a horror movie.

We divided up the chore. Dr. Buultgens worked on one side, taking nerve specimens every two inches or so for later study under the microscope. The technician wrote detailed labels and put each piece of nerve in its own bottle of formalin. I worked on the opposite side and took no specimens. I wanted to see the nerves whole and in detail in relation to the bones and muscles. The fast, crude procedures of autopsy went against all my surgical instincts, but I knew this body held only one thing of value for us: nerves. After making long lateral cuts along the arm and leg, I peeled back skin, fat, and muscle, clamping the tissue to the side as I proceeded.

For at least three hours we dissected at a brisk pace, cutting deep to the nerves, snipping samples, clamping back tissue. We hoped to expose every peripheral nerve from hands and feet, all the way past the elbow and shoulder, thigh and hip, on to the nerve roots that emerged from the spinal column. Not until we had retrieved some samples from all the nerves affected by leprosy could we begin to relax.

The three of us barely spoke. The only sounds were the clicking of the instruments and the high-pitched whine of cicadas outside. After finishing the man's arms, we moved on to the legs and finally the face. My mind flashed back to the my project in Cardiff, Wales, but this time I exposed only the fifth and seventh facial nerves, in search of some clue as to why eyelids suffer early paralysis.

At last we had accomplished our goal. I stood up straight, and felt as if I had just been stabbed. The tension of the trip, combined with my stooped-over posture from the autopsy, had taken its toll on my back. I had not slept in twenty-four hours, and my eyes stung from the constant drip of perspiration. I breathed deeply a few times, my nose by now inured to the rancid odor in the tiny room.

Light from the kerosene lantern flickered over the body, and the fresh, exposed nerves gleamed white in contrast to the dark body tissue. The first gray light of dawn was creeping over the hills, filtering through the open doorway. I mopped my brow with a handkerchief and stretched the cramping muscles in my back and fingers. The rising sun suddenly climbed above the hills and streamed in the door, illuminating in one broad view all that we had seen thus far in feeble circles of flashlight. My eyes traveled up and down each arm and leg, reviewing our handiwork. I was not looking for anything in particular, merely taking a break to gather strength for the final phase of the autopsy.

And then I saw it. "Look at the nerve swellings," I said to Dr. Buultgens. "Do you see the pattern?" A striking abnormality was easily visible. She leaned over the side of the body I had worked on, visually tracing the full lustrous length of the nerves, and then nodded enthusiastically. At certain places—behind the ankle, just above the knee, and also at the wrist—the nerves swelled up to many times normal size. Swellings also bulged slightly on the facial nerve branches at the chin and cheekbone, and were most marked just above the elbow on the ulnar nerve.

We both knew that nerves swelled in reaction to an infestation of leprosy germs, but now we saw clearly that nerve swellings tended to occur in just a few sites. Indeed, swellings arose only where the nerve lay close to the skin surface, and not in the deep tissues. The ulnar nerve, which suffered paralysis, swelled hugely at the elbow. The median nerve, a mere inch away, seemed fine—perhaps because it was located an inch deeper, beneath muscle tissue.

For the first time I sensed some rationality behind the mystery of leprosy-induced paralysis. There was a pattern after all: a thin white nerve gradually distending as it nears the elbow, then shrinking down to normal size as it plunges deep among the forearm muscles, swelling again as it courses around the wrist, and tapering slightly in the carpal tunnel into the hand. The same pattern applied in the leg: every time a nerve came near the surface it bulged, and whenever it lay under muscle fibers it returned to normal. Dr. Buultgens and I speculated aloud as to what might cause the swelling. "Perhaps nerves closer to the surface are more subject to impact damage?" she suggested.

In any case, the glimpse of that overall pattern cleared up one abiding mystery: muscles controlled by nerves located deep in body tissue did not seem endangered. Even in an old man riddled with leprosy, those muscles remained a rich, healthy red. In contrast, muscles controlled by nerve twigs that passed close to the skin surface were pinkish and shriveled from atrophy. The presence of healthy muscles in a man in such an advanced state of infection confirmed my hunch that the disease always left certain muscles unaffected. I could now identify forearm muscles for use in reconstructive surgery—possibly to transfer over to replace the paralyzed muscles—with no fear that they might become paralyzed later. We had a simple guideline to use in selecting "good" muscles: choose those muscles whose motor nerves had not been near the surface of a limb.

I felt a second wind of energy and enthusiasm. I took photographs of the long, exposed nerves and we snipped off more segments for later study. These samples would contain our best clue into how the disease destroyed nerves. I had the vague sense that we had just stumbled onto a medical secret of very great import, but what was it?

After the autopsy, pathologists at Vellore took up the arduous task of examining cross sections of our samples, staring at what Hansen had called the "frog spawn" masses of leprosy nodules, searching for the tiny rod-shaped bacilli stained red by our chemicals. Years would pass before we unraveled the full mystery, but we would eventually learn that leprosy's predilection for knees, wrists, cheekbones, and chins had nothing to do with impact damage or any other conjecture we had made that night in the death hut. The solution, when it came, was a simple one: to multiply, leprosy bacilli prefer the cooler temperatures that prevail close to the surface (this also explains why they seek refuge in testicles, earlobes, eyes, and nasal passages).

As leprosy bacilli migrate to nerves in the cooler regions, such as around the joints, the body's immune system dispatches platoons of macrophages and lymphocytes which swarm in, swelling inside the nerve's insulating sheath and choking off vital nourishment. The nerve swellings we were gazing at in the flickering light were in fact evidence of the body's own defensive response to an invasion.

We did not fully appreciate what we had discovered in that stifling makeshift mortuary in Chingleput. If we had, perhaps we would have celebrated with some dramatic gesture (Pythagoras, when he proved a theorem, sacrificed a hundred oxen to the gods who sent him the idea!). Instead, we stitched up the corpse, trudged over to Bob Cochrane's house for breakfast, and borrowed a car to take us back to Vellore, passing by our charred wreck of a Land Rover on the way.

8
Loosening the Claw

—◦—◆—◦—

The hand is the visible part of the brain.
Immanuel Kant

After the Chingleput autopsy I could hardly wait to attempt reconstructive surgery on claw-hands. There was a chance, just a chance, that by transferring the strength of the "good" muscles left untouched by leprosy, we could free clenched fingers and restore movement to damaged hands.

When I sought the Vellore hospital's permission to perform such surgery, though, roadblocks went up. Even staff who were supportive of our efforts questioned the wisdom of admitting leprosy patients. "We're already short of beds, Paul," said one administrator, "and you know good and well that leprosy patients can't pay for services." (This was true in a Catch-22 sense: they could not pay because paralyzed hands made it impossible for them to earn a decent living—the very condition I wanted to address.) The hospital maintained some free beds for charity cases but, as the administrator reminded me, these were reserved for urgent cases who had the prospect of a cure. Orthopedic leprosy patients did not qualify.

Appealing to their sympathies, I told other hospital staff about some of the leprosy patients I had met. In a nation with a five-thousand-year tradition of caste, leprosy victims occupied the lowest rung of the social ladder. Their own families usually evicted them, with good reason: otherwise, the village would run the entire family out of town. I examined one young boy with nodules all over his body who had been locked in an upstairs room for seven years. Another teenager had, before going to the Chingleput sanatorium, kept his left hand in his pocket to hide the telltale skin patches: below the tan line his hand was soft and pale like a baby's, and very weak from disuse. Leprosy strikes twice as many males as females—no one knows why—but in India I heard the most poignant stories from young girls who contracted the disease. Unable to find husbands or jobs, many of them ended up begging on the streets, assigned to a patch of pavement by a gang chieftain who exploited their earnings. Some served time in a brothel until the disease became noticeable to customers.

"Paul, these are moving stories, but we can't help them medically," a respected physician on the hospital staff responded. "They have bad flesh. That's the nature of the disease—even accidental wounds don't heal. If you proceed with your plans to operate on leprous flesh, the surgical wounds will never heal properly. If you find a good muscle and fix it today, it will likely be paralyzed next year. The disease will only progress. Don't waste your time."

One objection to admitting leprosy patients probably lay at the root of the staff resistance. "If word got out that we were treating lepers here," an administrator told me bluntly, "other patients would flee the hospital in fear. We can't risk that. Why not go and treat leprosy in leprosy centers where it belongs?"

Nevertheless, after much lobbying the hospital did grant permission for us to open a "Hand Research Unit"—we dared not use the word leprosy—in a mud-walled storeroom attached to the outer wall of the hospital compound. Leprosy patients began coming to our clinic right away, and they seemed grateful for any help. Their lack of anger or resentment over their plight amazed me. Moslem or Hindu, they accepted their condition with a spirit of melancholy fatalism. They had no expectations—no hope—of a better life. I wondered if, having been treated as inhuman for so long, they now saw themselves that way.

The Fear Barrier

As I began treating leprosy patients I had to confront my own deep-seated prejudice and fear. Patients presented the most horrible, purulent sores for treatment, and often the pungent odor of pus and gangrene filled the storeroom. Even though I had heard Bob Cochrane's assurances about the low contagion rate, I, like most people who worked with leprosy back then, worried constantly about infection. I began keeping a map of my hands. Whenever I pricked myself accidentally during surgery with a needle or sharp edge of bone, I marked the point on the map, noting the time and the name of the patient I had been treating so that if I contracted leprosy I would be able to track the source. I abandoned that policy after the total of pricks, cuts, and scratches reached thirteen.

My wife, Margaret, led the way in helping me overcome fear of close contact. One weekend when I was away, a cycle rickshaw pulled up to our house on the medical college campus. Out stepped a slim man in his early twenties, and Margaret went to meet him. She noticed that his shoes were open in the front, and his feet were heavily bandaged. White scars covered much of the surface of one eye, and he kept lowering his eyes to avoid the sun's glare. "Excuse me, Madam," the man said very respectfully, "could you tell me where I might find a Dr. Paul Brand?" Margaret replied that Dr. Brand, her husband, would not return until Tuesday, three days away. Obviously crestfallen, the man thanked her and turned to go. His rickshaw had already pulled off, so the man began walking back toward town in an awkward, hobbling gait.

My wife, who has a heart of gold, could not bear to turn away someone in need. She called him back. "You do have somewhere to go, don't you?" she asked. It took some coaxing, but in the next few minutes Margaret managed to extract Sadan's story, an all-too-typical story of rejection and abuse. He had first noticed skin patches at the age of eight. Kicked out of school, he became a social outcast. His former friends crossed the street to avoid him. Restaurants and shops refused to serve him. After six wasted years he had finally found a mission school that would accept him, but even with a diploma no one would hire him. He had managed to scrape together the fare for the train trip to Vellore. Once he arrived there, however, the driver of the public bus had refused to let him board. Sadan had then spent all his remaining cash to hire the rickshaw that brought him the four miles to the medical college. No, he had nowhere to go. Even if a hotel would let him in, he could not pay for the room.

In a flash Margaret invited Sadan to sleep on our veranda. She made a comfortable bed for him and he spent three nights there until I returned. I admit with some shame that I did not react well when the children came rushing out to tell me about our new guest, the nice man with leprosy. Had our children now been exposed to the disease? Margaret offered just this one-line explanation, "But, Paul, he had nowhere to go." A little later she told me just that morning she had read the New Testament passage in which Jesus said, "For I was hungry and you gave me something to eat, I was thirsty and you gave me something to drink, I was a stranger and you invited me in, I needed clothes and you clothed me, I was sick and you looked after me." In that spirit she had invited Sadan into our house, a decision for which I am now eternally grateful. Besides teaching us about our own exaggerated fears, Sadan became one of our dearest friends.

A missionary physiotherapist named Ruth Thomas helped us all surmount the fear barrier. She had recently fled China because of the Maoist revolution, booking passage from Hong Kong back to her home in England. Just before leaving, she heard that an orthopedist in India was doing experimental work with leprosy patients. At once she changed her plans and traveled to Vellore. Ruth set up a physiotherapy area in our clinic, equipping it with facilities for hot paraffin treatment and electrical stimulation of muscles. She was a pioneer, one of the first physiotherapists in the world to work with leprosy patients.

Ruth believed that vigorous hand-to-hand massage would help prevent hands from stiffening. Every day she sat in the corner stroking, stroking, stroking the hands of leprosy patients. "Ruth, this is intimate skin-to-skin contact!" I would warn her. "You really should be wearing gloves." She would smile, nod, and keep on stroking. Ruth Thomas achieved remarkable success with her simple therapy, success which I credit as much to her gift of human touch as to any massage techniques.

A few months after we opened the unit I was examining the hands of a bright young man, trying to explain to him in my broken Tamil that we could halt the progress of the disease, and perhaps restore some movement to his hand, but we could do little about his facial deformities. I joked a bit, laying my hand on his shoulder. "Your face is not so bad," I said with a wink, "and it shouldn't get any worse if you take the medication. After all, we men don't have to worry so much about faces. It's the women who fret over every bump and wrinkle." I expected him to smile in response, but instead he began to shake with muffled sobs.

"Have I said something wrong?" I asked my assistant in English. "Did he misunderstand me?" She quizzed him in a spurt of Tamil and reported, "No, doctor. He says he is crying because you put your hand around his shoulder. Until he came here no one had touched him for many years."

The First Cut

We settled on teenage boys as our primary target group for hand surgery. Teenagers seemed most likely to benefit from our surgeries, and there were far more male patients to choose from. Since no orthopedist had ever worked with leprosy, I had no specific manuals or case studies to follow. I felt very alone, as if I had just entered a foreign country without a guide.

First I pored over the newly released textbook on hand surgery by Sterling Bunnell, a book destined to become a classic. It comforted me that Bunnell had also begun with no special training in the field. He had specialized in gynecology before World War II, when he was assigned to the Medical Corps. On the battlefield he kept encountering paralysis of the hand caused by bullet wounds. Bunnell had no preconceptions about which procedures were appropriate, so he invented his own techniques, leading to his reputation as "the father of hand surgery." To treat paralysis resulting from ulnar nerve damage, for example, Bunnell used muscles and tendons supplied by the median nerve, cutting them free and moving them to new locations as a substitute for the paralyzed muscles. The operation became known as the "Bunnell tendon transfer," and a color illustration of that method formed the frontispiece of his first book on surgery of the hand.

Although my training as a general surgeon gave me little direct knowledge of the mechanics of the hand, at least my background in the building trade had provided a solid foundation in engineering. In medical school I had listened with amazement as Ilingworth Law, the hydraulics expert, explained the complex engineering behind hand movements. Now, seeking ways to repair damaged hands, I studied those processes with an increasing sense of awe. "In the absence of any other proof, the thumb alone would convince me of God's existence," said Isaac Newton. A single hand movement can involve as many as fifty muscles working together in concert. Even more impressive, the powerful and delicate movements of fingers are purely the result of transferred force. There are no muscles in the fingers (otherwise they would enlarge to a bulky and unwieldy size); tendons transfer strength from the muscles in the forearm.

For such an exquisite mechanism as the human hand, the surgery manuals were appallingly imprecise. "Attach tendon so that it exerts moderate force," they said. *Moderate* force! I could not imagine such imprecision in a set of instructions for building a bridge or even a garage. The difference of a few grams of tension and a couple of millimeters of leverage could determine whether a finger moved or not.

To gain surgical experience, I practiced in the autopsy room on deceased hospital patients. I had only a few hours to go in, open the hand, test some tendon movements, and then sew it closed before the body had to be prepared for burial. Fortunately, I managed to obtain a cadaver hand to practice on at a more leisurely pace. After negotiating with my wife for precious space, I stored it wrapped in foil in our tiny freezer compartment. (I gave the cook strict instructions to leave the package alone, but twice he pulled it out and asked Margaret suspiciously, "Ma'am, is it bacon?") I tried various techniques on the cadaver hand, transplanting tendons to new sites and anchoring them to different bones. The dissection gave me valuable experience, but in the end the cadaver hand proved to be of limited use because it lacked the counterbalancing forces of a living hand. I could test one tendon or one muscle at a time, but not the simultaneous interaction of scores of muscles. It became clear that only actual surgery on a living patient could tell me what I needed to know.

On my next trip to Chingleput I assembled a group of leprosy patients, preselected for their advanced state of paralysis. I wanted volunteers whose hands I could not make worse. "In the hospital at Vellore, we are planning some experiments that *might possibly* help a paralyzed hand," I told them. "We need a few volunteers. The procedures have never been tried, and there is no guarantee whatsoever that they will work. You'll have to come to the hospital for a long stay, involving several surgeries, and the rehabilitation process will be very strenuous. Again, we may find there's no improvement at all." I made the process sound as unappealing as possible in order to dampen expectations. When I asked for volunteers, to my astonishment every patient stood up. I could have my pick.

After consulting with Bob Cochrane, I examined and interviewed a Hindu teenager named Krishnamurthy. His overall health seemed good, but leprosy had ravaged his hands and feet. He had large ulcers on the soles of both feet, exposing bone. If nothing else, I thought, a hospital stay would certainly improve that condition. His fingers, nearly their original length, curled in to form a stiff claw. He had a strong grasping motion but could not open his fingers enough to hold what it was he wanted to grasp.

Cochrane told me Krishnamurthy could read six languages and was one of his brightest patients. I never would have guessed it. His dress was ragged, his head hung low, and his eyes were blank and lightless. Krishnamurthy spoke in a practiced beggar's whine and answered most of my questions in monosyllables. Mainly, he seemed interested in a free trip away from the sanatorium. I reiterated to him that his hand would probably need several different operations and we could make no guarantees. He shrugged and made a casual gesture, pulling the edge of one hand across his other wrist as if to say, "Cut it off if you wish. It's no use to me." We drove Krishnamurthy back to Vellore and smuggled him into a private room away from other patients.

Every muscle in Krishnamurthy's hand was paralyzed, plus a few forearm muscles. His thumb would bend quite strongly, since that muscle was supplied by the median nerve in the forearm. But the opposing motion was controlled by the length of median nerve dead below the wrist, and he could not get his thumb to stand up and face the other fingers, an essential part of grasping.

We decided to borrow a muscle in the forearm that normally helps bend the ring finger. A long tendon runs from that muscle down through the palm of the hand to the ring finger. I made an incision at the base of the ring finger, cutting the tendon free. Then I made another incision at the wrist and pulled the tendon fully out, so that it lay on the table like a long piece of sinewy string. Next I made a tunnel for this tendon under the heel of the palm, adjusted its length, and fastened it to a new site on the back of the thumb.

The surgery lasted about three hours, much of it consumed by my attempts to gauge how much tension to apply on the tendon. I used my best guess based on what I had learned from the cadaver hand, sutured the incisions, and wrapped the hand in a plaster splint.

For three weeks we waited. Krishnamurthy adapted well to his new environment. He loved the food from the hospital kitchen and the air of secrecy in the ward with the clandestine leprosy bed. All the attention made him feel very important. Meanwhile, bed rest and regular treatments were doing wonders for his foot ulcers.

I checked on him daily and found that Cochrane had judged his potential correctly. This "beggar" from Chingleput was coming alive.

Without doubt I was more nervous than Krishnamurthy himself on the day his bandages came off. He was the first leprosy patient in history to undergo such a procedure. Other physicians had groused that I was wasting my time trying to reverse progressive paralysis, and I wanted to prove them wrong. I slit through the plaster, unwrapped the gauze, and checked the sutures. The incisions had healed beautifully. *Aha, this will silence the doubters who claim that leprous flesh is "bad flesh,"* I thought to myself. Insensitive to pain, Krishnamurthy showed no signs of postoperative tenderness, and he let me move his fingers back and forth, up and down. The transplanted tendon seemed to be holding.

"You try it," I said, in the final test. He stared hard at the thumb, as if willing it to obey. It took his brain a few seconds to figure out a new pattern for thumb movement, but then it moved! Stiffly, minutely at first, but unmistakably. He grinned and the nurse beside me cheered aloud. Krishnamurthy wiggled his thumb again, basking in the spotlight.

I could only imagine what was happening inside that hand. For years he had worked to control his thumb. He had tried to pull it straight, using his other hand, but the thumb would always snap back into the clawed position before he could use it. It was a castoff, a vestigial appendage that neither moved nor felt sensation. Now, a part of his body long since given up for dead was coming back to life.

Branching Out

A few weeks later I operated again, transplanting other tendons to help liberate Krishnamurthy's index and middle fingers. (One-sixth of the muscles in the human body are devoted to hand movements, so we had plenty to choose from.) Progress came slowly, as laborious hours of physiotherapy had to follow each surgery. Ruth Thomas dipped his hands in warm paraffin wax to loosen the joints, and millimeter by millimeter coaxed each finger into a new range of movement.

Until Krishnamurthy mastered independent finger movements his claw-hand worked crudely, like a grasping hook worn by an amputee. He learned to hold a rubber ball, which he spent many hours squeezing, then a spoon, and even a pencil. After much practice, he could open and close his fingers at will, nearly forming a fist. One day he proudly called me in to demonstrate a new skill: he scooped up rice and curry from his food plate, formed it in a ball with the help of his opposing thumb, and dropped it in his mouth without spilling a single grain.

With each stride new aspects of Krishnamurthy's personality emerged. He laughed again, played practical jokes on the nursing staff, scoured the hospital library for books he had not read. The light returned to his eyes. He became a Christian and adopted the Christian name John. Before long he learned to type, and offered to translate some of our health materials into the local dialects. As I passed by his room one morning and saw him happily pecking away at a typewriter keyboard, I thought back to the bedraggled beggar boy who had once cowered like a wounded animal, his hands hanging useless at his side.

I knew the time had come for John Krishnamurthy to move on when I glanced through his window from the courtyard and caught him scratching his wounds with a stick. So that was why the sores on his feet never healed! The rascal, knowing we had depleted all our ideas on how to improve his hands surgically, had found a way to prolong his stay. Bed space was far too precious to allow long-term care, and other leprosy patients were clamoring for help, so a few weeks later we sent John packing with healed feet, passably working hands, and a fresh new identity to match his name.

After our initial success the hospital released two more isolation rooms for the use of indigent leprosy patients, and soon patients were streaming in and out of the ward. A fine young surgeon named Ernest Fritschi joined me, and together the two of us explored any technique that held out some promise for restoring damaged hands.

Ernest wondered whether we could fashion an artificial thumb for thumbless hands. We tried grafting bone from a toe and surrounding it with a tube of abdominal skin to form a thumb and to lengthen stumpy fingers, but these appendages rarely worked out. The patients proved no better at protecting their new fingers than they had been at protecting the originals. Rather mysteriously, the body appeared to absorb the transplanted bone and the thumb or finger shortened again. I had no explanation for these puzzling disappearances.

Tendon transfers showed much more potential, and through trial and error we arrived at the correct mechanical tensions. Attached too tightly, a muscle would cause a thumb to stick up like a lamp post; the patient could not retract it if he wanted. Or, if I bowstringed a tendon taut across a finger joint, the patient might be able to make a fist, but have trouble getting the one finger to unbend.

We found an improved way to correct the claw-hand, by borrowing a strong muscle tendon from the forearm high above the normal region of paralysis, a muscle that had previously served to move the wrist. Through a small incision near the wrist we pulled the tendon out, affixed a free graft from the leg, and tunneled the lengthened tendon all the way through the wrist and into the palm of the hand. Making another incision, we pulled the tendon out again, split it into four separate branches, and tunneled each branch to a different finger. The patient could then bend all four fingers simultaneously and straighten them where they had been clawed, utilizing the strength transferred from the powerful forearm muscle.

Patients sometimes requested custom treatment, which we tried to accommodate within reason. One man wanted us to adjust the angle of his flexed thumb so he could wind his watch. Another man, the owner of a rubber plantation, asked us to fix his stiff joints in an almost straight position; even though he might never be able to close his fingers into a fist, he preferred a hand that looked normal to a functional one. We enhanced the appearance of his hand by using fat grafts to plump up the hollows left by muscles that had permanently atrophied, a cosmetic improvement we soon began to offer other patients. A clarinetist requested that we spread his fingers apart to match the stops of his clarinet, then fuse the joints in place. "But you won't be able to eat rice—it will slip through your fingers," I protested. He was adamant: "I can always use a spoon. But if I cannot play my clarinet I'll have no money to buy the rice!"

Meanwhile, Ernest Fritschi turned his attention to the foot. In a survey at Chingleput he found that large numbers of patients suffered from "foot drop" due to paralysis in the muscles responsible for lifting the feet and toes. Each time one of these patients lifted a leg off the ground, the foot dropped and the heel would not go down. In time the Achilles tendon shortened, so that each step put enormous pressure on the downward-pointing toes. With the body's full weight coming down on the toes rather than on the heel designed to bear that weight, skin broke down and sores developed. Adapting what we had learned about tendon transfers in the hand, we were able to correct this problem in the foot as well, and soon Chingleput began to see a marked decrease in foot ulcers.

Those were heady days at the humble Hand Research Unit. We suffered failures, of course, as when the patient named Lakshamanan threw himself into a well and drowned after learning we could do nothing to save two of his fingers. But since we had selected a patient base with gross deformities and defects, most procedures we tried brought about a significant improvement. The patients themselves seemed honored that a medical team would lavish such care on them. Even if we improved their hands and feet only slightly, almost always they left Vellore with new enthusiasm and hope.

Reprogramming

"At the end of the mind, the body. But at the end of the body, the mind," said Paul Valéry. I saw those words acted out as if by parable as my leprosy patients struggled through the rehabilitation process. By surgically transferring tendons from one place to another, we were forcing the mind to adjust to a brand new set of realities.

Brain neurons are organized into fifty to one hundred specialized areas: one region controls lip sensation, another lip movement. Specific areas govern sensation and movement for the thumb, and the brain and thumb gradually "get to know one another" as a person matures, forming a rich association of nerve pathways. Because of its constant use, the thumb ends up with a huge area of representation in the cortex, one almost as large as the region dedicated to the hip and leg. I soon learned that when I surgically repair a damaged thumb I must take into account its specialized area within the brain as well.

Early on, I performed a tendon transfer on a patient who, like John Krishnamurthy, had a paralyzed thumb and claw-hand paralysis. I performed the same operation as I had for Krishnamurthy, moving a tendon from the ring finger over to his thumb. Evidently, I had not explained the results as carefully to him as I had to John. When we unwrapped the bandages several weeks after surgery I said to him, "Now you can bring your thumb forward." I could see him struggling, with a look of some consternation on his face, for I had promised him a movable thumb and nothing was happening. He was unable to get any movement at all out of that thumb.

"Well, try your ring finger," I said. His thumb leaped forward and he jumped backward! We laughed together, and I explained to him that he would have to retrain his brain to think *thumb* instead of *ring finger*. We had confused the brain by, in effect, rewiring the motor nerves. For days afterward when I passed his room I saw him sitting on a mat, studying his thumb, wiggling it, remapping the neural pathways in his brain.

In one respect the leprosy patients were fortunate. They could concentrate exclusively on remapping movement, since nerve damage had already blocked sensory messages of pain and touch that would further confuse the brain. Otherwise, they might find it impossible to adjust. Many hand surgeries fail because of resistance in the mind, not the injury site.

I once performed an "island flap transfer" on a sixty-year-old man whose median nerve had been damaged in a handgun accident. He had no sensation in his thumb and index finger, but his little finger and ring finger, fed by a different nerve, worked fine. The recommended surgery was to transfer two island flaps of the sensitive skin along with their nerve supply from the less important fingers over to the thumb and index finger. I did the procedure and several weeks later judged the operation a success. He now had sensation and a wide range of movement in his thumb and forefinger.

Yet after several months had passed, that tormented patient began to question whether he should have had the surgery after all. The problem lay in his mind. For sixty years his brain had stored away all messages from those two island flaps under the categories "ring finger" and "little finger." Now the actions his brain ordered did not match the sensations it received back, and the brain could not reorient itself. If the man picked up a hot poker and the brain gave an emergency order to let go, he relaxed his little finger, not his thumb. No matter how hard he tried, at his age he could not reprogram his brain to think "thumb" instead of "little finger."

The brain's isolation inside its ivory box of skull, which I had seen so graphically during the Cardiff dissection, is what makes reprogramming so difficult. The brain learns to count on electrical signals from *this* nerve to represent the thumb, and *that* one to represent the little finger. Touch is normally the most trustworthy of sensations. Vision may prove illusory and hearing may lie, but touch involves my self—it indents my skin. From the brain's perspective, it seems I am lying to myself if new sensations suddenly start streaming in from the "wrong" site. If someone mischievously rewired my house so that the switch that had always controlled the coffee maker now controlled my radio, I would learn to adapt after a few tries. But neural pathways are inside me, a part of me, and contribute fundamentally to my construct of reality.

The mind cannot easily trust signals that contradict its entire history, and a patient will never adapt unless he or she learns to overrule the sense of deception by reeducating the brain.* In a young person, I learned, it is possible to transfer a muscle to do an action opposite to what it originally did. For example, in John Krishnamurthy's case, we selected one of the two muscles used for bending the finger and reattached it so it would straighten the finger. His brain had to learn that one of the previous commands for "Bend!" still produced a bent finger while the other produced the opposite result. As people get older, such reprogramming changes in the brain become more and more difficult. Ultimately we had to stop performing radical tendon transfers for any of our leprosy patients over the age of sixty. If we tried to convert muscles to perform a completely new task, their older brains could not make the reprogramming adjustments.

I tried to encourage my leprosy patients in their reprogram-

---

*In the early days of microscope-guided surgery, hand surgeons buzzed with excitement. Now that they possessed the ability to reconnect individual tiny arteries and nerve fibers, they could reattach severed fingers and hands. Enthusiasm has moderated, though, even as the surgical procedures have been perfected. Some of my colleagues follow a policy of not transferring sensation and rarely reattaching amputated fingers or hands in elderly people. Reprogramming the mind is just too difficult.

Like a thick telephone cable, a single nerve bundles together thousands of axons that carry separate messages of heat and touch and pain. If the cable is cut, even with the aid of a microscope it is impossible to line up each individual axon in its original position. A young person can learn new pathways so that eventually the brain will automatically reinterpret sensations without a hitch. Elderly patients, however, rarely make the adjustment. They complain bitterly about odd tingling sensations and a feeling like "static" in the nerves. Their nerves are lying to them. Sometimes they may even ask that the finger or hand be reamputated.

ming efforts. "You have a kind of 'advantage,'" I said. "You can concentrate on movement. Just think how confusing it would be if you had to deal with false sensations, too." Yet I got the distinct impression that most of them would have preferred false messages to none at all. No matter how strongly I warned them in advance, they seemed disappointed to find that our surgeries did not restore sensation. Yes, they could now curl their fingers around a gummy ball of rice, but the rice felt neutral, the same as wood or grass or velvet. They gained the ability to shake hands, but could not feel the warmth and texture and firmness of the hand they were shaking. I had to teach them not to grasp someone else's hand too tightly; like the sandal-wearer in Chingleput, they could not even tell when they were hurting the other person. For them, touch had lost all meaning. And so had pain.

Shortly after I began attempting tendon transfers I received an unexpected visit from Dr. William White, a professor of plastic surgery in Pittsburgh, Pennsylvania. On tour after completing a visiting professorship in Lahore, Pakistan, he stopped by Vellore for a few days to investigate leprosy work. White kindly agreed to show me a new technique of tendon transfers. We prepared the patient, scrubbed, and set to work. I felt relieved to step aside and watch an experienced hand surgeon. The procedure took almost three hours, with White giving detailed explanations of every step.

The patient, insensitive to pain, needed little or no anesthetic and stayed alert, observing the whole process. We sutured him, White said a few encouraging words, and then held up his own hand in demonstration. "Soon you'll be able to move your fingers like this," he said, straightening his fingers. We watched dumbfounded as the patient, still reclining on the operating table, mimicked the doctor by straightening out his own fingers. Immediately his hand shrank back into the claw position. White laughed in chagrin as it dawned on him what had happened: the man, feeling no pain, had just ripped all the newly sewn tendons away from their attachments. We opened the wounds and settled in for another session to reattach the tendons.

That experience, and others like it, forced us to come up with rigorous safeguards for postoperative recovery. Normally, pain sets the limits: a person who has just undergone hand surgery will not flex his fingers, just as an appendectomy patient will not do sit-ups in bed. But our leprosy patients, without a pain reflex, had no built-in safeguards for repair and healing. We had to impose them from outside.

Most physiotherapists in hand surgery have to coax their recuperating patients to move their fingers a little more each day. Unless the patient pushes into the pain zone a little bit, the tendons and ligaments will become adherent, permanently impairing movement. In working with leprosy patients, we fought the opposite problem of preventing them from moving their fingers too much too soon. All day long I heard the words "Gently now" and "Just a little" from Ruth Thomas and the other physiotherapists. The same hand therapist treating two identical tendon transfer recipients, one due to polio and the other to leprosy, would urge one on to greater effort, and strive to hold the other one back. Several times I had to repair tendons that had been yanked out by an overeager leprosy patient.

Our therapists much preferred working with the leprosy patients, because they never complained about pain and their hands seldom stiffened from lack of movement. In recuperation from surgery, the strange quality of insensitivity to pain seemed at first like a blessing. But soon, in a terrible irony, I found painlessness to be the single most destructive aspect of this dread disease.

9
Detective Hunt

❦

If I were to choose between pain and nothing, I would choose pain.
William Faulkner

Father Damien, the Belgian priest in Hawaii, knew for certain he had leprosy when, shaving one morning, he spilled a mug of scalding water over his foot and felt no pain. That was in 1885. Leprosy workers had long recognized that the disease silenced pain signals, leaving the patient vulnerable to injury. Yet patients and health workers alike believed that leprosy caused even worse damage directly. Something about the disease made flesh rot away and die.

The more I worked with leprosy patients, however, the more I questioned the common view of how the disease accomplished its awful work. I learned early on that the scenes depicted in popular novels and movies (*Papillon*, *Ben Hur*) are based on myth: the limbs and appendages of leprosy patients do not simply drop off. Patients told me they lost their fingers and toes over a long period, and my own studies confirmed that gradual change. Even an inch-long finger stub usually retained the nail bed, which meant the outermost joint had not been severed from the rest of the finger. X rays revealed bones that had mysteriously shortened, apparently from sepsis, with the skin and other soft tissues shrinking back to the length of bone. Something was causing the body to consume its own finger from the inside.

I quizzed Bob Cochrane on this subject at Chingleput. "I've now examined hundreds of shortened fingers," I said. "Tell me, how can I know whether a finger has been hurt in an accident or whether leprosy has done the damage?" Cochrane replied that if he saw a hand with all its fingers shortened about the same length, he assumed the damage was due to leprosy infection. If one or two fingers were very short and the others normal, he judged that some accident or secondary infection had caused the injury.

That explanation satisfied me, although it seemed strange that something as unusual as the loss of a finger, a rarity in any disease, would have two different causes in leprosy. But then I started comparing finger measurements over a period of months and years. I found some of the most severe loss of digits was occurring in people who now tested negative for leprosy. In other words, tissue kept on wasting away long after the disease had been cured. With the leprosy dormant, why was normal tissue spontaneously breaking down?

No Bad Flesh

I had no solution to this riddle when I began the tendon transfer surgeries in the Hand Research Unit, and the continuing mystery dampened our enthusiasm over the early successes. We were still haunted by the predictions from other physicians that our efforts would ultimately fail. Although patients might realize some short-term benefits from the surgery, they said, eventually the fingers we had so painstakingly corrected would rot away. If these skeptics were right, I was wasting valuable staff time and cruelly raising the hopes of patients.

Even as I gained confidence from the speedy healing of our patients' surgical wounds, other signs gave me reason for concern. I heard an echo of the damning phrase "bad flesh" nearly every time I stopped by the clinic we had set up to treat foot ulcers. Typically a leprosy patient, insensitive to pain, would neglect to visit the clinic until the odor grew offensive, at which point the ulcer had already penetrated deep into the foot. We would clean out every sign of sepsis, trim away necrotic tissue, and bathe the wound in the antiseptic agent gentian violet. A week later, when the patient returned for a change of dressing, we saw no improvement. Once again we would meticulously clean and bind up the wounds and send the patient on his way—only to have him come back in another week with the ulcer in worse condition.

Sadan, the gentle young man who had slept on our veranda, exemplified this pattern. We had good success with his hands, and after a few months of surgery and recuperation he landed a job as a clerk/typist. But nothing we tried seemed to help his feet. He had come to Vellore as a last resort after several doctors had advised amputation of both legs below the knee. His feet had shortened almost by half, and an angry red ulcer persisted on the ball of each rounded, toeless foot. We experimented with ointments, magnesium sulfate, penicillin cream, and any other treatment that might help clear up the ulcers. They only seemed to get worse.

This frustrating cycle went on for months. Several times Sadan asked us to stop wasting time on his feet. "Go ahead and amputate them as the other doctors recommended," he said. I could not do it. Nor could I find a solution to his foot sores, however. It mystified me that surgical wounds on his hands healed on schedule while foot ulcers on the very same patient did not. Was "bad flesh" the explanation?

Sadan felt no pain from the foot ulcers, and he never complained. One day I changed his dressings for at least the tenth time. I could hardly bear to meet him and remove his socks. I had come to love Sadan, and I knew he loved me and clung to me as his last hope. It broke my heart that day to tell him that the other doctors were probably right. We might have to amputate, because we simply could not stop the spread of infection. Sadan received the news with sad resignation. I put my arm around him and ushered him down the hospital corridor to the door, trying to think of some word to encourage him. I had none to offer. I fully shared his sense of despair.

Instead of returning to my examining room, I stood and watched Sadan walk down the steps, cross a sidewalk, and head down the road. His head and shoulders sagged in a posture of defeat. Then for the first time I noticed something. He had no limp! I had just spent half an hour cleaning out a grossly abscessed wound on the ball of his foot, and he was putting his full weight on the exact spot we had so carefully treated. No wonder the wound never healed!

How could I have missed it before now? Gentian violet, penicillin, and every other drug stood no chance of helping Sadan as long as he, quite unintentionally and as a result of his lack of pain, kept the tissue in a continual state of trauma. At last I had found the culprit responsible for the nonhealing wound: the patient himself.

We tried to train patients with foot sores to limp, but they rarely seemed to remember. My assistant Ernest Fritschi came up with the best solution. "We use plaster casts on our hand patients and their surgical wounds heal properly," he said. "Why don't we apply the same treatment to foot ulcers?" This simple idea proved more valuable than all the other treatments put together. (Later, we read a report from Colombo, Ceylon, of a Doctor DeSilva who had used the same technique of plaster casts to heal ulcers on leprosy feet.) Encased in plaster of paris long enough, foot ulcers healed beautifully. Since we could not afford much plaster of paris, we had to swallow our misgivings and leave each cast on for a month. We learned to our surprise that a sore sheltered in a cast healed much better than a sore wrapped in dressings, even if the dressings were changed daily. Often the cast stank to high heaven when we removed it, but after wiping away dead material and pus we found healthy, shining, red tissue underneath.

Three or four months' rest inside hard plaster sufficed to heal the stubbornest ulcers. Like a medieval knight's armor, the full-limb plaster gave a hard shell of protection for tender tissue, providing an external substitute for the internal warning system of pain. Pain-sensitive patients needed no such protection, for the vanguard of pain would never let them rest their body weight on an ulcerous foot as Sadan had. Comparison studies soon revealed that our casted leprosy patients were healing as quickly as non-leprosy patients. The amputation rate among leprosy patients began to drop dramatically. Other doctors at the hospital, skeptical of our leprosy work, were astonished at these results. Where was the "bad flesh"?

I have often berated myself for not identifying the problem sooner. Medical training had attuned me to patients' complaints about pain, but nothing prepared me for the unique plight of people who do not feel pain. I had no idea how vulnerable the body becomes when it lacks a warning system. I soon noticed that we doctors and nurses who worked on insensitive patients lost our normally careful and tentative approach, almost as if the patients' lack of pain transferred itself to us. I had to learn not to use a metal probe too vigorously in exploring a patient's foot ulcer. The probe itself could cause harm, for patients who lacked the protective instinct of pain could not warn me when I went too far and damaged good tissue. (I once saw a nurse push a probe from the bottom of a patient's foot so far that it pierced through skin at the top of the foot. The patient did not flinch.)

Working with patients such as Sadan triggered the revolution in my thinking about pain. I had long recognized its value in informing of injury after the fact, but I had no real appreciation for the many loyal ways in which pain protects *in advance*. Healing ulcers proved to be a simple matter compared to preventing them in those who lacked this advance warning system.

Reluctantly, we had to insist that our patients wear shoes. Although I loved going barefoot, it became apparent that insensitive patients needed the extra barrier of protection against thorns, nails, glass, and hot sand. Even after we supplied sandals or shoes for all patients, the problems did not go away. One man walked all day with a tiny metal screw digging into his heel; he failed to notice the screw until he pulled the shoe off at night and found it imbedded in his heel. I optimistically assumed that the number of injuries would decline once the patients learned to check their shoes for such dangers. I was wrong.

It took our staff years of dead-end research—and our patients years of misery—before we fully comprehended a basic fact of human physiology: gentle stress repeatedly applied to the same spot can destroy living tissue. One clap of a hand does no damage; a thousand consecutive claps may cause pain and real damage. In walking, the mechanical force of the thousandth step is no greater than that of the first step, but by design foot tissue is vulnerable to the cumulative impact of force.* The foot's main enemy turned out to be not thorns and nails, but the normal, everyday stresses of walking.

Every healthy person knows something of this phenomenon. I buy a new pair of shoes, put them on, and start walking around the house and yard. For the first few hours they feel fine, but after a while the stiff leather begins to wear on my little toe and a rough edge grates against my heel. Instinctively I limp, shortening my stride and redistributing the stress to other parts of my foot. If I

---

*Repetitive stress only damages living tissue. If I clapped my hand against the hand of a corpse, even one who had died very recently, the dead hand would not change. After half an hour of continuously slapping a cadaver hand, my own hand would be red and swollen; after several hours my hand would probably have an open ulcer. But the cavader hand would look the same. This fact has complicated the science of physiology, because physiologists often use cadavers to test tissue strength and durability. Cadaver tissues simply do not respond to low-level repetitive stress, just as they do not heal a wound. In living tissues, the phenomenon of *inflammation* heightens the defensive response to repetitive stress even as it assists healing. Inflammation increases sensitivity to pain and thus prevents a person from clapping hands too long or walking too far in new shoes.

ignore the warning signals, a blister will pop up and I will experience acute pain. At that point, either I begin to limp more severely or, more likely, I remove the new shoes and put on some soft slippers for relief. On average it takes me about a week to break in new shoes, a process that involves adaptations in both the leather of the shoe and the leather of my foot. The shoe gets softer and more compliant to my foot's shape, while my foot grows extra layers of callus for protection at the stress points.

This entire process is foreign to a leprosy patient. Because he feels no pain from his little toe and heel, his stride never adjusts. After a blister rises, he still keeps walking, oblivious. The blister bursts, and an ulcer begins to form. Even so, he puts the shoes back on the next day, and the next, each time damaging more tissue. Infection may set in. If it goes untreated, that hot infection may spread into the bone, where it will not heal unless it gets complete rest. Studying a succession of X rays, we learned how pernicious a deep infection can be: tiny pieces of bone fragment break off and are extruded with the discharge from the wounds until eventually the infection leads to the loss of toes or even the entire foot. All this time, the leprosy patient may continue to walk on the injury site, showing not the slightest sign of a limp.

We had solved the mystery of missing toes—they are destroyed, little by little, because of infection—but how could we break the cycle? To combat the problem of repetitive stress on insensitive feet, we had to become shoe experts. Starting from total ignorance, I tested hundreds of models, trying them out on a regular walking route from the hospital to the railway station. We needed a soft material that would adapt to the shape of a patient's foot and spread out stress over a large area, combined with a firm sole that would keep a patient's foot from bending. We tried plaster casts, finely sanded wooden clogs, and plastic shoes formed from wax molds. I traveled to Calcutta to learn how to mix polyvinyl chloride and to England to test spray-on plastics. Finally we came up with the right combination: a microcellular rubber platform, a firm "rocker" bar to guide the walking motion, and a custom-fitted leather insole. Sadan was one of the first patients to get new shoes custom-shaped to his stubby feet.

Support for this project came from many sources, including the Madras Rubber Company and Bata Shoes. In time we built our own microcellular rubber factory and employed half a dozen apprentice shoemakers in a workshop near Vellore. We persevered because we knew we could benefit far more leprosy patients by training a few good shoemakers to help prevent deformities than by teaching scores of orthopedic surgeons to correct them.

Hand Signals

We were still working on the problem of foot ulcers when a potentially devastating problem surfaced among our first hand surgery patients. Some returned to the clinic with the dismaying news that their newly mobile fingers were shortening. Embarrassed, for they knew how much time and effort we had devoted to the Hand Research Unit, they admitted that their fingers were developing sores and ulcers at a faster rate now than before the surgery.

My heart sank as I examined their newly injured hands. "Don't waste your energy on leprosy, Paul," colleagues had warned me. Perhaps they were right. We had made much progress in surgical technique, but what good was a liberated hand if the patient ended up destroying it anyway? We dressed the wounds and wrapped them in plaster of paris. Months later the same patients returned with new signs of tissue damage.

The pattern baffled me for months, and threatened to derail our entire leprosy program. Before proceeding any further, we had to find the cause of hand injuries, just as we had with foot injuries. I decided to spend much more time with rehabilitated surgical patients in order to observe their normal routine. Many of the teenage boys were now living in a makeshift village of mud huts and thatch roofs near Vellore. We asked these boys, about twenty-five in number, to help us unravel the mystery of spontaneous wounds.

First I made a baseline survey, tracing outlines of the boys' hands on a piece of paper and noting every scar or sign of finger damage. For weeks, even months, I visited them nearly every day, examining and measuring their hands, watching them at work, studying every tiny abnormality. It did not take long to discover why boys who had managed to stay free of injuries before surgery sometimes got into more trouble afterward. With new mobility and strength in their hands, they were more likely to work harder and thus take more risks.

Some culprits I spotted right away. One young man was working as a carpenter. He had left our clinic in high spirits several months before, proud that his once-paralyzed fingers could again curl around the handle of a hammer, thrilled to resume an occupation he had thought lost to him forever. I, too, was excited that he had found a source of income. But neither he nor I had foreseen the hazards of carpentry without pain.

When a large blister appeared on his hand, I easily matched it to a splinter on the hammer handle: he had pounded all day with a wood splinter sticking in the flesh of his palm. I fashioned a thicker, padded handle for his hammer, solving the splinter problem. Then I noticed his fingertips beginning to show signs of abuse, so I taught him to hold the nails with a pair of pliers. I had to reach back in time to my days in construction to design casings that would protect his hands from the plane, saw, and other potentially dangerous tools. Ever since medical school I had wondered if I had misspent those five years in the construction field. Now I was thankful to find a redeeming purpose to my circuitous career path.

Each occupation had its own hazards. One young farmer used a hoe all day, not noticing a nail that stuck out from its handle into his palm. Another boy damaged his hand on a spade with a cracked handle that had been wrapped in baling wire. A barber lost his ring finger and nearly his middle finger through the repeated pressure from working a pair of scissors. A few simple design changes made these handles safer as well.

One of our most careful patients, a boy named Namo, experienced his first major setback when he volunteered to hold a floodlight for an American visitor who dropped by to shoot film footage of our work. Insensitive to heat, Namo didn't notice when the handle began to get hot (insulation around it had broken off). As soon as he set the light down, though, he saw shiny pink blisters already forming on his hands. He dashed out of the room and I followed him. Without thinking I asked, "Namo, does it hurt?"

I will never forget Namo's poignant reply. "You know it doesn't hurt me!" he cried. "I'm suffering in my mind because I can't suffer in my body."

All this time as I was tracking injuries, a suspicion was growing in my mind. One day I shared my idea with the patients. "We've seen that the people who talk about the 'bad flesh' of leprosy are wrong. Your flesh is as good as mine. The problem is that you don't feel pain and so it's easy for you to injure yourselves. You've already been very helpful in identifying the cause of many hand injuries. I have a theory I'll need your help to test. What if we assume that *all* wounds occur because of accidents—not because of leprosy itself?"

I asked the patients to join me in a detective hunt: together we would track down the cause of every single injury. We would meet as a group weekly, and each boy would have to accept responsibility for his injuries. Never could anyone say about a wound, "It just came by itself," or "That's what leprosy does." If I detected a new blister on the back of a knuckle or a spot of inflammation on the thumb, I wanted some explanation, no matter how far-fetched it sounded.

Some of the boys hid their wounds at first. Years of rejection had conditioned them to conceal injuries, and they found it shameful to acknowledge their wounds so openly. In contrast, a few (the "naughty boys," as we called them) seemed to take morbid delight in their painlessness. These rapscallions liked to shock people. One boy pushed a thorn through the palm of the hand until it poked through the other side like a sewing needle. Sometimes I felt like a schoolmaster, with the odd sense that I was introducing the boys to their own limbs, begging their minds to welcome the insensitive parts of their bodies.

It was easy to think of the boys as being careless or irresponsible until I began to understand their point of view. Pain, along with its cousin touch, is distributed universally on the body, providing a sort of boundary of *self*. Loss of sensation destroys that boundary, and now my leprosy patients no longer felt their hands and feet as part of self. Even after surgery, they tended to view their repaired hands and feet as tools or artificial appendages. They lacked the basic instinct of self-protection that pain normally provides. One of the boys said to me, "My hands and feet don't feel part of me. They are like tools I can use. But they aren't really me. I can see them, but in my mind they are dead." I heard similar comments often, underscoring the crucial role pain plays in unifying the human body.

As weeks went by, the message finally sank in and the group joined together in the detective hunt. Whenever we spotted a wound we examined it carefully in search of a cause, then applied a splint to keep the finger or hand out of action until it had healed. We uncovered both everyday and exotic causes of spontaneous wounds, feeling especially proud when we managed to solve a difficult case. For example, some of the boys had developed ugly sores between their fingers. We discovered that soap suds tend to get trapped in the crevices between partially paralyzed fingers and toes; the skin softens, macerates, and eventually cracks open.

Once we had ferreted out the origin of an injury, we could usually prevent it from recurring. It took us weeks to decipher blisters that sometimes appeared on the knuckles of patients during the night. One boy seemed especially susceptible. At night we examined him and found healthy, unmarked hands; by the next morning, a tiny row of blisters had mysteriously appeared. How could injuries occur during sleep? Were they pressure sores? We quizzed him on his sleeping positions, and searched his room for any knobs or sharp objects.

Finally, his keen-eyed roommates identified the problem. The boy with the blisters liked to read at night in bed. Just before retiring he would reach over and turn off the hurricane lamp by twisting a metal knob to withdraw the wick. As he did so, the back of his hand, insensitive to both heat and pain, rubbed against the glass globe, searing the flesh in a regular pattern along three fingers. We fitted large, long knobs on all hurricane lamps, and late-night readers no longer had to worry about blisters.

The patients learned to account for 90 percent of spontaneous wounds. By far the most mystifying injuries involved the sudden disappearance of almost a whole segment of a finger or toe. Every once in a while a leprosy patient would show up at our daily meetings and sheepishly display a raw, bleeding patch, with the flesh around an inch-length section of a finger or big toe missing and bare bone exposed. This oddity defied everything we had learned and, until we solved the mystery, it put our entire theory in jeopardy. I dared not tell other hospital personnel about the problem, for it seemed to confirm the worst myths about leprous fingers and toes simply "falling off."

Almost always, the afflicted person noticed the missing digit in the morning. Something ominous was taking place during the night. A patient solved the mystery by sitting up all night in an observation post from which he watched a scene straight out of a horror movie. In the middle of the night a rat climbed onto the bed of a fellow patient, sniffed around tentatively, nuzzled a finger, and, meeting no resistance, began to gnaw on it. The lookout yelled, waking the whole room and scaring away the rat. At last we had the answer: the boys' fingers and toes had not dropped off— they were being eaten!

This most repugnant cause of spontaneous wounds had an

easy remedy. First we set traps for the rodents and built barriers around the beds of our patients. When trouble continued, we settled on a more effective solution: we went into the cat breeding business, using the blood line of a proven Siamese male who was an excellent ratter. From then on, no leprosy patient could leave the rehabilitation center without a feline companion. The problem of missing pieces of fingers vanished almost overnight.

Never Free

I began leprosy work with a singular desire to repair damaged hands. Along the way I met with an even greater challenge: quite simply, to keep my leprosy patients from destroying themselves. New dangers sprang up, Hydra-like, to replace those we eliminated. We made lists of rules for the patients. Never walk barefoot. Inspect your hands and feet every day. Don't smoke (we frequently had to treat "the kissing wound," named for the adjacent burn marks a cigarette leaves if held too long between insensitive fingers). Wrap hot objects with a cloth. When in doubt, wear gloves. Use coconut oil to soften skin and prevent cracks. Don't eat in bed (so as not to attract rats and ants). On a bus or truck, don't sit near the hot engine or rest your feet on a metal floor. Always use a mug modified with a wooden handle.

In time we turned the tide of battle, and the incidence of spontaneous wounds plummeted. Indeed, my most careful patients were now keeping their hands and feet free of any serious damage. Even the most reluctant patients, those who had joined the group solely as a favor to me, caught the vision I had hoped for. More than promoting a cold, scientific theory, our little group at Vellore was fighting a crusade: to help overturn ancient prejudice against leprosy. Sulfone drugs could now arrest the disease; perhaps proper care could prevent the deformities that made it so terrible.

As we worked with the patients each day, we were most pleased to see that gradually, inexorably, the all-important sense of "self" began to extend to parts of their bodies they could no longer feel. They were indeed taking a kind of moral responsibility for their insensitive limbs, an attitude in welcome contrast to their earlier apathy. With that sense of self came hope and with hope came, sometimes, despair. The story of proud Raman comes to mind.

A wiry teenager of Anglo-Indian descent, Raman was one of our most diligent sleuths. Like many Anglo-Indians, he had a healthy dose of self-confidence, and he took great pride in his unmarked hands. We never had to encourage Raman's cooperation in our project—he delighted in informing on other patients who might be trying to conceal a wound.

One weekend Raman asked permission to visit Madras to spend a holiday with his family. "I want to go back to where I was rejected," he told me. Before, when his fingers had been drawn into a claw shape, people had treated him as an outcast. Now, with limber hands, he wanted to try out his new identity in the great city of Madras. We reviewed all the dangers he might encounter, and Raman excitedly boarded the train for Madras.

He returned two days later a pathetic, forlorn figure, a different Raman than I had ever seen. Thick gauze bandages covered both hands. His shoulders slumped, and he could hardly speak to me without crying. "Oh, Dr. Brand, look at my hands, look at my hands," he moaned. Some time passed before he could tell me the whole story.

His first night home, Raman had celebrated in a joyous reunion with his family. He told them he was now certified negative, and after a few more surgeries on his hands he could begin searching for a job. At last he felt fully accepted by his family. Happier than he had been in years, he retired to his old room, vacant for years, and fell asleep on the woven pallet on the floor.

The next morning Raman inspected his hands first thing, as we had trained him. To his horror he found a bloody wound on the back of his left index finger. The finger I had worked on now had no skin on the back side. Raman knew the telltale signs: drops of blood and marks in the dust confirmed that a rat had visited him during the night. He had not thought to take his cat along for a weekend visit.

All that day Raman agonized. Should he return to Vellore early? He shopped for a rat trap, but shops were closed for the holiday. He decided to spend one more night, this time with a stick at his side. He would force himself to stay awake to get revenge against that rat.

Sunday night Raman sat cross-legged on his pallet, his back against the wall, reading a book. He managed to keep his eyes open until four o'clock in the morning, when they grew heavy and he could no longer fight off sleep. Still in the sitting position, he dozed. The book fell forward onto his knees and his hand slid over to one side against the hot hurricane lantern.

And that explained Raman's other bandaged hand. When he awoke the next morning he saw that a large patch of skin had burned off the back of his right hand. He stared in disbelief and despair at his two hands. He who had admonished others about the dangers of leprosy had now failed to protect himself.

I tried my best to comfort Raman. This was no time for scolding. After months of soaring expectations in Vellore, one weekend trip to Madras had shattered his confidence. "I feel as if I've lost all my freedom," he told me when he could finally talk about the incident. And then, in tears, he asked a question that has stayed with me: "Dr. Brand, how can I ever be free without pain?"

Spreading the Word

For most people, preventing avoidable injuries takes no conscious thought. The pain reflex will jerk a hand away from a hot object, order a limp if shoes fit too tightly, and startle a sleeper awake if a rat even nuzzles a hand. Deprived of that reflex, leprosy patients must anticipate consciously what might harm them. Yet the conscious mind can do wonders to compensate for the loss of reflex. Our constant harping on the dangers finally had its effect: at the end of one year, we determined that not one finger had shortened among the boys in our experiment.

I had asked our patients to assume, just for the sake of our "detective hunt," the radical theory that all damage to hands and feet was related to their insensitivity to pain. They had become so skilled at tracking the causes of injury that I was now ready to go public with the theory that painlessness was the only real enemy. Leprosy merely silenced pain, and further damage came about as a side effect of painlessness. In other words, all subsequent damage was preventable.

I knew such a notion flew in the face of hundreds of years of tradition, and the medical community would likely greet a new theory with skepticism. But my patients—the carpenter, the boys with foot ulcers, Namo, Raman—had convinced me that painlessness, not leprosy, was the villain. We could now identify the underlying cause of virtually all injuries at Vellore, and all were secondary effects. We had removed forever the excuse patients used to give all the time, "The wound happened all by itself. It's just part of leprosy."

If we were right, the standard approach to leprosy treatment addressed only half the problem. Arresting the disease through sulfone drug treatments was not nearly enough; health workers also needed to alert leprosy patients to the hazards of a life without pain. We now understood why even a "burnt-out case" with no active bacilli continued to suffer disfigurement. Even after leprosy had been "cured," without proper training patients would continue to lose fingers and toes and other tissue, because that loss resulted from painlessness. I began to sense the time had come to carry that message to other leprosy centers.

I drove to a nearby leprosy mission hospital, Vadathorasalur, with some apprehension, for this would be my first attempt to persuade others to adopt the new approach to wound prevention. The director, a solidly built Danish nurse named Miss Lillelund, took pride in her hospital's Scandinavian standards of hygiene and efficiency, and she ruled patients and staff with absolute dictatorial powers. Her hospital specialized in the care of children with leprosy, and behind Nurse Lillelund's stern mask, I knew, there lay a deep love and concern for her children. I knew that if I could convince Nurse Lillelund of a new approach, the entire leprosarium would soon fall into step behind her.

Our surgical team visited Vadathorasalur every six weeks, and each time we followed a prescribed regimen. First came the welcoming ceremony: Nurse Lillelund had trained her patients to assemble in the courtyard in formation. Then we retired to the director's quarters for morning tea. For such occasions, she appointed one of the schoolboy patients to be the *punkah wallah*, or turner of the fan. The punkah fan consisted of a large woven mat attached to a block of wood that hung from the ceiling on two chains. The punkah wallah had the honorable and monotonous task of pulling cords and pulleys in such a way as to keep the woven mat moving back and forth at a steady pace, stirring up air in the room. As we sat talking to Nurse Lillelund over tea, the mat would move more and more slowly until suddenly she would call out, "Punkah wallah!" We started in our seats, the fan abruptly speeded up, and the conversation continued.

It was at one of these morning teas that I first presented our findings about leprosy to Nurse Lillelund. I described in detail the tests we had performed at Vellore and gave our preliminary conclusion that all tissue damage in leprosy patients could be prevented. "Their worst problem is that they lack pain," I said. "Our job is to teach them how to live without it."

Nurse Lillelund listened with interest, but I could see warning signs in her furrowed brow and the cloud forming behind her eyes. "Why don't we go into the cottages and wards and visit some of the patients," I suggested. She agreed, and as we strolled the immaculate corridors I noticed suspicious marks on hands and feet right away. I pointed to one ulcer on a boy's palm. "There's the kind of injury I've been talking about. You know, all the paths here are bordered with a thorny succulent bush. I wonder if that ulcer started to form when he climbed over a bush and grabbed a thorn without knowing it."

"No!" Nurse Lillelund said. Then she exploded: "No! No! My boys here never do that! Besides, if they get the slightest wound they report immediately to my clinic. These are leprosy *infections* we're looking at. They are not injuries." Now I sensed the real issue: Nurse Lillelund viewed as a personal affront any suggestion that her patients were somehow negligent in protecting themselves.

Fortunately, Nurse Lillelund also had a Nordic commitment to the scientific method. She agreed to let me survey her patients for significant hand injuries. Soon all were assembled in formation, standing at attention with their hands extended. I went up and down the rows, noting any problems. I counted 127 patients who showed signs of broken or inflamed skin. I suggested possible reasons as I examined them: splinters from rough wood, burns from a metal coffee cup or cooking pan.

At first Nurse Lillelund, at my side, tried to defend her patients. "Oh, that's nothing," she said about a small ulcer on the web of a boy's thumb. I remarked that small ulcers tend to develop into large ones, and told her of some patients who had lost their thumbs as a result of infections in that same spot. In a flash she turned on the child, "Why didn't you report this to me, young man?"

About halfway through the round, Nurse Lillelund became totally deflated. She no longer tried to defend her methods. The sight of so many hand injuries had convinced her of the importance of prevention, and she pronounced herself mortified, angry, and ashamed. "Believe me, I *will* restore order!" she vowed, and not for a moment did I doubt her. After we finished the survey she assembled all the patients and asked me to give a lecture on preventing injuries. I talked for half an hour, allowing Nurse Lillelund enough time to regain her composure and come up with a plan.

The leprosy patients stood respectfully in the courtyard as I spoke, evidently well accustomed to a lecture format. Most of them wore impassive expressions, and I wondered how many were grasping my message. I needn't have worried. Nurse Lillelund followed my lecture with a speech of her own.

"The reputation of our institution is at stake," she declared. "We should be ashamed! You boys are injuring yourselves, and you are not reporting it. From now on, I will hold a thorough personal inspection every three days. Anyone found to have a wound that has not been reported in advance will get no more home food rations. All meals must be taken in the canteen." A groan went through the crowd. Nurse Lillelund had seized on the single most effective deterrent. Everyone hated the bland cafeteria food and cherished the privilege of cooking private meals, Indian style, on charcoal stoves in the living quarters.

I left Vadathorasalur with mixed feelings, unsure whether we had accomplished our goal of communicating a spirit of hope and encouragement to the patients at Nurse Lillelund's hospital. But six weeks later, I saw undeniable results. We held another hand inspection and this time I found not 127 but 6 wounds, all of which were properly dressed in bandages or plaster. Nurse Lillelund beamed, and with good reason. I was overwhelmed by the results of her campaign. With a few more Nurse Lillelunds, we could change the course of leprosy.

10
Changing Faces

—◆◆◆◆—

. . . we are not ourselves
When nature, being oppressed, commands the mind
To suffer with the body.
Shakespeare, *King Lear*

In 1951 Vellore became the first general hospital to build an entire ward for the treatment of leprosy patients. When word got out that a hospital in Vellore could make a claw-hand work again, the grounds filled with patients, many of them desperately poor beggars who camped out in the courtyard and set up begging posts at the hospital gate. Even the new ward couldn't possibly accommodate all these people, and once again our emphasis on leprosy drew criticism from some of the staff.

This time we were helped by a powerful Indian politician, a champion of the independence movement who had worked with Mahatma Gandhi. Dr. T. N. Jagadisan initially came to Vellore as a leprosy patient, easily the most illustrious patient we had yet treated. He went home boasting about his "Brand new hands," and nominated me for the committee that managed the trust fund established after Gandhi's death. Gandhi had always shown great compassion for the Untouchable caste—he renamed them *Harijan*, or "children of God"—and for victims of leprosy, many of whom came from that caste. Breaking taboos, he had personally nursed a leprosy patient near his ashram. It was a fitting tribute, then, that some of the memorial contributions would go to the Gandhi Memorial Leprosy Foundation, headed by the Mahatma's son, Devadas Gandhi.

I was the only foreigner on the committee. We held our meetings in the hut where Gandhi had spent his last years, sitting yoga style on the floor in a circle around the great man's simple pallet. The others, all Gandhi disciples who had become leading politicians, wore rough cotton *dhotis* and, carrying on the Mahatma's practice, they would use a brass spinner to twist small wads of raw cotton into thread as we conducted our business.

When they heard of our needs, the Gandhi Foundation helped purchase a large house near the Vellore hospital to serve as a hostel for leprosy patients, alleviating the problem of beggars on the hospital grounds. At first neighbors, who did not relish living next to leprosy patients, threw rocks through windows and defecated on the threshold. In time, though, the neighborhood adjusted and our recuperating and prospective patients moved into "No. 10."

New Life

After we learned how to heal old wounds and prevent most new ones, I had hoped that our leprosy work would settle into a manageable routine of hand surgery and rehabilitation. But a new, unexpected crisis arose when some of our best patients began returning to Vellore, despondent. John Krishnamurthy, the very first surgical volunteer, was typical. When he showed up for an unscheduled visit several months after his corrective surgery, I greeted him warmly—and got a rather stiff response. "John, is something wrong?" I asked. "You certainly look well."

"Dr. Brand, these are not good hands," he announced, as if he had rehearsed the line for a speech. I waited, but he said nothing more.

"What can you mean, John?" I asked at last. "They look fine. You've obviously been doing the rehab exercises, and now you can move all ten fingers. You've taken care to avoid further injuries. We've both worked many months on those hands, John. I think they're beautiful."

"Yes, yes, but they're bad *begging* hands," John said. He explained that charitable Indians gave readily to beggars with the characteristic "leper's claw." By freeing his fingers from that claw position, we had spoiled his main source of income. "People don't give as generously now. And still no one will give me a job or even rent me a room." Though we had killed the active bacteria and repaired his hands, scars on his face gave him away as someone who had had leprosy.

My stomach twisted in a knot as John told me of the rejection he had encountered in the outside world. When he tried to board a public bus, sometimes the driver would physically throw him off. He, an educated man, was now unemployed and homeless, sleeping in an open plaza. He barely earned enough money from his begging to buy food. What had I done, repaired his body just enough to ruin his chance for a livelihood?

We found a clerical position in the hospital for John, but I knew that offered only a short-term solution for a single patient. What of all the other tendon transfer patients—had we ruined their lives as well? I checked and found that many had stories like John's. Clearly, our efforts to repair their hands and feet had not adequately equipped them for life beyond the hospital walls.

It became obvious that we needed a halfway house, a kind of decompression chamber to prepare patients for life on the outside. Thus the New Life Center was born. We selected a site on the shady grounds of the medical college campus four miles outside town. If we meant for patients to return to their villages, it made no sense to construct dwellings more elaborate than they would find at home and so, using a five-hundred-dollar bequest from a retiring missionary, we built five simple brick-and-mud huts, each divided into four rooms. We painted them white and covered them with palm-thatch roofs. The peaceful setting, tucked between wooded, rocky hills, made a great contrast to the bustle of downtown Vellore.

Thirty patients moved into the New Life Center in 1951. All were male, since leprosy affected so many more men than women and at that time mixing sexes would have been culturally unacceptable. We planted a large vegetable garden, raised chickens, and opened a weaving shop. I set up a carpentry workshop for the manufacture of wooden toys, and taught those who had lost fingers how to work a treadle jigsaw. Soon we were producing a line of toy animals, trains, cars, picture frames, and jigsaw puzzles for sale in the community. (Although these toys were better than anything available in the area, they did not sell well until we took the quite unnecessary precaution of storing the toys in formaldehyde vapor to "sterilize" them.)

One rundown building already existed on the site of the New Life Center, which I claimed for an operating facility. Eight feet square, with sun-dried brick walls and a tile roof, it bore little resemblance to the gleaming white room we had been using at the hospital in Vellore. It had no sink, so we had to scrub before entering the room. We added mosquito screens, beat a sheet of aluminum into the shape of a parabola to reflect shadowless light from a one-hundred-watt bulb, and modified a wooden kitchen table with arm supports and headrests for the surgeries. We purchased a pressure cooker and installed it over a kerosene Primus stove for use as our sterilizer (this worked fine until one day the cooker cranked up too much pressure and exploded, blowing a neat lid-size hole in the tile roof).

More and more of my time was spent in this tiny room. It was here that Ernest Fritschi and I settled on the best surgical procedures to correct claw-hand and drop-foot deformities, and here too that we began to comprehend fully the challenge first posed to us by John Krishnamurthy. In order to equip leprosy patients for life on the "outside," we would have to change our approach radically. We must lift our sights from the narrow field of surgery on hands and feet and bring the whole person into view.

Eyebrows

A young man named Kumar came to the center one day presenting a certificate that declared his leprosy inactive. I examined him quickly. We had worked on his hands, which now showed no sign of clawing or accidental injury, and his feet no sign of nerve paralysis.

Kumar's body had always given evidence of some natural resistance to the disease. Leprosy bacilli had followed the typical pattern of first infiltrating the cooler areas of his face (forehead, nostrils, and ears) and had even hid in the hair follicles of his eyebrows. For a time this had made his skin shiny and swollen. But the body's defenses, assisted by aggressive sulfone treatment, had killed off all the bacteria, and by now Kumar's facial skin had nearly returned to normal. Wrinkles creasing across the areas of former swelling made him appear slightly older than his twenty-five years.

I could spot only one visual reminder of the disease, naked patches where his eyebrows once grew, and these hardly seemed worth noting. It heartened me to see someone who had fought the disease so successfully, and I congratulated Kumar on taking care of himself. "Why have you come?" I asked, after completing my examination. "As you know, we specialize in surgery of the hands and feet, and yours seem fine." Kumar pointed to his eyebrows, or rather the places on his face where eyebrows used to grow, and told me his story.

Before contracting leprosy Kumar had tended a stall in the marketplace of his village. He sold packets of betel nut and tobacco that he hand-wrapped with a touch of slaked lime. Village people loved to chew this mixture, called *pan*, and a stop at Kumar's booth became routine for many shoppers. He exchanged jokes and news with them, busily wrapping more packets of betel in leaves as he talked.

Village people are often shrewder than doctors at detecting the early signs of leprosy, and when Kumar's skin began to show an unnatural sheen, customers spread the news and trade dropped off. Before long nobody bought his goods and few would stop to talk. Kumar, too proud to become a beggar, closed down his stall and headed for a nearby leprosarium.

When he returned to the village several years later, negative health certificate in hand, he assumed he could resume his trade. All signs of the disease had vanished except the naked eyebrows. For superstitious village folk, though, this feature alone gave enough reason to ostracize him. Showing a certificate did not matter. He had to look free of the disease. He had to grow eyebrows.

"No one will buy from a man without eyebrows," Kumar reported to me sadly. "Please, Doctor, can you make me some eyebrows? I can't stand having customers peer at me and look for hairs to see if I'm really clean."

I listened to Kumar with mixed emotions. Although his story moved me, I certainly had no desire to get into cosmetic surgery. We had a waiting list of candidates for corrective surgery, many of them with paralyzed hands that could be set free. A request for new eyebrows seemed almost trivial. And yet I remembered the lesson I had learned from John Krishnamurthy. Unless we could find a way to restore patients to a useful life in their villages, we would create a permanent class of dependents. If facial appearance created a barrier to acceptance, we had to find a way to knock it down.

Kumar stayed at the New Life Center a few days while I researched plastic surgery techniques that might help him. The Japanese had developed hair transplantation procedures in which they transplanted individual hairs, follicle by follicle, like young plants in a rice paddy. Another, less time-consuming procedure involved transferring eyebrow-shaped pieces of scalp to a new location. If we succeeded in preserving the blood supply, the transplant would guarantee Kumar bushy eyebrows—as bushy as the thick black hair on his head. I explained the process, and he enthusiastically consented.

The trick was to find a piece of scalp connected to blood vessels long enough to reach down to the eyebrow site. Before the surgery I clipped Kumar's hair very short and made him go for a run. Fifteen minutes later, when he climbed the stairs to my office, his heart was pounding and I could see arteries throbbing under his scalp. Using a marker, I traced the outline of his temporal artery, selected some long branches, and drew in two bold, wide eyebrow shapes, one on each side of his shaved head.

The next day Kumar lay on the wooden operating table. I cut out the eyebrow shapes I had marked and lifted them free of the skull. Still attached to an artery and vein, they hung down like two mice dangling by their tails. Next I removed the skin where his old eyebrows had been and made tunnels under the skin from each eyebrow up toward the opening in the scalp. Using long forceps I reached through the tunnel, grasped the dangling sections of scalp, and carefully pulled them across to their new sites crowning Kumar's eyes. Transplanted, the scalp sections looked so large that I was tempted to trim them a bit, but I feared cutting into the curving arteries that would keep the new eyebrows alive.

I need not have worried about their size. From the instant his dressings were removed, Kumar was delighted with his new eyebrows. As the hair began to grow, and kept on growing, his delight increased. When I explained that he would have to clip his new eyebrows or otherwise they would grow as long as scalp hair, Kumar insisted he wanted them long. Before he left Vellore, bushy eyebrows hung down over his eyes.

Eventually, of course, Kumar did trim his eyebrows. But in his home village their very luxuriance created a sensation. Former customers lined up to have a look at Kumar's eyebrows, and this time when he showed them his certificate of cure from leprosy, they believed him.

Noses

Our experience with Kumar's eyebrows opened up a whole new arena for corrective surgery: the face. Next we were confronted with noses. Bald eyebrow patches were a minor problem compared to the "saddleback noses" that disfigured many patients.

Because leprosy bacilli prefer cool areas, the nose becomes a major battleground. The body's response to the invaders causes inflammation, which, if it persists, may block the airways. In time the mucous lining ulcerates from secondary infections, and the nose may shrink away to almost nothing. The elevated ridge of cartilage disappears, leaving a collapsed patch of skin and two flared nostrils that open directly outward. It is rather disconcerting, to say the least, to look at the face of a person who has leprosy and see into the nasal cavities.

Everyone in India recognized the collapsed nose as a sign of leprosy—some believed that noses "rotted off" like toes and fingers—and any person so afflicted faced a life of stigma and ostracism. A woman with such a nose stood no chance of marriage, even if she was certified negative and bore no other marks of the disease.

As more of these patients with facial deformities came to our clinic, I felt grateful that I had had some exposure to plastic surgery during war days in London. One of the pioneers in the field, Sir Archibald McIndoe, had gained national acclaim in World War II for his heroic efforts to reconstruct the burned faces of Royal Air Force pilots, and I did some follow-up study on some of these downed airmen.

In those days before microvascular surgery, skin grafts from the abdomen and chest had to be transferred in two stages, with the arm serving as a temporary host. A plastic surgeon would slice away a swath of skin on, say, the belly, leaving one end attached to the old blood supply and connecting the other end to the arm at the wrist. The arm was strapped to the abdomen for three weeks, allowing time for a new blood supply to grow between the graft and arm, at which point the surgeon cut the flap of skin free of the abdomen and moved it up to the new site on forehead, cheek, or nose, again strapping the arm in place. Eventually a blood supply would develop on the facial graft site and the skin could be cut free of the arm. To a young medical student, the scene in Archie's wards was at once bizarre and thrilling: arms seeming to grow out of heads, a long tube of skin extending from a nasal cavity like an elephant trunk, temporary eyelids formed of skin flaps too thick to open.

Our clinic followed Archie's method for a while, using two-stage grafts to construct noses for leprosy patients. In many ways abdominal skin was inherently unsuitable for rhinoplasty: thick and unwieldy, it offered little visual improvement over the saddleback nose. Yet although these first crude attempts may not have produced beautiful noses, at least the new ones did not look like leprosy deformities, so the patients went away satisfied.

Then I learned about a new technique which had much in common with my eyebrow transplants. We lifted the whole of the forehead skin as a single flap, keeping the blood supply intact, and swung it down to form a new nose, attaching it to the cut edges where the old nose had been. (We used split skin grafts from the thigh to fill in the raw area left on the forehead.)* Patients seemed even more pleased with the new noses that resulted, but those of us on the surgery team did not share their enthusiasm. We left a permanent scar on the forehead, and the bulky edges of the new nose did not merge perfectly with the fine skin of the cheek. It sometimes looked as if someone had pressed a clay nose onto a face.

Another British plastic surgeon, Sir Harold Gillies, taught us a much better way. He had come to Bombay near retirement age

---

*I learned this method from Jack Penn, a renowned plastic surgeon in South Africa, who had adapted a procedure first performed by the ancient Hindu surgeon Susruta eleven centuries before Christ. Hindu warriors sometimes punished their vanquished enemies by cutting off their noses with a saber, and Susruta devised a remarkably advanced technique of transplanting a section of skin from the forehead down to the nose area.

An odd event in 1992 revealed just how common this ancient form of vengeance used to be. To right a historical wrong, Japan agreed to return twenty thousand noses that its army had amputated from Korean soldiers and civilians during a military invasion in 1597. The noses, along with some heads of Korean generals, had been preserved in a special memorial for nearly four hundred years.

I actually treated an Indian landlord whose tenants had risen against him and administered this ancient punishment cutting off his nose and upper lip with a saber. A rather inexperienced surgeon had tried to use Susruta's method of moving a flap of forehead skin down to form a new nose and upper lip for the man. In order to get a long enough flap of skin, he included a patch of the hair-growing scalp beyond the forehead, folding the skin double to form the underside of the lip. (Having shaved the scalp first, he may not have realized that he had included this hair-growing scalp.) Now, a year later, the patient came to us in agony. Bristly scalp hair was growing inside his mouth, scraping across his swollen, bleeding gums every time he spoke or ate. That hairy skin had to be replaced with mucous membrane grafts from the underside of his cheeks, a procedure which made the former landlord much happier.

at the invitation of Dr. N. H. Antia, a local plastic surgeon who had studied in England. Encountering leprosy patients in Bombay, Gillies remembered a technique he had tried on leprosy patients many years before, on a trip to Argentina. Gillies was probably the first surgeon ever to operate on a leprosy nose, and at Dr. Antia's suggestion the two of them journeyed to Vellore to teach us the technique.

In Argentina, Gillies had observed that leprosy embeds itself in the mucous lining of the nose, damaging that inside lining much more severely than it damages the skin. The resulting inflammation destroys cartilage, and without cartilage to support it the expanse of skin collapses like a tent without poles. "Why bother to transplant skin when you have perfectly good skin sitting there unused?" Gillies asked. "The mucous lining has been destroyed, but you can always replace it with grafts once you reshape the nose out of its original skin."

We prepped a patient for surgery. Looking at his shrunken nose, I found it hard to imagine that anything worthwhile could be salvaged from that shriveled patch of skin. Gillies picked up a scalpel and demonstrated. Peeling back the upper lip, he cut inside the mouth between teeth and gum and lip until he could lift the lip high enough to expose the nasal cavity. He freed the whole upper lip and then the nose from its attachment to facial bones. "Now watch," he said. He took a roll of gauze and stuffed it inch by inch into the cavity of the shrunken nose. As if by magic the skin spread apart, stretched, and plumped up to form a quite respectable nose. I could hardly believe it. The outer layer of nasal skin had expanded like a bubble blown from a small wad of chewing gum. Gillies assured us that if properly supported the nose would retain its new shape.

Over the next few years we experimented with various supporting structures. We used nose-shaped plastic splints, then acrylic, then bone grafts from the pelvic rim. For those patients who had insufficient blood supply in the nasal tissue to sustain a bone graft, we borrowed material from the dentists. We learned to fashion a soft warm mold of wax to virtually any shape. The patient, awake, could choose his or her nose on the spot: "A touch longer and not quite so wide, please." From that wax model we formed a permanent support made of the hard pink substance used for dentures. Dental wire attached to the teeth held the structure in place.

Today, many leprosy patients in India and around the world walk around with noses that look perfectly normal from the outside but are supported by an artificial under-nose insert. The new noses serve them well as long as they follow a rather bizarre maintenance procedure: they must take out the artificial support periodically for cleaning in order to remove foreign matter and guard against infection. Because of the way we line both sides with mucous membrane, the gap between upper lip and jaw does not reclose, and it is a simple matter for the patient to peel back the upper lip and slide out the bright pink under-nose. The outer nose collapses back into its flattened, wrinkled shape, only to reinflate when the clean under-nose is again inserted.

Like the transplanted eyebrows, our artificial noses had an immediate effect on the patients' social acceptance. I remember one very pretty young woman who came to Vellore with no marks or nodules on her face, but a fully collapsed nose. Her family had tried earnestly to find a groom for her, to no avail. She chose exactly the nose she wanted, a fine, dainty nose which she assured us was much better looking than the original. A few months later she sent me a photo of herself dressed up in wedding finery. Her disease had been cured; now the stigma was healing as well.

Eyelids

All this time, as we experimented with various ways to reconstruct hands and feet and improve our patients' facial appearance, we were neglecting one of leprosy's worst afflictions: blindness. When I first started working with leprosy patients, old-timers told me that blindness, like paralysis and tissue destruction, was a tragic but unavoidable consequence of the disease. Eighty percent of leprosy patients experience some eye damage, and health experts estimate that leprosy is the fourth leading cause of blindness in the world.

As I have mentioned, blindness presents an unusual hardship for leprosy patients who have also lost the sense of touch and pain. I once watched a blind patient who lacked sensation in his fingers. To get dressed, he bent over the clothing and touched it with his still-sensitive lips and tongue for orientation, feeling out the location of sleeves and buttons and buttonholes. It took him about an hour to dress. A person both blind and insensitive also cannot read Braille, or learn a friend's face by touching it with his fingertips.

He will have difficulty maneuvering through a room crowded with furniture. An everyday task like cooking becomes almost impossible for someone who can neither see nor feel the dangers.

Without doubt, blindness is the most feared complication of leprosy. I have been told that at some institutions the fear of blindness leads many patients to attempt suicide. One of our patients, who had already lost sight in one eye, said quite openly, "My feet have gone and my hands too, but that didn't matter much as long as I could see. Blindness is something else. If I go blind, life will mean nothing to me and I shall do all I can to end it."

My wife made one of the first systematic studies of the onset of blindness in leprosy patients. Margaret, who had come to Vellore with experience in family practice, took up ophthalmology when the medical college was extremely short of staff and had no one else to cover that specialty. She quickly became proficient at cataract surgery and soon organized assembly-line "eye camps" in nearby villages. Working in a borrowed school building, or even outdoors under a tree, the surgical team performed as many as 100 to 150 cataract surgeries in a single day. It was in one of these camps that she first became aware of the eye problems of leprosy patients.

"I had just finished the active surgery and was loading equipment in the van for our trip home," she recalls, "when I noticed a group of people sitting on the ground about forty yards away. I asked one of the workers if they were patients who had come late and needed attention. 'Oh, those are just leprosy patients,' he said. I offered to examine them anyway, much to my assistant's—and the patients'—surprise.

"I had seen all sorts of eye problems in India, but never in my life had I seen eyes like these. The surface of the eye, normally moist and transparent, was clouded over with thick layers of white scar tissue. I shone a penlight into the eye and got no response whatever. Most of these people were totally, irremediably blind. Two of the younger ones were well on the way but not quite blind, and I persuaded these two to come to Vellore with me for hospitalization."

From that one encounter, Margaret's life work began to take shape. She knew that leprosy bacilli liked to gather in the cornea, one of the coolest parts of the body, and that anti-leprosy drugs could help slow the damage to the eye. Cortisone drops helped to control acute inflammation and sometimes saved an eye. Also, by tattooing small droplets of India ink into the white scar tissue on the cornea, she could reduce the bright glare that tormented some leprosy patients. All these measures, however, paled beside the most important observation Margaret made as she surveyed hundreds of leprosy patients: many were going blind from not blinking.

The blink reflex is one of the wonders of the human body. No pain sensors are more sensitive than those on the surface of the eye: a stray eyelash, a speck of dirt, a flash of light, a puff of smoke, or even a loud noise will trigger an instantaneous muscular response. The eyelid slams shut, pulling a protective skin covering over the vulnerable eye and trapping any foreign particles in the eyelashes.

Even more impressive, the intermittent blink reflex operates at a maintenance level all day long, opening and closing the eyelid every twenty seconds or so to assure that the eye stays lubricated. The splendid mixture of oil, mucus, and watery fluid that we know as tears provides the cornea with a constant supply of nourishment and cleansing. Without that lubrication, the surface of the cornea dries out and becomes much more susceptible to damage and ulceration.

Margaret noticed that some leprosy patients never bothered to blink at all. They had an unsettling stare, and their tears gathered in a pool in the lower eyelids until they spilled over. In the dusty atmosphere of India, a trail of wasted tears ran down the faces of these leprosy patients, their corneal cells deprived of the wind-shield-washer benefit of a blinking eyelid.

She found that leprosy interfered with the blink reflex in two ways. We already knew the first way, for I had studied segments of these swollen nerves after the Chingleput autopsy. Because of nerve damage, some leprosy patients (about 20 percent) experienced paralysis of the eyelid muscle, losing the ability to blink. These patients slept with eyes wide open, and before long the cornea dried out and began to deteriorate. Margaret showed me the effect of partial paralysis on one boy: his left eye blinked on schedule, while the right stayed open.

We did not realize, however, that many more patients suffered from the familiar nemesis of painlessness. Try to go without blinking and after a minute or so you will feel a mild irritation. Pain whispers before it shouts. Keep your eyes open, though, and that irritation will gradually turn into intense pain, forcing you to blink. Insensitive leprosy patients do not perceive these pain signals. Just as the bacilli damage nerves in fingertips and toes, they also damage the hair-trigger pain sensors that provoke blinking. Numbed, the sensors on the surface of the eye never initiate the blink reflex.

Early on, Margaret saw a vivid illustration of the kind of abuse that can happen to a patient whose eyes are insensitive to pain: a man reached up and vigorously rubbed his open eyes with a hand covered with huge, crusty calluses. Little wonder her patients were going blind!

Margaret's research confirmed that most leprosy blindness was not an unavoidable consequence of infection but rather a by-product caused by a breakdown in the nerves. She chose to work first with the insensitive patients who had not lost their motor nerves. For this large group, the solution seemed simple: she needed only examine them regularly and train them to blink consciously rather than by reflex. If she educated the younger patients to the danger, surely they could learn to blink every minute or so. The alternative was blindness.

With great hope, Margaret began an education campaign among these patients, drilling them to blink every time she held up a flashcard. They followed her lead enthusiastically for an hour or two, but later in the day as she walked among them she noticed the same wide-eyed, unblinking stare. She tried egg timers, buzzers, and other timing devices. These too worked for a while, but patients either lost interest or became inured to the signal. She put goggles on the patients to protect their eyes against foreign objects, but still they were missing the essential benefits of blinking.

In desperation, we researched surgical procedures that might help. Sir Harold Gillies had devised an elegant technique to aid people with Bell's palsy, who also have problems with the blinking muscle. His innovative procedure held out promise even for those with complete eyelid paralysis. It involved detaching one end of part of the temporalis muscle, which controls clenching of the jaw and chewing, and connecting it to a strand of fascia running through the eyelids. This adjustment made it easier for patients to blink consciously, for now the same muscle controlled both the motion of chewing and lid closing. Margaret only had to teach her patients to clench their teeth periodically—or, better yet, chew gum—and the eye would get the lubrication it needed.

The procedure worked well, and is still used widely in India.

If a patient chews gum vigorously every time he goes outdoors on a dusty day, his eye should get the protection it needs. The surgery produces some unusual side effects—a person blinks rapidly as he chews on a piece of meat—but a conscientious patient could literally keep blindness at bay simply by chewing.

Alas, we were reminded never to underestimate the contribution of pain. Solving the motor problems to restore a patient's ability to blink did not solve the much more difficult sensory problems. Even our most eager patients, who held within their conscious power the ability to forestall blindness, would lapse. Unless they retained some residual pain sensation on the surface of the eye to alert them to a feeling of soreness or dryness, they would forget to blink or chew. They had simply lost the motive; for them to blink with perfect regularity, it had to hurt. They needed the compulsion of pain.

When a patient lacked all sensation of pain, we had to revert to a much less satisfactory procedure. Using thread and needle, we stitched the upper and lower eyelids tightly together in the corners, leaving enough of an opening in the center to permit vision. Because so little of the eye was exposed, lubricating tears collected around the cornea and bathed it even though the patient never blinked. Patients hated the overall effect on their appearance, as they hated anything that made them look unnatural, but at least it preserved their sight. Even today, this simple procedure, albeit a poor substitute for silenced pain cells, serves as a remarkable sight saver for leprosy patients.

11
Going Public

—◆◆◆—

You purchase pain with all that joy can give,
And die of nothing but a rage to live.
Alexander Pope

My work with leprosy patients gradually overwhelmed other
teaching and orthopedic duties at the hospital. Often I lay awake
at night thinking of the patients. What new surgical innovations
might reduce the stigma they faced? How could I improve the
quality of their lives? More and more, leprosy work became for me
a vocation, not mere avocation.

In 1952 I received a generous and quite unexpected offer
from the Rockefeller Foundation. "Your work with leprosy shows
good potential," their representative told me. "Why don't you travel
around the world and get the best advice possible. See anyone you
want—surgeons, pathologists, leprologists—and take whatever time
you need. We'll foot the bill."

The offer was a godsend. I had operated on many hands and
feet, and a few noses and eyebrows, but always with the gnawing
awareness that I had not been properly trained for such procedures. Now I had the freedom to study under world-class experts.
Furthermore, I could visit neuropathologists who might be able to
shed light on how leprosy damaged nerves. Our own study had led
nowhere. From the time of the Chingleput autopsy I had known
that nerves became swollen in odd places, leading to paralysis and
loss of sensation, but I had no clue as to what was actually killing
the nerves. I eagerly unpacked the tiny vials we had collected at
the autopsy and selected some segments to stain and mount on
microscope slides to take with me.

Sir Archibald McIndoe, my first contact in London, seemed

intrigued by the tendon transfers we had done at Vellore. He lined up a meeting with the Hand Club, an elite group of thirteen hand surgeons, and nominated me for a lecture at the Royal College of Surgeons. My appearance at these two meetings opened the door to every hand surgeon of note in London and, like a wide-eyed young intern, I went to some of them and observed their work.

I had far less success, though, with the second goal of the trip, figuring out the nerve pathology of leprosy. At various research centers I displayed my collection of autopsy slides and described the mysterious pattern of swellings I had found in nerves of the elbow, knee, and wrist. "It's beyond me what's killing that nerve," said one expert, in a typical response. "I've never seen anything like that pathology."

After completing the rounds in England, I carefully repacked my boxes of slides and specimens and boarded the ocean liner *Queen Mary* for my very first visit to the United States. I had appointments with leading hand surgeons and neurologists, and even hoped to examine my nerve specimens under the powerful electron microscope at Washington University in St. Louis.

For me as a surgeon, the high point of the trip was the month I spent in California studying under Sterling Bunnell, "the father of hand surgery" himself. From there I went to the only remaining leprosarium in the continental United States, the Public Health Service Hospital in Carville, Louisiana, and met with Dr. Daniel Riordan, the only surgeon outside India who had operated on hands in leprosy. Dan and I had a grand time swapping ideas, but in Carville I also got a foretaste of the resistance we would soon face as we publicized our theories about leprosy and nerve damage.

Carville led the world in experimental drug therapy for leprosy, but the staff seemed uninterested in our findings about insensitivity to pain. In a lecture I described how we had succeeded in overturning the "bad flesh" myth and stressed that injuries to the feet, hands, and eyes could be greatly reduced if patients learned a few basic precautions. As I stepped down, the director gave this cryptic response: "Thank you very much, Dr. Brand, for telling us about your work. We have all noticed that you use the word leprosy. Here at Carville we call it Hansen's disease." He sat down, and I had my first lesson on the importance of using politically correct language in America. Then the director took me aside and said in a patronizing tone, "Your people in India seem to be doing some interesting work. I agree that injury and stress may cause damage to patients' hands. But I've been in this business a long time, and I can assure you that Hansen's disease itself causes these fingers to shorten."*

I got one last rebuke at Carville when I inquired about some nerve biopsies. On my trip west I had stopped in St. Louis to use the electron microscope, only to learn that nerves fixed in formalin would not work. I needed fresh nerves. I thought I would find a solution at Carville: if any surgeries were scheduled, I could simply ask the surgeon to collect some small twigs of nerves that had gone dead and were no longer of any use. Our patients in India gladly donated dead nerves for our study. But this was the United States, not India, and the staff greeted my request with shock. "Our patients are very conscious of their rights and would not agree to being used as guinea pigs!" they said. I had much to learn about the American concept of personal rights.

Denny-Brown's Cats

The Rockefeller-sponsored trip accomplished nearly everything I wanted, even without the electron microscopy. As it turned out, one serendipitous meeting in Boston helped solve for me the baffling mystery of nerve destruction. All but one of the neurology experts I met with gave the same puzzled reaction to my nerve specimens ("I've never seen anything like that pathology"). The

---

*Years later, when I moved to the United States, I learned the peculiar American custom of addressing a problem by changing its name. There are certainly settings in which I will use the term *Hansen's disease* to avoid offense (although I find that when I am delivering a lecture and use the term I often get puzzled stares; when I stop and explain that I am referring to leprosy, the audience understands, and interest quickens). But I believe the stigma surrounding leprosy does not relate so much to the name as to the disease and the misconceptions surrounding it. Other countries, such as Brazil, have found that changing the name away from a stigmatized word does not in itself affect the social stigma. I would much rather change the stigma by educating people of the reality of the disease caused by the organism *Mycobacterium leprae:* that most people have built-in immunity, that it can be easily treated, and that with proper care it need not lead to serious complications. In India the Tamil and Hindi names for leprosy also carry heavy stigma, but where effective rehab programs have been in effect, stigma has melted away, with no change of name.

one exception was Dr. Derek Denny-Brown, a New Zealander and a brilliant neurologist who practiced at a charity hospital in Boston.

Without a doubt, Denny-Brown's office was the most cluttered office I visited in America, a jumble of boxes, file folders, slide containers, and X-ray negatives. Typically, the physicians I visited would steal a glance at their watches every half hour or so. Not Denny-Brown. When I presented a problem, his instincts went on full alert and he became oblivious to time. He was a pure scientist.

I briefly described our research on insensitivity. "We've traced almost all the destructive side effects of leprosy to the root cause of nerve damage. But I cannot establish any theory or convince others unless I come up with an explanation of *how* leprosy damages the nerve. So far, none of the specialists I've visited have recognized this pattern of nerve pathology."

Denny-Brown rose to the challenge. "Let me have a look," he said. He spent a very long time in silence, hunched over a microscope, poring over the specimens from the Chingleput autopsy. "You know, Brand, these specimens remind me of my cats," he said at last. He began rummaging through the boxes of microscope slides on his shelves, and as he did so he told me about his experiments with cats—the kind of experiments performed before the days of animal rights activism.

"I used to anesthetize cats and then expose a nerve, usually the nerve controlling the right front foreleg. I'd put a little steel clip right on that nerve surface, like a paper clip on a wire. If the clip was tight enough, I found, the pressure would damage the nerve and the leg would become paralyzed. Permanent nerve damage. Next I tried putting a tiny cylinder, a steel sheath, around the nerve, but I could never get the cylinder tight enough to cause any problems. Then I tried trauma. I struck the exposed nerve with a blunt instrument. The cat was anesthetized, of course, so she didn't feel anything, but the trauma caused the nerve to swell up to double its normal size. Despite the swelling, though, I noticed that no paralysis occurred. The nerve kept functioning.

"Finally, I got the idea of hitting the nerve first and *then* encasing it in the tiny steel sheath. The nerve started to swell, but this time it had nowhere to expand because of the cylinder. I really got a reaction then. Very quickly the cat lost all sensation and movement in muscles supplied by that nerve. I learned a lot about nerve damage, but I didn't know what to make of those findings, so I just set them aside. That was more than ten years ago. But somewhere around here I've got some specimens."

I was impressed by Denny-Brown's visual recall of a pattern he had seen many years before. At last he located a dusty box of microscope slides, pulled them out, and put them side by side with the Chingleput nerve specimens. Under the microscope, they matched perfectly. We now had two independent demonstrations of the same mysterious pattern.

"Well, now, that tells you something," Denny-Brown said with obvious pride. "Your leprosy nerves are being damaged by ischemia. Something's causing them to swell, and the nerve sheath [a fat-protein sleeve resembling the insulation around a wire] restricts the swelling. What happens is that pressure inside the sheath becomes so tight that it squeezes shut the blood supply and causes ischemia. Like any tissue, a nerve will die if it's cut off from blood supply long enough."

That afternoon with Denny-Brown proved to be the most valuable session of my entire four-month trip to America. Ischemia I knew about firsthand, for that was what I had experienced as one of Sir Thomas Lewis's volunteers back in medical school. I remembered the agony I had felt as the blood pressure cuff shut off all incoming blood and my muscles went into spasm. Ironically, the very same mechanism that had caused me such pain was now doing the opposite in my leprosy patients: it was destroying their sense of pain. If I had kept the pressure cuff on long enough, hours instead of minutes, I too would have damaged the nerves in my arm, leading to paralysis and loss of sensation.

For the first time, I had a sensible explanation of leprosy's assault on the nerve. As the leprosy bacilli invade nerves, the body reacts with a classic response of inflammation, causing the nerve to swell. Bacilli multiply, the body sends in reinforcements, and before long the expanding nerve is pressing against its sheath. Just as Denny-Brown's steel sheaths had constricted the swelling of the cat nerves, the leprosy-invaded nerve's own sheath acts as a constrictor, and eventually the swollen nerve squeezes shut its own blood supply and dies. A dead nerve will no longer carry the electric signals for sensation and movement.

As I peered through the microscope lens in Denny-Brown's cluttered office, some of the final pieces of the leprosy puzzle clicked into place. For centuries, medicine had focused on the visible harm that leprosy did to toes, fingers, and face—hence the "bad flesh" myth. My own work with patients, as well as the Chingleput autopsy, had convinced me that the real problem lay elsewhere, in the nerve pathways, but until that moment I had not understood how the nerves were damaged. Denny-Brown's explanation of ischemia solved the puzzle.*

At last I was beginning to piece together an overall picture of leprosy as, primarily, a disease of the nerves. Bacilli do proliferate in cool places such as the forehead and nose, provoking a defensive response, but those invaders do mostly cosmetic damage. The truly devastating symptoms come about when bacilli invade nerves close to the skin surface. Each major nerve is a conduit for motor and sensory fibers, and a failure in the nerve affects both. Motor axons no longer carry messages from the brain, and the hand or foot or eyelid muscle becomes paralyzed; sensory axons no longer carry messages of touch, temperature, and pain, and the patient becomes vulnerable to injury. When an injury does occur, an infection often sets in, and the body's reaction may cause the bone to be destroyed or absorbed, resulting in shortened fingers and toes.

I thought back to my first contact with the victims of leprosy, the beggars in the streets of Vellore. Their symptoms—blindness, marred faces, paralyzed hands, stumpy fingers and toes, ulcers under the feet—certainly pointed to a disease of the skin and extremities. It had taken me a long time to be more precise in assigning blame. Now I had confirmation that most of the gross deformities and dreaded symptoms of leprosy had the same cruel source: damaged nerves.

Oasis

I returned from the Rockefeller-sponsored trip armed with new surgical skills and loaded with ammunition for our theories on painlessness, but I also brought back the sobering knowledge that we were on our own in India. None of the top neuropathologists had ever studied leprosy-damaged nerves, and of the noted surgeons I visited only one had ever worked with its victims. By default, Vellore itself was the pioneering outpost in the campaign for leprosy rehabilitation.

---

*Years later, Dr. Tom Swift identified another, less common cause of paralysis that occurs when leprosy sometimes invades nerves directly amd destroys the myelin coating of the fibers.

Our program still lacked an important element: a full-scale leprosy hospital and dedicated research center, long the dream of Bob Cochrane. The same year as my Rockefeller trip, the state government offered a 256-acre site in a rural area called Karigiri, fourteen miles from the medical college. I remember all too well the dismay I felt inspecting this gravelly, parched site for the first time. Hot winds swept across the sere landscape, and as I stepped from the jeep they hit me in the face like exhaust from a blast furnace. No one on earth would choose to live in such a blighted place, I thought to myself. But leprosy patients rarely have the luxury of personal choice: neighbors had blocked our purchase of several lovely sites closer to town. We accepted the land gratefully and broke ground. Plans called for an eighty-bed hospital, a well-equipped research laboratory, and a training facility.

Karigiri soon named Dr. Ernest Fritschi to the post of chief surgeon and later to medical superintendent, wise moves for reasons beyond his medical skills. Fritschi's father, a Swiss agricultural missionary, had taught his son basic principles of botany and ecology, and Ernest now adopted the wasteland at Karigiri as his most challenging "patient." He built dirt trenches, contour dams, and percolation dams in an effort to control erosion and raise the water table. He sought out drought-resistant plants to stabilize the thin soil. He planted as many as a thousand trees a year, nourishing seedlings in his own house, transplanting them carefully, and watering them with a bullock-drawn water tanker.

Karigiri was gradually transformed. I visited there weekly, and at first the gray and white buildings of the research center stood stark and tall against the shimmering horizon of the desert. Over time, a lush green forest grew up to shield those buildings, lowering the ground temperature and taming the whipsaw winds. I began to look forward to my visits as a welcome relief from the heat of town. Birds returned, as many as a hundred different species, and I stashed a pair of binoculars in my briefcase.

The research work at Karigiri kept pace with the physical improvements. Once we had identified the hazards an insensitive person might encounter, we were able to reduce dramatically the number of injuries. Mobile teams went out every working day to educate leprosy patients in the villages.

Meanwhile, I began publishing papers and traveling around the world, trying to communicate what we had learned about leprosy treatment. Doctors who had experience in leprosy work seemed sometimes indifferent and occasionally hostile to our findings. I remember one conversation with a stubborn, elderly doctor in South Africa. As I explained our theories, I pointed to the large blisters on the palm of one of his leprosy patients. "No doubt those blisters came from burns," I said. "He probably picked up a metal cooking pot. And he had no pain messages to warn him to let go."

The doctor bristled. "Young man, you've been at this disease for less than a decade. I've been doing leprosy work all my life, and I *know* leprosy produces blisters in the palm of the hand." He scoffed at my rebuttal. To him, the diagnosis was clear-cut: leprosy followed a predictable pattern of tissue destruction which no treatment could reverse.

The World Health Organization named leprosy as one of its five priority target diseases and began pumping millions of dollars into research and treatment, but even WHO showed little regard for rehabilitation. Once drugs had killed off the active bacilli in a patient, WHO pronounced that patient cured. Subsequent damage to eyes, hands, and feet was regrettable, but not really their concern.

We at Karigiri argued that patients have different standards of "cure" than WHO, and the patient's view often determines whether treatment is effective. "We are treating a person, not a disease," I said, "and therefore our programs must include training and rehabilitation. If a man who is taking drug therapy continues to find ulcers on his foot and hand and eye, he may simply stop taking the pills." My patients viewed leprosy in terms of obvious damage to their bodies, not live bacterial count. A person free of active leprosy who is left with crippled hands and feet hardly thinks of himself as cured, no matter what WHO or any doctor claims.

Finally, in 1957 an Italian filmmaker helped provide the breakthrough I was looking for. Carlo Marconi, then living in Bombay, agreed to produce a documentary on our work, funded by the Leprosy Mission in London. The result, *Lifted Hands*, depicted the life story of a downcast village boy who came to us with badly clawed hands and after extensive surgery left with restored hands and a new lease on life. Marconi, a perfectionist, spent many weeks with us, creating havoc with our normal schedule but delighting the villagers whom he employed as extras and assistants.

Lifted Hands proved its worth almost immediately. Finished just in time, the film made a vivid impression at a Tokyo conference attended by leprosy experts from forty-three countries. At last they seemed to grasp the importance of preventing and correcting deformities. Only one dissenter, a strict scientist who insisted on rigorous data, stopped the committee from adopting a new policy. "We have no proof of the accuracy of Dr. Brand's assertions about the role of insensitivity in leading to deformities," he said. "We must not pass any resolutions without a thorough investigation."

Ironically, that dissent proved decisive in our campaign. An investigating team of hand surgeons, leading medical scientists, and leprologists descended on Vellore for the inquiry. Fortunately, we had kept meticulous records on each of our surgical patients. We followed a standard procedure of dictating nineteen descriptive paragraphs for each operation (1, the external site before procedure; 2, preparation of skin; 3, anesthesia; 4, incision, and so on). In addition, we had made a complete photographic record of each hand to demonstrate its progressive range of motion and flexibility: six photos before surgery, six photos after surgery, six photos after postoperative physiotherapy, and follow-up photos after one year and five years. We opened all these files to the experts and also let them examine our long-term patients.

For the first time ever we had world-class surgeons and leprosy experts in a room together focusing on the same medical issues, and the mixture was explosive. The hand surgeons got excited about what could be done for a paralyzed hand; the leprologists got excited about our success rate in healing wounds and preventing injuries. The entire group caught the vision for rehabilitation that had been motivating us since our earliest days in the mud-walled hand clinic. With great enthusiasm, this committee issued an official report endorsing our approach to rehabilitation. Soon afterward WHO hired me as a consultant, and Karigiri became a regular stopping place for international leprosy experts and for all new trainees sponsored by WHO.

Indeed, in the next few years surgeons and physiotherapists from more than thirty countries found their way to the tiny town in the desert of South India. They could study medicine and epidemiology elsewhere, but no other place offered practical experience in the surgery and rehabilitation of leprosy patients. On my weekly visits to Karigiri, I would usually eat dinner in the guest dining room, where I would join health workers from perhaps a dozen countries. Bob Cochrane's original dream of an international training center at Karigiri was coming true at last.

Restoration

For those of us who knew Karigiri in the early days, what transpired in the desert looked like a miracle of nature, an oasis of beauty and new hope sprouting in a landscape of death. I saw in that transformation a metaphor of what we hoped to accomplish in our patients. We were attempting to reshape the lives of human beings, many of whom had come to us barren of all hope. Could loving care do for them what it was doing for the land? Over the next few years, the metaphor moved closer to reality.

My mother, Granny Brand, was still active in the mountains and she brought us some of our most challenging cases. Two or three times a year she would show up after a twenty-four-hour journey by horseback, bus, and train with a miserable specimen of humanity in tow, usually a half-starved beggar with severely paralyzed limbs, missing fingers and toes, and open sores on hands and feet. I would explain to her that we had no vacant beds and that we had to choose our patients carefully on the basis of who showed the most potential. Mother would smile sweetly and say, "Oh, I know, Paul, but just this once for your old mother. And pray about what Jesus would want you to do." As always, she won the argument.

The elaborate care at Karigiri often went to "nobodies" like these. But the staff—many of whom we had hired from local villages—did not shrink back or turn their faces. Fear and superstition had melted away as they understood the nature of the disease. They listened to the new patients' stories, unrevolted, unafraid. They used the magic of human touch. A year or so later I would see these patients, Lazarus-like, walk out of our hospital and proudly head for home or the New Life Center to learn a trade. A grant from the Swedish Red Cross soon made possible a medium-size factory specially designed to employ workers with leprosy, polio, and other disabling diseases.

As knowledge about leprosy spread and barriers of stigma fell, we had occasional success in restoring leprosy patients to their former status in life. Vijay, a trial lawyer from Calcutta, was one of our least typical patients because he came from a high caste. He had enjoyed a successful career in court until the day he discovered signs of leprosy. He sought medical advice and took several months off work in order to undergo intensive treatment with sulfone drugs. Soon the infection was under control and Vijay received a certificate of negativity. Even though he now posed no danger, other lawyers in the court drew up a petition of disbarment to block his return to practice. Claw-hands would be a disgrace in the courtroom, they protested.

Vijay telegraphed me in desperation and I urged him to come immediately to our hospital. He flew to Madras and took a train to Karigiri. "The court hearing to determine my future is in five weeks," he said. "I must have new hands by then." I had never before operated on both hands of a patient at the same time—we always left one hand free for eating and other essentials—but Vijay's case was different. We operated on all his fingers and thumbs of both hands at the same time, bandaged him up, and put him in plaster casts. Totally helpless with both hands in plaster, he had to be fed and dressed by nurses and assistants. Three weeks later we removed the casts and gave him an accelerated course in physical therapy. On the last day of the five-week deadline, we drove Vijay back to the train—practicing his finger exercises all the way—for a return trip to the Madras airport.

Vijay had a flair for courtroom drama. At the hearing, as he later told me, he kept his hands hidden until all the complaints had been made. When his turn came he spoke at length about the bigotry of those who looked upon a physical defect as something that might detract from the dignity of the court. He waited until the concluding paragraph to mention his own case. "As for my own situation, my accusers have complained about my deformed hands. I ask this court, what deformities are they talking about?" He removed both hands from his pockets and raised them aloft, fingers stretched out straight, revealing no sign of clawing. The accusing lawyers crowded forward in amazement. The case was dismissed.

Over the next decade, as I worked with patients like Vijay in the new, expanded facilities at Karigiri, I realized that I had never felt a greater sense of personal fulfillment. Quite unexpectedly, the leprosy work had brought together all the stray vectors of my life. I had all the surgery I could handle, a fine laboratory in which to conduct research, and even the opportunity to reach back in time and resurrect skills from construction days. I remember feeling an intense stab of déjà vu as I sat with a dozen boys in the New Life village, supervising them on how to use their reconstructed hands in carpentry. Suddenly I was transported back to the workbench where I had apprenticed, with my supervisor guiding me. I had a sharp, numinous sense of the hand of God leading me forward, down paths I had once thought to be blind alleys.

The process of following patients through the whole rehabilitation cycle ultimately challenged my approach toward medicine. Somewhere, perhaps in medical school, doctors acquire an attitude that seems suspiciously like hubris: "Oh, you've come just in time. Count on me. I think I'll be able to save you." Working at Karigiri stripped away that hubris. We could not "save" leprosy patients. We could arrest the disease, yes, and repair some of the damage. But every leprosy patient we treated had to go back and, against overwhelming odds, attempt to build a new life. I began to see my chief contribution as one I had not studied in medical school: to join with my patients as a partner in the task of restoring dignity to a broken spirit. That is the true meaning of rehabilitation.

Each of our patients was acting out a lead role in a personal drama of recovery. Our mechanical rearrangement of muscles, tendons, and bones was but one step in rebuilding a damaged life. The patients themselves were the ones who traveled the difficult path.

12
To the Bayou

———◆———

Pain has an element of blank;
It cannot recollect
When it began, or if there were
A day when it was not.

It has no future but itself,
Its Infinite realms contain
Its past, enlightened to perceive
New periods of pain.
Emily Dickinson

In 1965, after nearly twenty years in India, we made the difficult decision to move on. Skilled Indian personnel had assumed control of most branches of the leprosy work and, since I spent several months each year traveling internationally, my ties to Karigiri had begun to loosen. The Brand family now included six children, some nearing college age, and it seemed a good time for us to relocate. We returned to England expecting to make our permanent home there.

Those plans changed when a lecture tour took me back to Carville, Louisiana, where this time I had a most cordial reception. Dr. Edgar Johnwick, the director of the leprosy hospital, sat entranced as I described the program at Karigiri. I must have stirred his American competitive instincts, for he pulled me aside that afternoon. "It's quite apparent your patients in India get a better rehabilitation program than our patients in the United States," he said with obvious concern. "As an officer of the U.S. Public Health Service, I can't accept that. Would you consider coming here and setting up a similar program?"

My wife and I, British subjects who had served in India, were reluctant to introduce yet a third culture into our children's lives. But Dr. Johnwick proved to be the consummate salesman. Carville would create a position in ophthalmology for Margaret, he promised, and the USPHS would fully support all my consulting work overseas. "It's the least we can do," he said, after a few phone calls to Washington for authorization.

I talked into a tape recorder for half an hour, describing the opportunities at Carville and my impressions of the Louisiana bayou country, and sent the tape to London. When it arrived, Margaret and all six children sat around playing and replaying the tape and searching for Carville on a map. (The hospital sits along an oxbow of the Mississippi River approximately a third of the way down from Baton Rouge to New Orleans.) All six children had a vote and all six voted that the family should move to America, though our oldest daughter, Jean, elected to stay in London to complete nursing school.

In January 1966 the Brand family entered the alien world of Cajun cooking, Huey Long–style politics, and riverboat legends as we moved into a wooden frame house on hospital grounds beside the Mississippi River levee. Immersion in a new culture presented many adjustments. For some time Margaret and I resisted family pleas for a television, but finally yielded to overwhelming pressure ("We're the only people in America who don't have one!") and bought a black-and-white set. Our children, accustomed to British schools in which students stand when the teacher enters the room or calls on them, were shocked at the casual behavior of American schoolchildren. Attending school in the American South in the late 1960s, they also found themselves caught up in a swirl of civil rights issues.

In Seclusion

Our family, however, was more attuned to a different kind of prejudice. Initially the Carville hospital had been operated by an order of nuns as a haven of refuge for beleaguered patients from New Orleans. Later, under state and then federal administration, it went through a long history of discriminatory treatment of leprosy patients, and our children were surprised to find official policy less enlightened than what they had known in India. As recently as the 1950s, patients arrived at the hospital in chains. All outgoing patient mail had to pass through an oven sterilizer, an absurd and medically useless practice which the hospital administration had long opposed but the Washington bureaucracy had not yet changed.* The hospital also had rules forbidding patients to visit staff homes and banning children under sixteen from patient areas, both of which our children found ways to break.

My daughter Mary balked at holding her wedding reception in the old Carville plantation hall because patients would not have been admitted to that building. Another daughter, Estelle, ended up marrying a former patient and moving to Hawaii. My youngest daughter, Pauline, took a different approach, preferring to tease exaggerated fears of the disease. Carville was well known in the Louisiana area, and tourists sometimes drove by the hospital fence, craning their necks for a look at the "lepers" inside. Pauline would stand by the fence until she saw a car slowing down, at which point she would scrunch up her fingers, distort her face, and do her best to fulfill the stereotype, in hopes of scaring the gawkers away.

The old-timers at Carville regaled us with tales of the hospital's dark past. The stigma of leprosy imposed on the hospital was once so great that many patients had adopted new names to protect their families on the outside. (I heard stories about the deceased "Ann Page," who had chosen her name from a local grocery store brand.) For a long time leprosy patients, like felons, were denied the right to vote. They were required to dip pocket money in a disinfectant before spending it. "This place used to be like a prison," one patient told me. "Like many of these folks, I had a wife and children. But back then leprosy was legal grounds for divorce and incarceration, and one day the sheriff came along

*A physiotherapist friend in India claims that, paradoxically, more educated societies are more likely to stigmatize disease. He cites New Guinea and Central Africa, which tend to be more accepting of leprosy patients than Japan, Korea, and the United States. I used to argue with him, but a U.S. government policy adopted just after the Vietnam War gave me pause. Tens of thousands of "boat people" refugees were then seeking asylum in the United States, and we in the Public Health Service strongly recommended that they be tested for leprosy. Vietnam has a moderately high incidence of leprosy, and it seemed foolish in the extreme to admit active carriers without screening them and arranging for treatment. But the government turned down our request. It was too risky, they said. If word leaked to the press that some boat people had leprosy, the general public would turn against the whole project.

and sent me to Carville. I could have slipped under the wire, I suppose. But anybody caught escaping from Carville risked a prison
term. And it's hard for a leprosy patient to hide."

Thanks to Dr. Johnwick's superb leadership, however, modern Carville was emerging from its shadowy past. Quarantine laws
for leprosy had been abolished. The barbed wire around the hospital grounds had come down, and tours were offered to visitors
three times a day. Johnwick died of a sudden heart attack just
before we arrived, but his humane reforms were well under way
and the last discriminatory barriers soon fell.

I loved the setting at Carville: long lines of oak trees draped
in Spanish moss, horses and cattle grazing in open fields of grass
and goldenrod. With the yellow quarantine flag down, Carville
was now an attractive place for patients to live. They had individual rooms, a softball field, a lake stocked with fish, and a nine-hole
golf course. They could roam the four-hundred-acre plantation
grounds, stroll along the levee, or even catch a ferry across the
river to visit a crawfish café.

A pleasant environment, free room and board, excellent
health care, government-funded recreation and entertainment,
air-conditioned buildings—my patients' comfort level in this
plantation setting far exceeded anything I had known in India.
But leprosy finds a way to work its peculiar pattern of destruction
regardless of the setting.

When I arrived in Carville in 1966 the most celebrated
patient was a man named Stanley Stein. Born in 1899, he was
older than the century, although the leprosy scars on his face made
it difficult to judge his age. Stanley was a genteel, sophisticated
man who had toyed with a career in acting before becoming a
pharmacist. At the age of thirty-one he was diagnosed with leprosy
and whisked off to Carville, where he spent the rest of his life. He
had written a poignant autobiography, *Alone No Longer*, and had
founded *The Star*, a patient newspaper that drew subscribers from
all over the world. It was from Stanley that I heard many of the
stories of Carville's past.

By the time I met him, Stanley had lost all sensory contact
with his hands and feet and had recently gone blind. Scars and
ulcers covered his hands, face, and feet, bearing mute witness to
the unintentional abuse his body had endured because it lacked
the sensation of pain. Stanley told me that when his eyes first
began to dry out he had sought relief by covering them with wet-

pack compresses. He would stand at the sink and let the water run until he thought it had reached the proper temperature. Unfortunately, because he had lost sensation and could not judge the temperature, he sometimes scalded his hands and his face, resulting in scarring and more deformity.

Blindness greatly complicated Stanley's life, and more and more he simply stayed in his room. He managed to carry on his responsibilities with *The Star* by having articles read to him and by using a Dictaphone for his own writing. Stanley had a keen mind, and I loved to visit him. Sensitive to my slightest inflection of voice, he was quick to perceive the meaning behind what I said. He questioned me about attitudes toward the disease in different countries and wanted to hear of any new advances in leprosy treatment.

As the disease progressed in Stanley's own body, however, the bacilli developed a resistance to our best drugs and his doctors had to turn to streptomycin, a powerful antibiotic that has the occasional side effect of causing nerve deafness. Tragically, Stanley Stein began to lose his hearing, his last link with the outside world. He could no longer listen to newscasts and talking books, and conversation with friends became extremely difficult.

Unlike Helen Keller, Stanley could not even use tactile sign language, for leprosy had destroyed his sense of touch. I remember entering Stanley's room, wanting to make my presence known. He could not see me and was so insensitive to touch that I would have to grab his hand and shake it vigorously for him to feel anything. His face brightened when he realized he had a visitor, and he would reach over to a bedside table and fumble vainly for his hearing aid. I would find it for him and then shout at close range directly into the hearing aid, and for a time we could still communicate. But soon the deafness closed in.

A visit to Stanley during the last months of his life was nearly unbearable. Unable to see, unable to hear, unable to feel, he would wake up disoriented. He would stretch out his hand and not know what he was touching, and speak without knowing whether anyone heard or answered. Once I found him sitting in a chair muttering to himself in a monotone, "I don't know where I am. Is someone in the room with me? I don't know who you are, and my thoughts go round and round. I cannot think new thoughts."

I got a haunting sense of Stanley Stein's absolute loneliness. "Acute loneliness," wrote Rollo May, "seems to be the most painful kind of anxiety which a human being can suffer. Patients often tell us that the pain is a physical gnawing in their chests, or feels like the cutting of a razor in their heart region." For the lack of pain, Stanley Stein suffered even greater pain. His brain, with all its liveliness and wit and erudition, was still intact. But pathways to the brain had dried up as, one by one, the major nerves went dead. Even the sense of smell disappeared when leprosy invaded the lining of Stanley's nose. Except for taste, all inlets from the outside world were now blocked off, and the ivory box of bone that had been the mind's armor became its prison.

With all the resources of the U.S. Public Health Service at our command, we could do little but make Stanley Stein's last days as comfortable as possible. He died in 1967.

New Tools

I came to the United States at a propitious time for scientific research. The government generously funded medical programs even when, as in our case, they primarily benefited people elsewhere. (The registered leprosy population in the United States was—and is still today—only about six thousand.) Carville had nearly as many staff members as patients and we were able to obtain research equipment which would have seemed lavish in India. For example, I soon learned of an exciting technology, thermography, which showed promise for medical applications, and ordered a $40,000 unit for our clinic. The thermograph was an elaborate machine for measuring temperature.

In India we had recognized the importance of monitoring the temperature of patients' feet and hands. Insensitive to pain, they do not usually know when they have damaged tissue beneath the surface, but the body responds anyway by rushing an increased blood supply to the damaged area. A spot of infection in the foot, for instance, requires three to four times the normal blood supply in order to heal the wound and control the infection. I had trained my hand to detect these "hot spots," practicing so that eventually I learned to perceive a change in temperature as small as one and a half degrees Celsius and sometimes even one and a quarter degrees. If I felt a warm spot on a patient's foot, I knew that it probably meant inflammation and thus I kept a careful eye on it. If the high temperature persisted, I would take an X ray to see whether the underlying bone had cracked.

Now, on the thermogram monitor or on a printout, I could see an entire foot at once, displaying variances in temperature as small as one-quarter of a degree. Cool areas of the skin showed up as green or blue; warmer areas appeared violet, orange, or red; the hottest areas glowed yellow or white. The thermograph was fascinating and fun to operate because it produced such colorful maps of the hand or foot. We experimented with the machine for several months before realizing its true potential: the thermograph's precision allowed us to detect problems at such an early stage that it helped compensate for the loss of pain.

Normally, the instant a foot makes contact with a tack and starts to put pressure on it, pain endings howl, preventing you from sustaining a serious injury. My leprosy patients, lacking this advance warning system, would keep walking and drive the tack into the foot, a problem we had learned to address by aggressively treating these visible injuries right away. Far more difficult was the damage caused by pressure sores: these developed under the surface and only broke open into an ulcer at a later stage. The thermograph offered us, for the first time, the ability to peer under the skin and observe such inflammation before it exposed itself on the skin surface. Now we could actually *prevent* ulcers, by arresting tissue breakdown sooner.

If the thermograph revealed a warm spot on a hand or foot, we could immobilize the limb for a few days, or at least reduce weight-bearing, to protect the patient from further harm and heal the commencing problem. Compared to a healthy pain system, of course, the high-tech thermograph was rather crude, for it detected a problem after the fact, not before (the beauty of pain is that it lets you know right away when you are harming yourself). Nevertheless, it gave us new precision in monitoring potential problems. I began requiring Carville patients to come for regular hand-and-foot checkups with the thermograph.*

The first few months of these clinics proved frustrating. I

---

*Mostly we used the thermograph to look for hot temperatures, which signified inflammation. But in one case it proved valuable in revealing cool temperatues. I had a patient who was a heavy smoker. Like many insensitive patients, he often hurt his fingers by inadvertently letting the cigarettes burn down too far. I warned him that, besides causing these chronic sores, the cigarettes were bad for him in more serious ways. The nicotine he inhaled reduced the circulation of blood to his fingers by constricting the blood vessels. Yet his fingers needed a good blood supply to repair the many injuries remember my first thermograph session with José, a "certified negative" patient who came from California for monitoring once every six months. Jose's toes had shrunken as a result of bone absorption, and pressure sores kept the infection from ever clearing up. Yet he stubbornly refused to wear orthopedic shoes. "They're too ugly," he said. José had a clean, unmarked face and no one suspected him of being a leprosy patient. "I have a good job selling furniture. If I wear the ugly shoes, someone may guess I have a disease. And then I will lose my job."

I had high hopes that the thermograph might persuade José to swallow his pride. He had never taken our warnings very seriously because his feet looked fine on the surface. Now I could show José on a thermogram exactly where the inflammation was developing. "Look at the hot white spot on your smallest toe. Do you see where your narrow shoe is pressing too tight?" He nodded, and I felt encouraged. Together we looked at his foot. "You can't see anything yet, and you don't feel pain. But that white color is a severe danger sign of problems under the surface. You'll have an ulcer there very soon." I used my sternest tone of voice. "José, mark my words, you may lose that toe if you don't do something."

José listened politely, but still refused to wear the therapeutic shoes. "Well, then," I said, "go shopping for some new shoes that you like. Buy the next largest size, and let me build up around the pressure points with a soft padding that will spread out the stress." He agreed to this plan, but when he left Carville I had no confidence that he would actually wear the new shoes.

Sure enough, six months later José returned with an open

---

that tend to afflict leprosy hands. He took no notice of my advice until one day I asked him to come to the clinic without having smoked for the past few hours.

I had set the thermograph to register the color blue at about two degrees cooler than his normal finger temperature. He held his hands up before the machine and, at my instruction, lit a cigarette and began inhaling deeply. The image of his fingers started off as green, then turned blue in about two minutes. After five minutes they disappeared off the screen altogether! The sudden high level of nicotine had constricted his arteries and capillaries, cooling his fingers to a temperature below the minimum setting for the thermograph. My patient was so astonished at the sight of his fingers vanishing on-screen that he threw away his pack of cigarettes and never smoked again. He lived among patients who had no fingers left, and the experience convinced him that he had better give his fingers a good blood supply to keep them as healthy as possible.

ulcer on his small toe. The toe had visibly shrunk, and X rays revealed progressive bone absorption from the chronic infection. José received this news with nonchalance. Because his feet did not hurt him, he ignored them. Nothing I said convinced him to care. During the next few years I watched with a feeling of total helplessness as José let other bones in his toes become absorbed. He ended up with two severely shortened stumps with little bumps where his toes had been, solely because he refused to wear different shoes. The thermograph could give us a visual warning, yes, but one which lacked the compulsion of pain.

I also faced initial resistance from the Patients' Federation, whose officers objected to any screening that might threaten patients' jobs. One of the early screenings revealed a hot spot of inflammation on a patient's thumb. After questioning him, I learned that his job included the task of raking up grass behind a mower. "You must stop that for a time, until this inflammation settles down," I advised him. He promptly reported our conversation to the Patients' Federation. Neither he nor the Federation could understand why I was concerned about a thumb that did not appear to be injured and did not hurt.

In time, however, the thermograph proved itself. Our clinic worked with the Patients' Federation in finding substitute jobs for endangered patients, and we began seeing a marked reduction in ulcers and chronic infections. Our investment in the machine paid for itself many times over.*

---

*I published articles on the diagnostic benefits of thermography, describing it as "an objective indication of pain." This led to a rather curious excursion into the field of animal rights. A government veterinarian who saw one of my articles in an obscure journal asked if I would help him prosecute some millionaire horse owners. Certain trainers of Tennessee Walker horses were gaining an unfair advantage through a cruel (and illegal) practice known as "soreing." The trainers applied mustard oil to the horses' front legs, then placed heavy metal bracelets around the leg joints. As the horses walked or trotted, irritation and pain from the heavy bracelets caused them to rear back and put more weight on their hind legs, jerking their front legs higher, which served to enhance the high-stepping gait that judges admire in Tennessee Walkers. Rubbing on the hot mustard oil caused inflammation and even more pain. The trainers took care to prevent the skin from breaking, however, so that no one could prove they had been using the illegal training technique. At show time, the lead bracelets were removed, and the approving audience never suspected that the horses' prancing was actually a response to pain.

Cries and Whispers

Thanks to generous government grants, we hired nine additional staff members in the rehabilitation department at Carville. Working as a team, engineers, scientists, computer experts, and biologists thoroughly investigated all aspects of the hazards produced by insensitivity to pain. In most cases, as with the thermograph, we were not breaking new ground, but rather adding sophistication and precision to the principles we had learned in India.

Gradually, a new understanding of how pain protects normal limbs emerged, and I began to view painlessness as one of the greatest curses that can befall a human being. In India we had relied mainly on visual cues—blisters from a lamp, rat bites—whereas in Carville the tools at our disposal allowed us to solve the more obscure mysteries of tissue breakdown. I gained an ever-increasing sense of awe and gratitude for the extraordinary ways in which pain daily protects every healthy person. Our research confirmed there are at least three basic ways in which danger constantly presents itself to a pain-insensitive person: direct injury, constant stress, and repetitive stress.

Direct Injury

Many direct injuries were familiar when we arrived at Carville, for we had tracked them extensively at the New Life Center in Vellore. I recognized the fingers of smokers by the

---

"Horse trainers with a conscience are being driven out of the business," the veterinarian told me. "We've taken some unscrupulous owners to court—some of them have mob connections—but can never get a conviction. We have no way of proving that the horses are suffering. Can you help us?"

With the permission of a cooperative trainer, I lugged our thermograph machine to a horse farm near Baton Rouge and made baseline measurements. Then we ran a few "soreing" tests, and the damage immediately became apparent on the thermograms. The temperature in a horse's foreleg went up as much as five degrees Celsius after treatment with the mustard oil and the lead bracelet. I had no doubt the horses were in pain from the inflammation. Armed with these test results, the government went back to court. In three successive court cases, the veterinarian ran thermograms on horses that were suspected victims, and then announced that the author of the article on "objective indications of pain" was willing to testify in court. Defendants in all three cases changed their pleas to guilty. Some horse show rings installed thermographs, and gradually the cruel practice died out.

"kissing wounds," and the fingers of cooks by burn marks from cooking pots. Some direct injuries at Carville were new to me. In one case that my wife, Margaret, treated, a woman named Alma hurt herself by using eyebrow liner. Characteristically, she had lost her eyebrows and eyelashes because of leprosy bacilli invasion. Each day she painted mascara on both areas with a brush, but because her hand and eye were insensitive she often missed the eyelid margin and stabbed the pigment into her eye. Margaret warned her strongly that she would soon damage her eye irreversibly. Alma ignored all these admonitions, and one day she explained why. "You don't understand," she said. "It's more important how the world sees me than how I see the world."

As a hand surgeon, I was called upon to treat a steady procession of direct injuries. A. E. Needham, a British biologist, estimates that the typical person suffers one minor wound a week, or about four thousand in a lifetime. The fingers and thumbs account for 95 percent of these wounds: paper cuts, cigarette burns, thorns, splinters. Leprosy patients, without the safeguard of pain, experience wounds much more frequently, and, because they keep on using the affected hand, severe damage often results. At least 90 percent of the insensitive hands I examine show scars and signs of deformity or injury.

Direct injuries were relatively easy for us to deal with. Patients understood them because they could see the damage. We merely had to keep the finger in a splint until it healed and then, just as we had at the New Life Center, teach patients the need for constant vigilance. We urged them to take responsibility for parts of their bodies they could not feel, relying on other senses for their clues. "Test your bath water with a thermometer in advance," I cautioned. "And never grip the handle of a tool without looking first to see if there's an edge that might cut you, or a splinter to stick into you." We put up posters illustrating the most common hazards.

The incidence of direct injuries at Carville began to decrease, especially as we relied on tools like the thermograph to monitor the early problems under the skin. Just as important, the patients improved at caring for wounds after an injury. A foot wound will heal if a patient tends to it. If, however, the patient keeps walking on the injured foot, infection may set in and spread through the foot, destroying bones and joints and making amputation inevitable. In the six years before we began the campaign against injuries, twenty-seven amputations had been performed at Carville; over the next few years the rate was zero.

Constant Stress

Other damage was much harder for us to track down. Human skin is tough: normally, it takes more than five hundred pounds of pressure per square inch to penetrate the skin and cause injury. But a constant, unrelieved pressure as low as one pound per square inch can do damage. Press a glass slide against your fingertip and the skin will blanch. Hold it there for a few hours and the skin, deprived of blood supply, will die.

A healthy person can sense the rising danger from constant stress. At first the finger or toe feels perfectly comfortable. After perhaps an hour a feeling of irritation sets in, followed by mild pain. Finally, intolerable pain intervenes just before the point of real damage. I can observe this cycle at work whenever I attend a banquet. The culprit is fashion: when women dress for special occasions they fall under the evil spell of shoe designers who favor narrow, pointed shoes and high heels. I glance under the table after an hour or two of dinner and speeches and observe that half the women have kicked off their fashionable shoes; they are giving their feet a few minutes of unimpeded circulation before subjecting them to another round of bloodlessness.*

I learned much about constant stress from a friendly pig named Sherman, who made an ideal subject for our experiments because pig skin has properties similar to those of human skin. We would anesthetize Sherman, put him in a plaster half-cast to keep him still, and apply very slight pressure to designated spots on his back. A cylindrical piston kept the pressure at a low but constant level for five to seven hours. Subsequent thermograms clearly showed that this very slight pressure caused inflammation in and under the skin. The pressure spot turned red, and hair perma-

---

*A Boeing engineer once received a call from a cargo company inquiring about transporting an elephant in a Boeing-designed plane. "Will we need to reinforce the floor?" the cargo executive asked. The engineer laughed and replied, "Don't worry. We design our floors for a woman in a stiletto heel." He went on to explain that a 100-pound woman standing on a heel that tapers down to a quarter-inch diameter (one-fourth-inch-by-one-fourth-inch) exerts a force of sixteen hundred pounds per square inch, far more than what an elephant exerts on his broad footpads.

nently stopped growing there. If we had kept up the pressure longer, an ulcer would have developed on Sherman's back.

I have many photographs of the pressure spots on Sherman's back, which neatly illustrate the process behind bedsores, the bane of modern hospitals. I have treated many bedsores, and some are as horrible as any surface wound you might find in a battlefield hospital. All bedsores trace back to the same cause: constant stress. A paralyzed or insensitive person tends to lie on the same spot hour after hour, shutting off the blood supply, and after about four hours of unrelieved pressure the tissue begins to die. People with a well-functioning nervous system do not get bedsores. A steady stream of quiet messages from the pain network will keep an active body tossing and turning in bed, redistributing the stress among the body's cells. If these quiet messages are ignored, the distressed region sends out a louder cry of real pain that forces the person to shift a buttock or turn over on one side to relieve the pressure.

(I notice a clear pattern whenever I deliver a lecture. As long as I manage to hold the audience's attention, I see much less restless activity. They are consciously attending to what I am saying, and thus squelching or ignoring the subtle messages of discomfort. As soon as my lecture gets boring, though, their mental concentration wanders and instinctively they tune in to the faint messages of distress from cells that have been sat on for too long. I can judge the effectiveness of my speech by watching how frequently members of the audience cross and uncross their legs and shift about in their seats.)

Our studies of constant stress helped us understand why a leprosy patient has such difficulty fitting shoes. When I came to Carville, I was surprised to find that U.S. patients had about the same incidence of amputated feet as their counterparts in India, many of whom went barefoot. The problem, we discovered, was that they were wearing shoes designed for patients who can feel pain. The risk of constant stress from poorly designed shoes is every bit as dangerous as the risk of direct injury from going barefoot. If my own shoes feel too tight, I loosen the laces or take them off and put on soft slippers. The leprosy patient, who feels no pain, leaves a tight shoe on even after pressure has shut off the blood supply. José, the California furniture salesman, lost some of his toes because of the quiet tedium of constant stress. Carville therapists began to require patients to change shoes at least once every five hours, a simple measure that, if followed, will prevent ulcers from ischemic pressure.

Repetitive Stress

In retrospect, the most valuable product of two decades of pain research was new insight into how ordinary, "harmless" stresses can cause severe damage to skin if they are repeated thousands of times. We first became aware of this syndrome in India while testing different kinds of footwear, but the research labs at Carville gave us the tools to discern exactly how repetitive stress does its work.

For several decades I had puzzled over why the simple act of walking represented such a threat to a leprosy patient. How is it, I wondered, that a healthy person can walk ten miles without injury while a leprosy patient often cannot? In an attempt to answer this question, Carville engineers rigged up a repetitive stress machine that reproduced the stresses of walking or running. The machine's tiny mechanical hammer repeatedly strikes the same area with a force calibrated to what a small region of the foot may endure while walking.

We used laboratory rats for these experiments, putting them to sleep and strapping them to the machine which proceeded to tap their footpads with a steady, rhythmic force. While the rats slept, their feet went for a simulated run. The results proved conclusively that a "harmless" force, repeated often enough, does indeed cause tissue breakdown. If we gave a rat enough rest between runs, it could build up layers of callus; if not, an open sore would develop on the footpad.

Several times I tested the machine on my own fingers. The first day I put my finger under the hammer, I felt no pain up to about one thousand strokes. The sensation felt rather pleasant, like a vibro-massage. After one thousand strokes, though, I began to feel tenderness. The second day it took far fewer strokes of the tiny hammer for me to sense tenderness. On the third day, I felt pain almost immediately.

I now knew that tiny pressures, if repeated often enough, could damage tissue, so that under certain circumstances the common act of walking might indeed prove dangerous. Yet I still had not answered the underlying question: What made the feet of leprosy patients more vulnerable to repetitive stress? I could walk ten miles without injury; why couldn't they?

Another invention, the slipper-sock, helped us solve that mystery. I had heard about a new way of applying herbicides to cultivated fields by using water-soluble microcapsules: the same rain that stimulated weed growth also dissolved the capsules, releasing a herbicide to kill the weeds. This clever invention gave me the idea of hiring a chemical research company to develop a tiny microcapsule that would break down as a result of pressure, not water. After many false starts we ended up with a slipper-sock made up of a thin foam that incorporated thousands of microcapsules of hard wax. The capsules contained bromphenol blue, a dye which turns blue in an alkaline medium. It took quite a lot of force to break the capsules, but the wax—exactly like human skin— would also break when subjected to the repetitive stress of many small forces. Now I had a convenient way to measure the pressure points involved in walking.

We built our own machines for making the microcapsules and suspended the dye in an acid medium to make it yellowish. The sur-rounding sock was alkaline, so that when the capsule broke, the dye would spill out and turn blue right away. Volunteer staff put on these socks, then their shoes, and started walking. After they had gone a few paces we removed the shoes and noted which were the highest-pressure points—the first spots to turn blue. As they walked farther, the blue areas spread wider, and the initial pressure points deepened in color. After fifty paces or so we had a good picture of all the danger areas. Then we tried the slipper-socks on patients.

After poring over thousands of used slipper-socks, I learned a lot about walking, but nothing more important than this: a person with an insensitive foot never changes his stride. In contrast, a healthy person changes his stride constantly.

A physical therapist in my office volunteered to run eight miles around the cement floor corridors of the Carville hospital in his stocking feet, pausing every two miles to let me take thermographic readings and test his stride in a slipper-sock. The first slipper-sock impression showed his normal walking pattern, a long stride with a high lift and a push from the great toe. The thermogram taken after two miles revealed a hot spot on his overworked great toe, and the slipper-sock showed that the main pressure point was on the inner side of his sole. After four miles, the signs of pressure shifted as his stride spontaneously adjusted. Now the outer side of his foot was outlined in bright blue, showing that his weight had shifted to the outside, away from the great toe, as the inner side took a long rest. By the time he ran the last two miles both the thermogram and the slipper-sock confirmed that he had again changed the way he put his feet to the ground: now the outer edge of his foot was getting hot and breaking the microcapsules.

The full set of thermograms and slipper-socks revealed a startling phenomenon: taken together, the socks portrayed a complete map of his foot, with strong blue dye at many different points. While the therapist himself was concentrating on jogging, his foot was sending out subconscious messages of pain. Although these tiny whispers from individual pressure and pain cells never made it all the way to his conscious brain, they did make it to his spinal cord and lower brain, which ordered subtle adjustments in his stride. Over the course of his run, the foot distributed pressure evenly, preventing any one spot from receiving too much repetitive stress.

I have never sent a leprosy patient on an eight-mile run, for that would be totally irresponsible. The reason shows up vividly in my slipper-socks taken from a patient's shorter runs: impressions before and after the run are virtually identical. The leprosy patient's stride never changed. Its pain pathways silenced, his central nervous system never perceived a need to make adjustments and so the same pressure—ten, twenty, or even sixty pounds per square inch—kept pounding on the same square inches of foot surface. If I had sent a leprosy patient on an eight-mile run, the thermogram would have shown just one or two areas of angry hot spots, the signs of damaged tissue. A few days later, I would likely see a plantar ulcer on the sole of the foot. Healthy long-distance runners seldom get plantar ulcers; leprosy patients often do.

Nowadays, repetitive stress injuries are widely recognized as a major problem in high-technology environments. More than 200,000 U.S. office and factory workers each year are treated for such conditions, accounting for 60 percent of the country's occupational illnesses. The frequency has doubled in less than a decade, mainly because technology tends to reduce the variety of movements required and thus increase repetitive stress. For example, so innocuous an action as typing, or operating a video game joystick, can by constant repetition subject the wrist to pressures that produce carpal tunnel syndrome. Computer keyboards are far more likely to cause injury than mechanical typewriters because the typist no longer has the relief of reaching up to move the carriage or pausing to change the paper. In the United States, repetitive stress injuries currently cost about $7 billion a year in lost productivity and medical costs.

Tuning In

It took many years of research to put together a full picture, but at last I understood. Pain employs a wide tonal range of conversation. It whispers to us in the early stages: at a subconscious level we sense a slight discomfort and change positions in bed, or adjust a jogging stride. It speaks louder as danger increases: a hand grows tender after a long stint at raking leaves, or a foot grows sore in new shoes. And pain shouts when the danger becomes severe: it forces a person to limp or even to hop or else quit running altogether.

Our research projects at Carville were giving us ever more powerful ways to "tune in" to pain, not unlike the astronomers who aim ever more powerful radio telescopes at the heavens. Our own instruments were aimed at the incessant hum of intercellular conversation that we so blithely take for granted—or even despise. As a result of our experiments, I made a conscious effort to begin listening to my messages of pain.

I love to take mountain hikes. Living in Louisiana curtailed that activity, but whenever I had the chance, on a trip back to the rocky hills of India or in the mountains of the American West, I took a hike and tried to pay closer attention to my feet. Normally I began the day with a long, energetic stride, lifting my heel and pushing off vigorously from my toes. As the morning wore on, I could sense the stride shortening a little, and the weight shifting from my great toe to the outer toes. I had taken many slipper-sock impressions of my own feet, so it was easy for me to visualize the changes taking place. After lunch, I noticed, I moved with an even shorter stride. Toward the end of the day, I was hardly lifting my heel at all, merely picking up a flat foot and putting a flat foot down—an old man's stride. That type of stride used the whole surface of my sole for every step, thus keeping the pressure low on any one spot.

Before, I had always thought of these adjustments as evidence of muscular fatigue. As our research had shown, they were in fact due much more to fatigue of the skin than of muscle. I now understood the changes as my body's loyal way of distributing stresses, sharing the burden of walking among different muscles and tendons and across different areas of skin. Occasionally I developed blisters. Instead of resenting them, I now understood them as my body's loud protest against overuse. Their very discomfort forced me to act, to take off my shoes and rest, adjust my stride even further, or add a layer of socks to relieve the friction.

Once, back at the leprosarium, I had an abrupt encounter with a loud "shout" of pain. I was walking along the sidewalk with my eyes lifted high, searching the treetops for the source of a lovely birdsong, when, *crash*, the next thing I knew I was lying face down on the path. I felt an instant flush of embarrassment and looked around quickly to see if anyone had seen me fall. I felt irritated, even angry. But then, as I rose to my feet and checked myself for injuries, I realized what had happened. As my eyes gazed upward toward the bird, my foot had wandered over to the edge of the sidewalk. I was in the process of putting all my weight on the foot, which hung precipitously over the concrete edge. My ankle began to twist until the tiny collateral ligament of the ankle sensed itself being stretched to the breaking point. Without consulting me, that little ligament set in motion a powerful pain message that forced the immediate slackening of the major muscle of my thigh. In the most peremptory fashion, that action deprived the knee of its muscular support and it collapsed. In short, I fell.

The more I reflected on the fall, the more I felt pride, not irritation. A minor ligament at the lower level of hierarchy had somehow commandeered my entire body. I felt grateful for its willingness to make me look a fool for the sake of the body, saving me from a certain ankle sprain and perhaps worse.

As I consciously tuned in to pain during such experiences, a different perspective began to take form and replace my natural aversion. Pain, my body's way of alerting me to danger, will use whatever volume level is necessary to grab my attention. It was their very deafness to this chorus of messages that caused my leprosy patients to destroy themselves. They missed the "shouts" of pain, leading to the direct injuries that I treated every day. And they also missed the whispers of pain, the dangers of the ordinary that come from constant or repetitive stress.

Without this chorus of pain, a leprosy patient lives in constant peril. He will wear too-tight shoes all day. He will walk five, ten, fifteen miles without changing gait or shifting weight. And, as

I had seen so often in India, even if sores break open inside his shoe, he will not limp.

I once saw a leprosy patient step on the edge of a stone just as I had on the sidewalk in Carville. He turned his ankle completely over so that the sole of his foot pointed inward—and walked on without a limp. I later learned that he had ruptured the left lateral ligament, severely damaging his ankle. At the time, he did not even glance at the foot. He lacked the indispensable protection of pain.

13
Beloved Enemy

───◆───

With the help of the thorn in my foot,
I spring higher than anyone with sound feet.
Søren Kierkegaard

I must confess that I sometimes question my crusade to improve the image of pain. In a society that routinely portrays pain as the enemy, will anyone listen to a contrarian message extolling its virtues? Does my own outlook merely reflect the oddity of a career among patients with the bizarre affliction of painlessness? The United States government eventually began asking these same questions. Why should Carville research money go toward restoring and enhancing pain when researchers elsewhere were focusing on how to suppress it?

In the early years our grant proposals for thermograph machines, ink-filled slipper-socks, and pressure transducers were usually approved. Visionaries in Washington supported basic research into pain even though it had immediate practical relevance for only a few thousand leprosy patients (and some Tennessee Walker horses). In the late 1970s, however, a new belt-tightening spirit made such research increasingly hard to justify. Each year the U.S. Public Health Service scrutinized the budget of the Carville hospital, weighing whether they could afford to invest so much money in research that would primarily benefit leprosy patients in other countries.

About this time, quite by accident I stumbled across a new practical application for what we had learned about pain at Carville, a fortunate turn of events that soon validated our entire investment in basic research. Although only a few thousand leprosy patients live in the United States, millions of diabetics live here, and we found that our ideas about pain had direct relevance to them as well.

Late one evening as I was scanning a medical journal I noticed the phrase "diabetic osteopathy." It struck me as odd: since when did diabetes, a disease of glucose metabolism, affect bones? Turning the page, I saw X-ray reproductions which looked exactly like X rays of the bone changes in the feet of my insensitive leprosy patients. I wrote to the authors, two doctors in Texas, who graciously invited me to visit them and discuss the topic.

A few months later I found myself in their Houston offices, involved in a good-natured contest of "dueling X rays." They would place an X ray of deteriorating bone on a light table, and I would rummage around in my briefcase until I found a matching X ray of bone absorption in a leprosy patient. We compared X rays of all the bones of the foot, and almost without exception I could duplicate each osteopathic problem they presented. The demonstration made a great impression on the doctors and interns assembled, for most of them had no experience with leprosy patients and thought they had described a syndrome peculiar to diabetes.

The Sugar Club

Next, the Texas doctors invited me to speak to the Southern Sugar Club, a genteel group of diabetes specialists from southern states who meet regularly to review the latest findings on diabetes. I addressed the subject of feet, challenging their assumption that the common problem with diabetic feet—ulceration so severe that it frequently leads to amputation—was caused primarily by diabetes itself or by the loss of blood supply that occurs in diabetes. My own observations had convinced me that the wounds were, like those of leprosy, caused by the loss of pain sensation.

In a vicious cycle, nerves die off because of the metabolic problems of diabetes,* the patients injure themselves because of the lack of pain, and the resulting wounds do not easily heal

---

*There is a striking difference in how nerve damage occurs in leprosy compared with diabetes. As I have said, leprosy germs congregate in cool areas, destroying nerves closest to the skin and producing an erratic pattern of paralysis. Diabetes, not a germ disease, alters the metabolism of sugar and the *longest* nerves suffer the nutritional deficit first. The critical feature seems to be the length of the axon that extends to the nerve endings. The toes tend

because the patient continues to walk on them. True, the reduced blood supply caused by diabetes complicates healing, but I had concluded that the typical diabetic foot still has plenty of blood supply to control infection and heal the wounds, as long as it is protected from further stress.

I recounted for the Sugar Club our long history of tracking similar injuries among leprosy patients in India, and then summarized our Carville findings on repetitive and constant stress. "I have examined the X rays of diabetics," I told them, "and frankly I think most of the foot injuries you see are preventable. They're caused by mechanical stress that goes unnoticed because the patient has lost pain sensation. Walking on wounded feet drives the infection deeper so that it involves the bones and joints, and with continued walking the bones are absorbed and the joints dislocate. We have found with our leprosy patients that resting the injured foot in a plaster cast will speed recovery. Fitting the patient with proper shoes will prevent further injury. I can almost guarantee you that proper shoes will dramatically reduce the number of foot injuries you see."

The chairman of the Sugar Club made a few remarks after my speech. "A fascinating lecture, Dr. Brand. I'm sure we have much to learn from your experiments at Carville. But of course you must recognize that diabetics have certain unique problems. I'm speaking especially of vascular loss. Diabetics simply lack the healing properties of your leprosy patients." My mind flashed back to gatherings of leprosy specialists where I had heard about "non-healing flesh." Wherever I went, it seemed, I met with skepticism over the far-reaching dangers of painlessness.

Returning to Carville, I informed local physicians that our foot clinic would offer consultation to any of their diabetic patients with foot problems. In addition to testing sensation, we also evaluated the overall blood supply to the feet. Their infected feet felt warm to the touch, and the thermograph revealed that

---

to be affected early on; then more of the nerve axon dies up the foot toward the ankle, creeping gradually up the leg. By the time the loss of sensation reaches as high as the knee, the longest axons in the arm are about the same length as the residual axons in the leg. At that point, nutritional deficit begins to affect the axons in the arm: the tips of the fingers go numb, then ultimately the hand, wrist, and forearm. The nerve damage progresses slowly, and most diabetics will have died before experiencing severe problems in the hand. But loss of foot sensation is very common.

ulcers in most diabetics produced hot spots almost as regularly as those in leprosy patients. Such evidence confirmed that most of these diabetic patients had plenty of blood available for healing.

Sensitivity tests verified that all the diabetics who had ulcers had indeed lost sensation: some of those with the worst ulcers had no sensitivity to pain on the soles of their feet. Furthermore, the ulcers on diabetic feet tended to occur at the same places as those on leprosy patients. It seemed clear to us that the fundamental cause of the ulcer was the same in both cases, a breakdown in the pain system. Apparently, nothing alerted the diabetics when they crossed a danger threshold, and they continued to walk on inflamed and damaged tissue, causing further harm. When I tested diabetics in slipper-socks I found a familiar pattern. Just like my leprosy patients, they walked with an unvarying stride, pounding the same foot surface over and over with repetitive stress. I now knew that diabetics were destroying their feet for the same reason as my leprosy patients: they lacked the sense of pain.

I studied the medical literature on diabetes. It advised doctors to expect injury and infection in the diabetic foot, often blaming poor circulation. Surgeons assumed that diabetics, with their reduced blood supply, had wounds that would not heal. I felt another wave of déjà vu, recalling the "bad flesh" arguments against treating leprosy patients that I had encountered in India. As had been the practice among leprosy specialists, when an ulcer became infected in a diabetic foot the surgeons often took off the leg below the knee before gangrene had time to spread.

I was astonished to read that diabetics were undergoing 100,000 amputations each year, accounting for half of all amputations in the United States. A patient over sixty-five had nearly a one in ten chance of foot amputation. If our theories were correct, tens of thousands of people were losing their limbs needlessly. But how could I, with a background in the rather obscure field of leprosy, get the attention of experts in another specialty?

A physician in Atlanta, Georgia, provided the solution. Dr. John Davidson, a renowned expert on diabetes, had attended the Southern Sugar Club, and I remember well our conversation after my speech. "Dr. Brand, I run the diabetic clinic at Grady Hospital, a charity hospital that treats over ten thousand diabetics a year," he said. "I must tell you, I'm skeptical about what you say. I haven't seen nearly the number of foot injuries you say I should. And I doubt seriously whether all the damage that I do see results from the loss of pain. But I want to be open-minded and so I'll check out your theories."

Back at his clinic in Atlanta, Davidson hired a podiatrist and instituted a simple rule: all patients had to take off their shoes and socks each time they came for a diabetic checkup. The podiatrist examined every foot, even if the patient had no complaints about feet. A few months later, Davidson called me, and this time I heard enthusiasm, not skepticism, in his voice. "You won't believe what I found out," he began. "I discovered that 150 of our patients had amputations last year, most of which we didn't even know about!

"It works like this," he explained. "They come into my office for a routine checkup, walking on an ulcer, and don't bother to mention it. Patients see me for regulation of insulin, urine tests, weight monitoring, and the like. When they get a foot injury, they visit a surgeon instead. The problem is, most of these patients don't report ulcers or ingrown toenails in the early stages because they don't feel any pain. By the time they visit the surgeon, the foot sore is in bad shape. And that accounts for all the amputations. The surgeon checks their charts, finds out they're diabetic, and says, 'Oh, we'd better amputate right away, or that leg will grow gangrenous.' All this time, I don't even know my patients have foot problems! The next time I see them for a checkup, they may be walking on an artificial leg, which they don't bother to mention either."

With a podiatrist now on staff, Davidson's clinic was able to interrupt the sequence. Detecting foot problems at an earlier stage, he could treat the sores and prevent serious infection. By the simple measure of requiring patients to take off their shoes and socks for a visual inspection, the clinic soon managed to cut its patients' amputation rate in half.

John Davidson became the number-one supporter of our foot clinic. He sent his entire staff of doctors, nurses, and therapists to Carville for training. He asked me to write a chapter on insensitive feet in his diabetes textbook and began reprinting our pamphlets on proper shoes and foot care. The Carville foot clinic got new life and, later, a formal name, the Foot Care Center. Its budget, instead of being slashed by the Public Health Service, was increased. Therapists, orthotic shoemakers, and physicians from around the United States began coming to Carville for regularly scheduled training conferences. A society of orthotic shoemak-ers—they call themselves "pedorthists"—developed standards of certification for providing footwear appropriate to insensitive feet.

Eventually the diabetic patients at our foot clinic outnumbered the leprosy patients. In most cases, the notion of "nonhealing wounds" proved as much a myth in diabetes as it had in leprosy. Our simple technique of keeping wounds in plaster casts for protection worked almost as well for diabetics. Ulcers chronic for years often healed within six weeks of the plaster cast routine. (Unlike in leprosy patients, in a minority of diabetic patients the blood supply is so reduced that healing is delayed and gangrene may set in even with good treatment.)

We also found that sores on diabetics' feet, like those on leprosy patients' feet, are preventable. Soaking the feet daily in a basin of water and using moisturizing cream does much to inhibit deep keratin cracks in the skin. And when we outfit diabetics in special footwear and teach them proper foot care, the ulcers tend not to recur. For a time the government considered issuing free shoes to needy diabetics, but, like other proposals that focus on prevention and not cure, that project never got approval. As a rule, I have found it is easier in the United States to obtain good artificial limbs than good shoes.

Wholly Indifferent

The Foot Care Center, now frequented by diabetics as well as leprosy patients, treated an endless parade of damaged feet. Wrapping gauze around a hundred foul, infected wounds caused by self-inflicted injury makes an impression, and I noticed a gradual change in perspective among the Carville nurses and therapists. When a new patient appeared for evaluation, we would first map out the range of insensitivity. I began to see the staff's faces brighten whenever they found a patient who retained sensation. Pain was good—the more potential for pain a patient had, the easier it was to keep that patient free of injury.

One memorable leprosy patient, a Hispanic man named Pedro, had retained a single spot of sensitivity on the palm of his left hand. That hand became for us an object of great curiosity. Thermograms revealed the sensitive spot to be six degrees hotter than the rest of the hand, hot enough to resist the invasion of cool-seeking leprosy bacilli. We noticed that Pedro approached objects with the edge of his hand, much as a dog leads with its searching nose. He picked up a cup of coffee only after testing the temperature with his feeling spot. Thanks to that single sensitive spot, the size of a nickel, Pedro had managed to keep his hand free of damage for fifteen years. (After much speculation we learned from Pedro that years before a doctor had burned off a birthmark there; a tangle of arteries under the surface continued to carry an increased blood supply to that one spot.)

The most difficult patients of all were those with the rare condition that made them totally insensitive to pain. In the opening chapter of this book I told the story of Tanya, a patient who had this malady. There were three such patients at Carville when I arrived, all originally misdiagnosed as having leprosy because of their deformities. (I have since learned when visiting a leprosy hospital for the very first time to ask to see the most deformed young patients in the hospital. The staff brings out a few children who are missing parts of hands and feet, and perhaps wearing an artificial limb. Typically I find that these children do not have leprosy but rather, like Tanya, suffer from a congenital defect of painlessness. In leprosy, it takes some years for sensation to be lost, so young children rarely damage themselves severely. When I find these misdiagnosed children I can get them released from the leprosarium, but they usually do better staying under the close supervision of an institution. Outside, life without pain is too dangerous.)

More than a hundred cases of congenital painlessness have been written up in medical literature. In the 1920s the painless Edward H. Gibson went on vaudeville tour as the Human Pincushion to demonstrate his "talent," inviting members of the audience to stick pins in him. Indeed, an aura of freakishness hangs over all accounts of this strange malady. A teenager dislocated his shoulders at will to entertain his friends. An eight-year-old girl pulled out all but nine of her teeth and poked both eyes out of their sockets. Another youngster bit his tongue in half while chewing gum.

For the painless, danger lurks everywhere. A larynx that never feels a tickle does not trigger the cough reflex that relocates phlegm from the lungs to the pharynx, and a person who never coughs runs the risk of developing pneumonia. The bone joints of insensitive people deteriorate because there are no whispers of pain encouraging a shift in position, and soon bone grinds against bone. Strep throat, appendicitis, heart attack, stroke—the body has no way to announce these threats to the painless person. Often the attending physician gets the first clue to the cause of death at the time of autopsy.

On a visit to McGill University in Canada I saw the specimens from one such autopsy on Jane, a female student who had just turned twenty. Like the segments of an old tree, her body gave a visible record of natural disasters of the past. I saw signs of frostbite, probably from the recent harsh winter. The inside of Jane's mouth was scarred, no doubt from being scalded by hot drinks and food. Some of her muscles had torn, unavoidable for someone who never felt the muscle soreness that warns against overuse. Her hands and feet resembled the plaster models I had made of my most deformed leprosy patients, with many missing and shortened digits.

Dr. McNaughton, the chief neurologist, told me some of Jane's history. "Jane was usually very careful, our prize patient. As you know, twenty is a ripe old age for someone with this condition. Her recent problems started with an auto mishap. Her car slid off an icy road into a ditch, and when she gunned the engine the tires spun. She must have panicked, because she got out of the car and foolishly tried to lift a wheel to slide a traction mat under it. Something went wrong—she heard a cracking sound—and she lost strength. Of course, she felt nothing.

"When she freed her car, she drove straight here for a checkup. We X-rayed, and found that her backbone had cracked right through. Imagine—a broken back and she didn't feel a thing! We put her in a plaster cast."

Insensitivity often affects sympathetic nerves as well, interfering with the ability to sweat. After a few weeks, Dr. McNaughton said, Jane began to feel hot in her plaster cast, so hot that she ripped it off with her bare hands, tearing her fingers in the process. The back healed improperly, with a false joint between vertebrae (he showed me X rays of the misaligned joint). One day when Jane bent over, the false joint slid across the spinal cord, severing it. The last few months of her life, Jane was paralyzed.

People do not die of paralysis, though, so it was not the back injury that killed Jane. She died of a simple urinary infection. Complicated by incontinence and her inability to feel any warning signs of pain, the infection did irreversible damage to her kidneys.

I returned to Carville determined to use Jane as an object lesson for my own painless patients. "Never let up!" I warned them. "You must be diligent all day long. Never stop thinking about ways in which you might be hurting yourself."

I wish I could report success in my education campaign, but in truth I cannot. Not long after the trip to Canada, I found James, a congenitally painless patient, straddling a hot automobile engine with his two amputee stumps, putting all his weight behind a sharp-edged wrench in an attempt to loosen a nut. I have never found a way to communicate to painless people the lessons that are taught so innately and compellingly by a healthy pain system.

Muffling Pain

Tanya, James, and others like them dramatically reinforced what we had already learned from leprosy patients: pain is not the enemy, but the loyal scout announcing the enemy. And yet—here is the central paradox of my life—after spending a lifetime among people who destroy themselves for lack of pain, I still find it difficult to communicate an appreciation for pain to people who have no such defect. Pain truly is the gift nobody wants. I can think of nothing more precious for those who suffer from congenital painlessness, leprosy, diabetes, and other nerve disorders. But people who already own this gift rarely value it. Usually, they resent it.

My esteem for pain runs so counter to the common attitude that I sometimes feel like a subversive, especially in modern Western countries. On my travels I have observed an ironic law of reversal at work: as a society gains the ability to limit suffering, it loses the ability to cope with what suffering remains. (It is the philosophers, theologians, and writers of the affluent West, not the Third World, who worry obsessively about "the problem of pain," and point an accusing finger at God.)

Certainly, the "less advanced" societies do not fear physical pain as much. I have watched Ethiopians sit calmly, with no anesthetic, as a dentist works his forceps back and forth around a decaying tooth. Women in Africa often deliver their babies without the use of drugs and with no sign of fear or anxiety. These traditional cultures may lack modern analgesics, but the beliefs and family support systems built into everyday life help equip individuals to cope with pain. The average Indian villager knows suffering well, expects it, and accepts it as an unavoidable challenge of life.

In a remarkable way the people of India have learned to control pain at the level of the mind and spirit, and have developed endurance that we in the West find hard to understand. Westerners, in contrast, tend to view suffering as an injustice or failure, an infringement on their guaranteed right to happiness.

Shortly after I moved to the United States I saw a commercial that blatantly expressed the modern attitude toward pain. The sound turned down, I sat before the television set and watched images flicker across the screen. First, a man in a laboratory coat pointed excitedly to a large drawing of the human head. Bright red streaks, like cartoon lightning bolts, converged on the head just above the eyes and at the base near the neck region. The announcer, who wore a perpetual smile, was describing a headache.

Next I saw a laboratory bench. Blank white paper covered two oversized bottles; the third was boldly marked with a brand name. As the man in the lab coat picked up the bottles, one by one, the camera switched to a large bar graph showing how many milligrams of pain reliever each product contained. Not surprisingly, the brand-name bottle had the most milligrams.

Next the camera showed a large green clock with a single hand, the second hand, sweeping across its face. The man pointed to the clock and back to the labeled bottle. The camera zoomed in on a closeup of the bottle and these words appeared on-screen: "More pain reliever. Faster acting."

In the modern view pain is an enemy, a sinister invader that must be expelled. And if Product X removes pain thirty seconds faster, all the better. This approach has a crucial, dangerous flaw: once regarded as an enemy, not a warning signal, pain loses its power to instruct. Silencing pain without considering its message is like disconnecting a ringing fire alarm to avoid receiving bad news.

I long for a commercial that at least acknowledges some benefit to pain: "First, listen to your pain. It is your own body talking to you." I too may take an aspirin to relieve a tension headache, but only after pausing to ask what brought on the nervous tension that provoked the headache. I have taken antacid for stomach pain, but not before considering what I might have eaten to give me such pain. Did I eat too much? Too fast? Pain is no invading enemy, but a loyal messenger dispatched by my own body to alert me to some danger.

Frantic attempts to silence pain signals may actually have a paradoxical effect.* The United States consumes thirty thousand tons of aspirin a year, averaging out to 250 pills per person. Newer and better pain relievers are constantly introduced, and consumers gulp them down: one-third of all drugs sold are agents that work on the central nervous system. Americans, who represent 5 percent of the world's population, consume 50 percent of its manufactured drugs. Yet what does this obsession gain? I see little evidence that Americans feel better equipped to cope with pain and suffering. Addiction to drugs and alcohol, a primary means of escaping grim reality, has mushroomed. In the years I have lived here, more than one thousand pain centers have opened to help people battle the enemy that will not surrender. The emergence of "chronic pain syndrome," a phenomenon rarely seen in non-Western countries or in medical literature from the past, should set off alarms for a culture committed to painlessness.

With all our resources, why can't we "solve" pain? Many people hope for a solution that will give us the ability to eliminate pain, but I dread what might happen if scientists ever do succeed in perfecting a "painlessness" pill. Already I see worrisome signs, as technology finds more effective ways to muffle the din of pain. Two examples, one from professional sports and one from a frostbite treatment center, give an ominous preview of the consequences.

Professional sports trainers excel at overriding pain signals. Injured football players disappear into the locker room for a painkiller injection, then return to the field with a broken finger

---

*A possible explanation for this phenomenon can be found in the human body's desire to conserve energy. Stop using a muscle and it will atrophy. Likewise, if I inject artificial doses of adrenaline and cortisone into a patient the adrenal gland, which normally produces those hormones, will cut back; over time it may shut down production completely. Some pain researchers believe that an addiction to painrelieving medications may have a similar effect on the brain. If we suppress the need for brain endorphins (the body's natural painkillers) by providing artificial substitutes, the brain may "forget how" to produce the natural substances. Heroin addicts show the final result: an addict's brain demands more and more artificial substances because it can no longer satisfy the cravings of its own opiate receptor sites. Long-term heroin addicts sometimes develop a hypersensitivity to pain after they come off the drug. The slightest pressure of a sheet or clothing causes intense pain because the brain no longer manufactures the neurotransmitters that deal with such routine stimuli.

or rib wrapped in tape. In one NBA basketball game a star player, Bob Gross, was asked to start despite a badly injured ankle. The team doctor injected Marcaine, a strong painkiller, into Gross's foot in three different places. During the game, as Gross was battling for a rebound, a loud *snap!* could be heard throughout the arena. Oblivious, Gross ran up and down the court two times, then crumpled to the floor. Although he felt no pain, a bone had broken in his ankle. By canceling out pain's warning system, Gross had laid himself open to an injury that caused permanent damage and prematurely ended his basketball career.

The second example comes from a visit I had in the 1960s with Dr. John Boswick, an authority on frostbite at Chicago's Cook County Hospital. He led me to a large, open ward where thirty-seven victims of severe frostbite lay, their bedsheets pulled back to expose seventy-four ugly blackened feet. (In treating frostbite, doctors leave the affected part open to the air so that it can dry off; the body soon walls off necrotic tissue, which can then be removed.) The sickly odor of gangrene hung in the air. I had seen nothing quite like that scene anywhere, and I was appalled. "I would think a city like Chicago would provide a shelter for these homeless people!" I said.

Boswick laughed. "These aren't homeless people, Paul. They all have access to shelters, and some of them are middle-class. They're either alcoholic or addicted to drugs. They go out and party, and can't find their way home. Or maybe somebody drops them off at their front door but they're too drunk to work the key in the lock. So they lie down and fall asleep on their own doorstep, or maybe lean into a snowdrift. Alcohol has dulled all sensation of pain and cold by then, and the snow feels fine. It feels quite good, really. They fall asleep, and next morning the family finds them in the front yard, sleeping contentedly. I deal with the damage that results from the numbed pain cells. Look at these fellows—some of them may lose a whole foot."

These two examples serve as a warning metaphor for modern society, depicting in the extreme what can happen when pain is silenced. I have lived many years among people who do not feel pain, and they are to be pitied, not envied. Rather than trying to "solve" pain, by eliminating it, we must learn to listen to it, and then manage it. That shift will require a radical change in outlook, one that cuts across the grain of Americans' we-can-fix-it optimism.

A Poor Substitute

During one period I conducted two regular clinics each week, one in Baton Rouge attended mainly by rheumatoid arthritis patients, the other at Carville for diabetes and leprosy. Rheumatoid arthritis is an autoimmune disorder in which the joints swell up in painful inflammation and the body attacks its own tissue. Sometimes I used the leprosy patients as an object lesson for those with rheumatoid arthritis, in an effort to convince them of pain's value. "Look at these leprosy patients," I said. "Do you envy them? Your disease is far more destructive to the body than leprosy infection itself. [In rheumatoid arthritis the bone grows soft and fragile, the ligaments give way and detach from joints, the muscles stretch and misalign.] And yet look at your fine hands! You have all five fingers intact. You've done a much better job protecting yourself than the folks over there with leprosy—simply because you feel pain. They have strong bones and joints, but notice all the missing fingers. Thank pain. It prevents you from abusing your fingers."

My sermonettes fell on deaf ears. Rheumatoid arthritis patients do not often express gratitude for the pain that saves their hands and feet; instead, they beg me to relieve their pain. Some, in search of relief, take steroids in such massive doses that their bones decalcify and their finger knuckles wobble, jointless. One overweight, bedridden patient took so many steroids that when she finally ventured from bed her foot bones crumbled like chalk. Rheumatoid arthritis often presents its victims with a classic dilemma: whether to silence pain and destroy the body, or listen to pain and preserve the body. In an even contest, pain rarely wins.

Why? For me, that was the conundrum of pain, in a nutshell. Why would our own minds inflict on us a state that we automatically choose against? I could easily demonstrate the overall benefit of pain: I need only take a skeptic on a guided tour of a leprosarium. But certain objections to the pain system, which I had distilled down to two questions, were not so easily resolved.

The first question—Why must pain be unpleasant?—I knew the answer to, an answer that underlay my entire approach to pain. The very unpleasantness of pain, the part we hate, is what makes it so effective at protecting us. I knew that answer theoretically, but the debilitating effect of pain on patients sometimes made me wonder. A related question followed: Why must pain persist? Surely we would better appreciate pain if our bodies came equipped with an on-off feature, allowing us to switch off the warning at will.

These two questions bothered me for many years. I kept returning to them, as if fingering an old scar. Despite my crusading efforts to improve the image of pain, I never fully resolved the two questions in my own mind until I embarked on a new research project, our most ambitious project to date at Carville.

My grant application bore the title "A Practical Substitute for Pain." We proposed developing an artificial pain system to replace the defective system in people who suffered from leprosy, congenital painlessness, diabetic neuropathy, and other nerve disorders. Our proposal stressed the potential economic benefits: by investing a million dollars to find a way to alert such patients to the worst dangers, the government might save many millions in clinical treatment, amputations, and rehabilitation.

The proposal caused a stir at the National Institutes of Health in Washington. They had received applications from scientists who wanted to diminish or abolish pain, but never from one who wished to create pain. Nevertheless, we received funding for the project.

We planned, in effect, to duplicate the human nervous system on a very small scale. We would need a substitute "nerve sensor" to generate signals at the extremity, a "nerve axon" or wiring system to convey the warning message, and a response device to inform the brain of the danger. Excitement grew in the Carville research laboratory. We were attempting something that, to our knowledge, had never been tried.

I subcontracted with the electrical engineering department at Louisiana State University to develop a miniature sensor for measuring temperature and pressure. One of the engineers there joked about the potential for profit: "If our idea works, we'll have a pain system that warns of danger but doesn't hurt. In other words, we'll have the good parts of pain without the bad! Healthy people will demand these gadgets for themselves in place of their own pain systems. Who wouldn't prefer a warning signal through a hearing aid over real pain in a finger?"

The LSU engineers soon showed us prototype transducers, slim metal disks smaller than a shirt button. Sufficient pressure on these transducers would alter their electrical resistance, triggering an electrical current. They asked our research team to determine what thresholds of pressure should be programmed into the miniature sensors. I replayed my university days in Tommy Lewis's pain laboratory, with one big difference: now, instead of merely testing the in-built properties of a well-designed human body, I had to think like the designer. What dangers would that body face? How could I quantify those dangers in a way the sensors could measure?

To simplify matters, we focused on fingertips and the soles of feet, the two areas that caused our patients the most problems. But how could we get a mechanical sensor to distinguish between the acceptable pressure of, say, gripping a fork and the unacceptable pressure of gripping a piece of broken glass? How could we calibrate the stress level of ordinary walking and yet allow for the occasional extra stress of stepping off a curb or jumping over a puddle? Our project, which we had begun with such enthusiasm, seemed more and more daunting.

I remembered from student days that nerve cells change their perception of pain in accordance with the body's needs. We say a finger feels tender: thousands of nerve cells in the damaged tissue automatically lower their threshold of pain to discourage us from using the finger. An infected finger seems as if it is always getting bumped—it "sticks out like a sore thumb"—because inflammation has made it ten times more sensitive to pain. No mechanical transducer could be so responsive to the needs of living tissue.

Every month the optimism level of the researchers went down a notch. Our Carville team, who had made the significant findings about repetitive stress and constant stress, knew that the worst dangers came not from abnormal stresses, but from very normal stresses repeated thousands of times, as in the act of walking. And Sherman the pig had demonstrated that a constant pressure as low as one pound per square inch could cause skin damage. How could we possibly program all these variables into a miniature transducer? We would need a computer chip on every sensor just to keep track of changing vulnerability of tissues to damage from repetitive stress. We gained a new respect for the human body's capacity to sort through such difficult options instantaneously.

After many compromises we settled on baseline pressures and temperatures to activate the sensors, and then designed a glove and a sock to incorporate several transducers. At last we could test our substitute pain system on actual patients. Now we ran into mechanical problems. The sensors, state-of-the-art electronic miniatures, tended to deteriorate from metal fatigue or corrosion after a few hundred uses. Short-circuits made them fire off false alarms, which aggravated our volunteer patients. Worse, the sensors cost about $450 each and a leprosy patient who took a long walk around the hospital grounds could wear out a $2,000 sock!

On average, a set of transducers held up to normal wear-and-tear for one or two weeks. We certainly could not afford to let a patient wear one of our expensive gloves for a task like raking leaves or pounding a hammer—the very activities we were trying to make safe. Before long the patients were worrying more about protecting our transducers, their supposed protectors, than about protecting themselves.

Even when the transducers worked correctly, the entire system was contingent on the free will of the patients. We had grandly talked of retaining "the good parts of pain without the bad," which meant designing a warning system that would not hurt. First we tried a device like a hearing aid that would hum when the sensors were receiving normal pressures, buzz when they were in slight danger, and emit a piercing sound when they perceived an actual danger. But when a patient with a damaged hand turned a screwdriver too hard, and the loud warning signal went off, he would simply override it—*This glove is always sending out false signals*—and turn the screwdriver anyway. Blinking lights failed for the same reason.

Patients who perceived "pain" only in the abstract could not be persuaded to trust the artificial sensors. Or they became bored with the signals and ignored them. The sobering realization dawned on us that unless we built in a quality of compulsion, our substitute system would never work. Being alerted to the danger was not enough; our patients had to be forced to respond. Professor Tims of LSU said to me, almost in despair, "Paul, it's no use. We'll never be able to protect these limbs unless the signal really hurts. Surely there must be some way to hurt your patients enough to make them pay attention."

We tried every alternative before resorting to pain, and finally concluded Tims was right: the stimulus had to be unpleasant, just as pain is unpleasant. One of Tims's graduate students developed a small battery-operated coil that, when activated, sent out an electric shock at high voltage but low current. It was harmless but painful, at least when applied to parts of the body that could feel pain.

Leprosy bacilli, favoring the cooler parts of the body, usually left warm regions such as the armpit undisturbed, and so we began taping the electric coil to patients' armpits for our tests. Some volunteers dropped out of the program, but a few brave ones stayed on. I noticed, though, that they viewed pain from our artificial sensors in a different way than pain from natural sources. They tended to see the electric shocks as punishment for breaking rules, not as messages from an endangered body part. They responded with resentment, not an instinct of self-preservation, because our artificial system had no innate link to their sense of *self*. How could it, when they felt a jolt in the armpit for something happening to the hand?

I learned a fundamental distinction: a person who never feels pain is task-oriented, whereas a person who has an intact pain system is self-oriented. The painless person may know by a signal that a certain action is harmful, but if he really wants to, he does it anyway. The pain-sensitive person, no matter how much he wants to do something, will stop for pain, because deep in his psyche he knows that preserving his own self is more significant than anything he might want to do.

Our project went through many stages, consuming five years of laboratory research, thousands of man-hours, and more than a million dollars of government funds. In the end we had to abandon the entire scheme. A warning system suitable for just one hand was exorbitantly expensive, subject to frequent mechanical breakdown, and hopelessly inadequate to interpret the profusion of sensations that constitute touch and pain. Most important, we found no way around the fundamental weakness in our system: it remained under the patient's control. If the patient did not want to heed the warnings from our sensors, he could always find a way to bypass the whole system.

Looking back, I can point to a single instant when I knew for certain that the substitute pain project would not succeed. I was looking for a tool in the manual arts workshop when Charles, one of our volunteer patients, came in to replace a gasket on a motorcycle engine. He wheeled the bike across the concrete floor, kicked down the kickstand, and set to work on the gasoline engine. I watched him out of the corner of my eye. Charles was one of our most conscientious volunteers, and I was eager to see how the artificial pain sensors on his glove would perform.

One of the engine bolts had apparently rusted, and Charles

made several attempts to loosen it with a wrench. It did not give. I saw him put some force behind the wrench, and then stop abruptly, jerking backward. The electric coil must have jolted him. (I could never avoid wincing when I saw our man-made pain system function as it was designed to do.) Charles studied the situation for a moment, then reached up under his armpit and disconnected a wire. He forced the bolt loose with a big wrench, put his hand in his shirt again, and reconnected the wire. It was then that I knew we had failed. Any system that allowed our patients freedom of choice was doomed.

I never fulfilled my dream of "a practical substitute for pain," but the process did at last set to rest the two questions that had long haunted me. Why must pain be unpleasant? Why must pain persist? Our system failed for the precise reason that we could not effectively reproduce those two qualities of pain. The mysterious power of the human brain can force a person to STOP!—something I could never accomplish with my substitute system. And "natural" pain will persist as long as danger threatens, whether we want it to or not; unlike my substitute system, it cannot be switched off.

As I worked on the substitute system, I sometimes thought of my rheumatoid arthritis patients, who yearned for just the sort of on-off switch we were installing. If rheumatoid patients had a switch or a wire they could disconnect, most would destroy their hands in days or weeks. How fortunate, I thought, that for most of us the pain switch will always remain out of reach.

In November 1972, about the same time I was reconciling myself to the failure of our project, I received word that my daughter Mary had delivered our first grandson. Some months passed before I could make my way to Minnesota to investigate this new phenomenon. When I arrived, Mary proudly presented a healthy boy named Daniel. I confess that for a few minutes I slipped back into my orthopedist's role, examining his finger joints, the curve in his spine, and the angle of his feet, all of which checked out splendidly. There was one more test to conduct, however, and I waited until Mary left the room before trying it.

With an ordinary straight pin, I performed a simple evaluation of the pain system on the tip of one finger. I was gentle, of course, but I had to do it. Daniel yanked his hand back, frowned, looked at the finger, and then looked at me. He was normal! His reflex worked according to design, and already at his young age he was learning an important lesson about straight pins. I held him close to my chest and prayed a prayer of thanksgiving for that tiny finger. The most elaborate glove we had developed at Carville included a grand total of twenty transducers and cost us nearly ten thousand dollars. This toddler came equipped with a thousand pain detectors in that one fingertip alone, each calibrated to a threshold specific to the fingertip. I felt a little grandfatherly pride, because my own personal genetic code was involved in the making of that little boy. As an engineer I had failed to create a pain system with my expensive electronic transducers, but my DNA had wildly succeeded.

It defied my comprehension that Daniel's miniature transducers would be able to sift through the many varieties of traumatic, constant, and repetitive stress and report in to the spinal column, with no short-circuits in the wiring and no need for outside maintenance, for a period of seventy or eighty years. More, these pain sensors would work whether he wanted them to or not; the switch was out of reach. The sensors were accurate, they were prompt, and they compelled a response, even from a brain too young to comprehend the meaning of danger. I ended my prayer with a familiar refrain, "Thank God for pain!"

Part Three

Learning to Befriend Pain

14
In the Mind

◆—◆—◆

English, which can express the thoughts of Hamlet and the tragedy of Lear, has no words for the shiver or the headache. . . . The merest schoolgirl when she falls in love has Shakespeare or Keats to speak her mind for her, but let a sufferer try to describe a pain in his head to a doctor and language at once runs dry.

Virginia Woolf

I am not a "pain expert" in the traditional sense. I have never worked in a pain clinic and have had limited experience in pain management. Instead, I came to appreciate the subtleties of pain by treating those who do not feel it. I certainly never said "Thank God for pain!" as a child in the Kolli hills, or in medical school during the Blitz; that outlook came after years of working among victims of painlessness.

Other patients, not to mention my own children, gave constant reminders of the more common attitude toward pain: "It hurts! How do I stop it?" Over the years, I have tried to fit together an approach that includes what I learned from the painless as well as from those of us who feel pain. We cannot live well without pain, but how do we best live with it? Pain is a priceless, essential gift—of that I have no doubt. And yet only by learning to master pain can we keep it from mastering us.

I divide the experience of pain into three stages. First there is the pain *signal*, an alarm that goes off when nerve endings in the periphery sense danger. My ill-fated project to develop "a practical substitute for pain" was an attempt to reproduce pain at this first, most basic level.

At a second stage of pain, the spinal cord and base of the brain act as a "spinal gate" to sort out which of the many millions of signals deserve to be forwarded as a *message* to the brain.

Damage or disease may sometimes interfere: if the spinal cord is severed, as in paraplegia, peripheral nerve endings below the break may continue to discharge pain signals, but those signals will not reach the brain.

The final stage of pain takes place in the higher brain (especially the cerebral cortex), which sorts through the prescreened messages and decides on a *response*. Indeed, pain does not truly exist until the entire cycle of signal, message, response has been completed.

A simple, everyday mishap—a little girl's fall while running— illustrates the interplay among these three stages of pain. When her knee first scrapes against the sidewalk, she rolls sideways to avoid further contact. This emergency maneuver, ordered by the spinal cord, takes place at the reflex level (stage one). Half a second passes before the girl becomes conscious of stinging sensations from her scraped knee. How she then responds will depend on the severity of the scrape, her own personality makeup, and what else is going on around her.

If the girl is running in a race with friends, chances are the noise and overall excitement of play will produce competing messages (stage two) that block the further progress of the pain. She may get up and finish the race without even glancing at her knee. When the race is over, though, and excitement dies down, pain messages will likely stream through the spinal gate to the thinking part of the brain (stage three). The girl looks at the knee, sees blood, and now the conscious brain takes over. Fear enhances the pain. Mother becomes important, and that is where the child turns. A wise mother first hugs her daughter, replacing the fear with reassurance. Then she fusses over the sore, washes away the blood, covers the wound with a decorative adhesive bandage, and sends the child back to play. The girl forgets about the pain. Later, in the night, when nothing is distracting the mind, the pain may return and her parents will be called back on duty.

All this time the actual pain signals have not changed much. Loyal neurons in the knee have been sending in damage reports all afternoon and evening. The girl's perception of the pain varies mostly by the extent to which the pain was blocked at stage two, by competing input, and, at stage three, by the parents' resourcefulness in calming anxiety.

In adults, who have a larger pool of experience and emotions to draw from, the mind plays a more paramount role. As a doctor I have gained an ever-increasing appreciation for the mind's ability to alter the perception of pain in one direction or the other. We can become adept at converting pain into the more serious state that we call *suffering*. Or, to the contrary, we can learn to harness the vast resources of the conscious mind to help cope with the pain.

The Orphan Sense

In medical school I mainly encountered pain at stage one. Patients came to me with specific complaints about signals in the periphery ("My finger hurts." "My stomach aches." "My ears are ringing."). No patient ever said to me something along this line: "Among the many transmissions entering my spinal cord, signals of pain from my finger have been judged of significant value to be forwarded on to the brain." Or "I am feeling pain in my stomach; could you please administer a morphinelike drug to my brain so that it will ignore the pain signals emanating from my stomach?"

Although I had to rely on the patient's report of stage one to help me diagnose the cause of pain, I soon realized the importance of responding to stage three from the start. Now I would probably rank the stages of pain in the reverse order, giving prominence to the third stage first. What takes place in a person's mind is the most important aspect of pain—and the most difficult to treat or even comprehend. If we can learn to handle pain at this third stage, we will most likely succeed in keeping pain in its proper place, as servant and not master.

I once knew a ballerina who felt severe pain in her foot every time she performed one particular maneuver on the point of her toe. Tchaikovsky's *Swan Lake* called for this maneuver thirty-two times in the course of the ballet, and for that reason she dreaded *Swan Lake*. Whenever the music came over the radio she would leap to her feet and switch it off. "I can actually feel the pain in my foot when I hear those chords!" she said. What took place in her mind affected what she perceived in her foot.

I first became aware of the power of the mind when I treated the soldier named Jake, the war hero with shattered legs who shrank in fear from a hypodermic needle full of penicillin. Later I learned that Jake's attitude at the front, strange as it seemed at the time, was a classic response to combat injury. Dr. Henry K. Beecher of the Harvard Medical School coined the term "Anzio effect" to describe what he observed among 215 casualties from the Anzio beachhead in World War II. Only one in four soldiers with serious injuries (fractures, amputations, penetrated chests or cerebrums) asked for morphine, though it was freely available. They simply did not need help with the pain, and indeed many of them denied feeling pain at all.

Beecher, an anesthesiologist, contrasted the soldiers' reactions to what he had seen in private practice, where 80 percent of patients recovering from surgical wounds begged for morphine or other narcotics. He concluded, "There is no simple direct relationship between the wound *per se* and the pain experienced. The pain is in very large part determined by other factors, and of great importance here is the significance of the wound. . . . In the wounded soldier the response to injury was relief, thankfulness at his escape alive from the battlefield, even euphoria; to the civilian, his major surgery was a depressing, calamitous event."

My study of the brain, especially in the dissection project in Cardiff, helped me understand why the mind plays such an important role in pain. The structure of the brain requires it. Only one-tenth of 1 percent of the fibers entering the cerebral cortex convey new sensory information, including pain messages; all the other nerve cells communicate one with another, reflecting, sifting through memory and emotion. Am I afraid? Is the pain producing something of value? Do I really want to recover? Am I getting sympathy?

Moreover, the conscious brain composes its response to this swirl of data inside the skull, secluded from the stimulus that caused the pain in the first place. Most sensations have a referent "out there," and we enjoy inviting others to share what excites our senses: "Look at that mountain!" "Listen closely, here comes the good part." "Feel his fur—it's so soft." But along comes the overpowering sensation of pain and each of us is orphaned. Pain has no "outside" existence. Two people can look at the same tree; no one has ever shared a stomachache. This is what makes the treatment of pain so difficult. None of us, doctor, parent, or friend, can truly enter into another person's pain. It is the loneliest, most private sensation.

How do you feel? How bad does it hurt? We can ask these questions, and form an idea about someone else's pain, but never with certainty. Patrick Wall, a pioneer in pain theory, states the dilemma: "Pain is my pain as it grows as an imperative obsession, a compulsion, a dominating reality. Your pain is a different matter. . . . Even if I have experienced a similar situation I only know my pain and guess at yours. If you hit your finger with a hammer I squirm as I remember how my thumb felt when I hit my own thumb. I can only assume how you feel." Wall says he has learned to respect a patient's own description, no matter how hazy, for despite what any high-tech diagnostic instruments may indicate, in the final analysis the patient's verbal report is the only possible account of the pain.*

And yet, although pain is an orphan sense that no one else can truly share, it seems to be indispensable in helping form one's personal identity. I hurt, therefore I am. The brain relies on a "felt image" of body parts to construct its inner map of the body; when nerve damage disrupts the flow of data to the brain, that puts the basic sense of self at risk. Speaking metaphorically, we use the word *dead* to describe a temporary state of painlessness, as when a dentist deadens a tooth or when we leave a leg crossed so long that it goes numb. Leprosy patients seem to regard their hands and feet as truly dead. The limb is there—they can see it—but with no sensory feedback to nourish the felt image in their brains, they lose the innate awareness that the numbed hand or foot belongs to the rest of the body.

I have seen this principle at work rather grotesquely in laboratory animals. For a while I used white rats to help determine the best design of shoes for the insensitive feet of leprosy patients. I would deaden a pain center in one hind leg and then imitate the stress of different types of shoes on the rat foot. I had to keep

---

*To help in the diagnosis of pain, Wall's colleague Ronald Melzack developed a pain chart based on the patient's perspective. He noted that patients tended to use certain combinations of words in describing particular ailments. Word like *dull, sore, aching,* or *heavy* describe a different kind of pain than *sharp, cutting, lacerating, burning, searing, scalding;* or *jumping, throbbing, thriving, pulsing.* Melzack admits these words are metaphorical, as is almost all our talk about pain. "It feels like someone is stabbing me in the eyes with knitting needles," a sufferer from migraine might say, or an injured runner might describe her leg as being "on fire," even though neither has experienced the actual pain of being stabbed in the eyes with knitting needles or having a leg held over a fire. We must rely on borrowed images to express the inexpressible. We report a "stabbing" pain, imagining a knife splitting flesh, although those who have been stabbed describe an entirely different sensation: not quick and violent penetration, but more like a blow that lands and does not let up.

these research animals well fed, for if they got hungry they would simply start to eat the deadened leg, a rat no longer recognizing it as part of self. Similarly, a wolf, its leg gone numb from the pressure of a trap and the cold, will calmly gnaw through fur and bone and limp away.

A Dominant Role

An amoeba, brainless, senses danger directly and galumphs away from harsh chemicals and bright lights. "Higher" animals perceive pain indirectly—the central nervous system reports to a brain isolated from the stimulus—and this in turn gives them much freedom to modify the experience. Almost a century ago the Russian scientist Ivan Pavlov trained a dog to overcome basic pain instincts by rewarding it with food just after applying electrical shocks to a particular paw. After a few weeks, instead of whining and struggling to get away from the shocks, the dog responded by wagging its tail excitedly, salivating, and turning toward the food dish. Somehow, the dog's brain had learned to reinterpret the negative, "It hurts!" aspect of pain. (Yet when Pavlov applied a similar shock to a different paw, the dog reacted violently.)

More recently, Ronald Melzack took Pavlov's experiments a step further. He raised Scottish terrier pups in individual, padded cages so that they would encounter none of the normal knocks and scrapes of growing up. To his astonishment, dogs raised in this deprived environment failed to learn basic responses to pain. Exposed to a flaming match, they repeatedly poked their noses into the flame and sniffed at it. Even when flesh burned, they showed no sign of distress. They also failed to react when he pricked their paws with a pin. In contrast their littermates, raised normally, yelped and fled after just one confrontation with the match or pin. Melzack was forced to conclude that much of what we call pain, including the "emotional" response, is learned, not instinctive.

In human beings mental powers reign supreme, and that is what gives us the ability to alter pain so dramatically. A cat that steps on a thorn instinctively begins limping, which will give the injured foot rest and protection. A man who steps on a rusty nail will also limp. But greater brain power allows him to reflect consciously, even obsessively, on the experience. In addition to limping, he may search for other coping aids: pain relievers, crutches, a wheelchair. If concern over the injury swells into fear, the pain will intensify so that it really does "hurt" the man more than it would presumably hurt a cat. He may worry about tetanus. If, like my patient Jake, this man has an exaggerated fear of needles, he may talk himself out of a tetanus shot and risk far greater pain. On the other hand, if he is paid ten thousand dollars a game to kick field goals in the National Football League, most likely the limper will bandage the foot, ignore the pain, and head for the practice field.

In my student days I saw vivid proof of how, through hypnosis, mental power can affect the experience of pain. Although not everyone is susceptible to deep hypnosis, pain threshold tests show the impact of hypnosis on some people. "I am not hurting you," the lab worker says, and a volunteer under deep hypnosis may not notice pain from a radiant heat machine even when the skin begins to redden and break into a blister. Conversely, if the researcher touches the hypnotized subject's skin with an ordinary pencil, telling her, "This is an extremely hot object," the skin site will redden and swell and a spontaneous blister may form! In each case the brain fabricates a response based on the sheer power of suggestion.* In a minority of people hypnosis can even be used to induce total anesthesia. The practice fell out of favor after the introduction of ether, but many major surgeries have been performed (some quite recently) with no anesthetic other than hyp-

---

*A hypnotized person with known allergies may have no reaction when touched by a poisonous leaf, if assured it is a harmless chestnut leaf. But if the researcher says, "I am now touching you with the poisonous leaf," and instead applies the chestnut leaf, the subject breaks out in an allergic skin rash!

Warts sometimes disappear overnight on command of a hypnotist, a physiological feat involving a major reordering of skin cells and blood vessels that medicine can neither duplicate nor explain. When I was in medical school I had extended contact with Dr. Freudenthal, a Jewish refugee from the Nazis who became a professor at University College. An authority on warts and melanomas, Freudenthal had concluded that the power of suggestion was slightly better statistically than any other treatment for warts. With a flourish, he would pass a black wand through a green flame, then tap the wart and speak strange words in another language. "The wart will fall off in exactly three weeks," he solemnly pronounced. Astonishingly, it often did just that. This "treatment" worked even on other scientists and physicians who gave no credence to such mumbo-jumbo magic techniques; the power of suggestion worked despite their skepticism and even hostility toward Freudenthal's methods.

notic suggestion. Hypnosis proves that under certain circumstances pain *response* at the third stage can overpower pain signals and messages from lower stages.

Whether consciously or subconsciously, the mind largely determines how we perceive pain. Laboratory tests reveal that, somewhat like Melzack's terriers, people reared in different cultural environments experience pain differently. Jews and Italians react sooner and complain louder than their Northern European counterparts; the Irish have a high tolerance for pain, Eskimos the highest of all.

Some cultural responses to pain nearly defy belief. Societies in Micronesia and the Amazon Valley practice a childbirth custom called *couvade* (from the French word for "hatching"). The mother gives no indication of suffering during delivery. She may break from work a mere two or three hours to give birth, then return to the fields. By all appearances it is the husband who bears the pain: during the delivery and for days afterward he lies in bed, thrashing about and groaning. Indeed, if his travail seems unconvincing, other villagers will question his paternity. Traditionally, the new mother waits on her husband and sits by his side to entertain the relatives who drop by to offer him congratulations.

Ronald Melzack tells of another cultural anomaly.

> In East Africa, men and women undergo an operation— entirely without anaesthetics or pain-relieving drugs—called "trepanation," in which the scalp and underlying muscles are cut in order to expose a large area of the skull. The skull is then scraped by the *doktari* as the man or woman sits calmly, without flinching or grimacing, holding a pan under the chin to catch the dripping blood. Films of this procedure are extraordinary to watch because of the discomfort they induce in the observers, which is in striking contrast to the apparent lack of discomfort in the people undergoing the operation. There is no reason to believe that these people are physiologically different in any way. Rather, the operation is accepted by their culture as a procedure that brings relief of chronic pain.

Have East Africans truly mastered the art of surgery without anesthesia? Whose pain is more "real," that claimed by a typical childbearing mother in Europe or a *couvade*-practicing father in

Micronesia? Both examples demonstrate the mysterious power of the human mind as it interprets and responds to pain.

Puzzles of Pain

If ever I had doubts about the mind's ability to modify and overrule messages of pain, three encounters—two from my days in India, and one from medical school in London—put such doubts to rest.

Lobotomy

In 1946, while I was completing surgical residency, an American neuropsychiatrist named Walter Freeman discovered a simplified way to perform a prefrontal lobotomy, a surgery on the brain first attempted by Italian doctors a decade before. The large frontal lobes in humans are involved in reflective thought and interpretation. The cerebral cortex handles a clear-cut response to pain, but the frontal lobes can modify that response—a process greatly affected by a prefrontal lobotomy.

After practicing on a cadaver, Freeman selected as his first patient a woman with schizophrenia. He used electroconvulsive therapy to stun the patient for a few minutes and chose as his surgical instrument an ice pick, the name "Uline Ice Company" clearly visible on its handle. He peeled back her right eyelid and slid the ice pick over the top of the eyeball. Meeting some resistance at the orbital plate, he punched through by tapping on the ice pick with a little hammer. Once inside the brain, he swung the instrument back and forth, shearing off neuronal pathways between the frontal lobes and the rest of the brain.

The woman awoke a few minutes later, and seemed so satisfied with the result that she returned in a week for the same treatment through the other eye socket. Freeman wrote to his son, laconically, "I have done two patients on both sides and another on one side without running into any complications, except a very black eye in one case. There may be trouble later on but it seemed fairly easy, although definitely a disagreeable thing to watch."

Freeman grew quite famous in the 1950s and 1960s, lecturing widely and demonstrating lobotomies to groups of psychologists and neurologists. He boasted that the procedure could help cure schizophrenia, depression, criminal recidivism, and chronic pain. Ever the showman, Freeman would sometimes reach in his pocket and pull out an ordinary carpenter's hammer for use. He got the procedure down to seven minutes, and once performed an "emergency lobotomy" to subdue an unruly criminal who was being restrained by policemen on a motel room floor. Psychosurgery only fell into disrepute after effective drugs reached the market. (Freeman, stung by the rising revulsion against his technique, scornfully labeled the new treatments "chemical lobotomy.")

I blanch now as I read the accounts of early psychosurgery, a field burgeoning just as I entered medicine. I have had limited contact with lobotomized patients, but while in India I did see in one patient dramatic evidence of lobotomy's effect on pain. A British woman from Bombay had for years sought relief from intractable vaginal pain. Initially she felt the pain during intercourse, which led to problems in her marriage, and over time she began to feel constant pain. She tried every available pain-relieving pill, and even underwent surgery to sever nerves, but nothing helped. Abject and in despair, she came with her husband to the hospital at Vellore. "I have no friends. My marriage is crumbling," she said. "Please, can you help me?"

A neurosurgeon on our staff had perfected a technique for lobotomy far enough forward in the brain that it minimized the dehumanizing impact but sometimes helped with psychiatric problems and chronic pain. He would drill holes on both sides of the skull, run a wire through them, and then, as if cutting cheese, use the wire to slice through nerve pathways and separate part of the frontal lobes from the rest of the brain. He explained the risks to the woman, who immediately agreed to the surgery. She was ready to try anything.

By all measures, the lobotomy was a great success. The woman emerged from surgery completely free of the suffering that had shadowed her for a decade. Her husband detected no difference in her mental capacity and only slight changes in her personality. Pain ceased to be a factor in their life together.

More than a year later I visited this couple in Bombay. The husband spoke enthusiastically about the lobotomy, and the woman herself seemed calm and content. When I inquired about the pain, she said, "Oh, yes, it's still there. I just don't worry about it anymore." She smiled sweetly and chuckled to herself. "In fact, it's still agonizing. But I don't mind."

At the time it startled me to hear words about agony coming from a person with such a placid demeanor: no grimace, no groan, only a gentle smile. As I read about other lobotomies, however, I found she was displaying a very typical attitude. Patients report feeling "the little pain without the big pain." A lobotomized brain, no longer recognizing pain as a dominating priority in life, does not call for a strong aversive reaction.

Lobotomized patients rarely ask for medication. As a German neurosurgeon who had performed many prefrontal lobotomies once told me, "The procedure takes all the suffering out of pain." Stages one and two of pain, the signal and message stages, proceed without interruption. But a radical change in stage three, the mind's response, transforms the nature of the overall experience.

Placebo

Placebos (Latin for "I shall please") have earned the medical establishment's grudging respect simply because they work so well. Nothing more than sugar pills or saline solutions, they nevertheless prove quite effective in relieving pain. Around 35 percent of cancer patients report substantial relief after a placebo treatment, about half the number who find relief from morphine.

Almost by definition, placebos work their magic at the mind-response level of pain control. Swallowing a capsule of sugar has absolutely no effect on neurons in the periphery or in the spinal cord. And placebos sneaked into a patient's milk or food without the patient's knowledge will have no effect either. What matters are the power of suggestion and the patient's conscious belief in the placebo's healing properties.

Recent tests indicate that placebos may trigger the release of painkilling endorphins, an instance of the higher brain's "belief" in the treatment translating into actual physiological changes. Placebos work best if the patient fully trusts their effectiveness. In one experiment, 30 percent of cancer patients claimed relief after a placebo pill, 40 percent after an intramuscular placebo injection, and 50 percent after an intravenous placebo drip! Some patients even grow addicted to placebos, and undergo withdrawal symptoms if treatment is halted.

While I was in medical school, Italian doctors were conducting a bizarre test—unlikely to be repeated—that suggests the act of surgery itself may have a placebo effect. In 1939 Italian surgeons learned that angina pectoris, heart pain, could be greatly reduced by tying off, or ligating, the internal mammary arteries, perhaps making more blood available to the heart. After this procedure the patients felt better, took fewer nitroglycerine pills, and for the first time could exercise without pain. Word spread, and soon surgeons worldwide were practicing the same technique and confirming the initial findings.

Meanwhile, the Italian innovators began wondering whether the success rate merely demonstrated a placebo effect.* They recruited a group of patients to participate in a study that, if proposed today, would raise serious ethical issues. Half the patients underwent surgery to have their internal mammary arteries exposed and ligated, and the other half simply had them exposed and not ligated. In other words, half the patients submitted to general anesthesia in order to have their chests cut open and then promptly sewn up! Amazingly, the two groups of patients showed comparable improvement after surgery: pain diminished, they took fewer pills, and they could exercise more. The Italians concluded that the very act of surgery had produced a placebo effect in their patients.

Health workers have learned to accept the placebo effect, and sometimes we use it to our advantage. Yet I confess that whenever I see the placebo effect up close, I marvel at the resourcefulness of a human mind that can fashion healing from a transaction of trust and deception.

*Given medicine's history of magic poultices, blood-letting, ice-cold baths, and other "cures," we should be grateful that at least doctors had the palcebo effect working in their favor. Dr. Franz Anton Mesmer (who gave us the epigram *mesmerize)* "cured" patients with his Animal Magnetism theories. Kings of England and France treated scrufulous patients with the Royal Touch for seven hundred years. Two nineteenth-century French physicians advocated directly contradictory methods of treatment. Dr. Raymond at Salpetriere in Paris suspended his patients by their feet to allow blood to flow to their heads. Dr. Haushalter at Nancy suspended his patients head upward. Their results: exactly the same percentage of patients showed improvement. Norman Cousins has remarked, "Indeed, many medical scholars have believed that the history of medicine is actually the history of the placebo effect. Sir William Osler underlined the point by observing that the human species is distinguished from the lower order by its desire to take medicine. Considering the nature of nostrums taken over the centuries, it is possible that another distinguishing feature of the species is its ability to survive medication."

In India our physician in charge of rehabilitation, Mary Verghese, always strove to keep up with the latest technology. We argued one day about the wisdom of investing in an ultrasound machine. I had never used ultrasound, which was being touted in medical literature and in advertisements as a breakthrough treatment for reducing scar tissue and relieving stiffness in joints. Mary wanted to order the machine right away; I remained skeptical.

Mary eventually won the debate, and soon the first ultrasound machine in all of India was humming away in her department. It caused a great stir of excitement. Partly to mollify me, Mary agreed to supervise a test on a hundred patients who had stiffness of the finger joints. All were to receive exactly the same physiotherapy and massage treatment, but only half would be exposed to the ultrasound machine. Their initial range of motion was recorded so that at the end we could compare objective results. Throughout the course of the test, Mary's physiotherapists insisted they were giving equal attention and encouragement to the ultrasound group and the control group.

When the day for evaluations finally arrived, I had to swallow my skepticism. The charts clearly showed that ultrasound treatment had worked in all the ways advertised. The patients' improvement was undeniable.

A few weeks later, a representative from the company that had sold us the machine dropped by to see if all was well. He listened to our reports with pleasure and discussed sharing our findings with other hospitals. He switched on the machine, it hummed, and he held a glass of water under the ultrasound applicator head. The surface of the water remained smooth, and a puzzled look crossed his face. He opened up the back of the machine, stuck his head in, and called out, "Hey, you've never had this thing working! When we ship it, we don't connect the ultrasound head, because it can get damaged. It's still unconnected."

Mary Verghese, quick to grasp the implications, was crestfallen. "But what makes the hum?" she asked at last.

"Oh, that's just a cooling fan," the technician said. "Believe me, you haven't been getting any ultrasound waves at all."

Our miracle cures had been yet one more expensive demonstration of the placebo effect. Somehow the therapists, thrilled with their new machine, had communicated an enthusiasm and hope that their patients' bodies had translated into actual improvement.

Phantom Limb

Most amputees experience at least a fleeting sensation of a phantom limb. Somewhere, locked inside their higher brains, a missing hand or leg perseveres in vivid memory. The limb may seem to move. Invisible toes curl, imaginary hands grasp things, a "leg" feels so sturdy that a patient rolls out of bed expecting to stand on it. The sensations vary: a feeling of pins-and-needles, a nagging awareness of heat or cold, the pain of phantom nails digging into phantom palms, or perhaps just an enduring sense that the limb is still "there."

Over time, these symptoms usually taper off. Sometimes sensations fade away only partially, so that the brain retains the perception of a hand—but no arm—dangling from a shoulder stump. Among an unfortunate few, this phantom limb sensation includes long-term pain, a pain like no other. They feel large nuts being screwed onto phantom fingers, razors slashed across phantom arms, nails pounded through phantom feet. Nothing gives a doctor such a sense of profound helplessness as phantom limb pain, for the part of the patient's body screaming for attention does not exist. What is there to treat?

I observed a strange encounter with severe phantom limb pain during University College days. The school administrator, Mr. Bryce, suffered from Buerger's disease, which restricted the blood flow in one of his legs. As circulation gradually worsened he felt constant, unrelieved pain in that leg. Smoking contributed to the thrombosis, and for Mr. Bryce a single cigarette would cause enough vasoconstriction to bring on excruciating pain.

Dr. Godder, Bryce's surgeon, was at his wit's end. An obstinate man, Bryce had adamantly rejected any thought of amputation, and Godder was struggling to keep his patient from overdependence on pain medication. (At that time, there were no effective grafting techniques for reestablishing blood supply to the leg.)

"I hate it! I hate it!" Bryce would mutter about his leg. After several months of this defiance, at last Bryce gave in. "Take it off, Godder, take it off!" he railed in his raspy voice. "I can't stand it anymore. I'm through with that leg." Godder scheduled surgery immediately.

The night before the operation Dr. Godder received a strange request from Bryce. "Don't send this limb to the incinerator," he said. "I want you to preserve it for me in a pickling jar, which I will install on my mantle shelf. Then, as I sit in my arm-chair in the evening, I will taunt that leg: 'Ha! You can't hurt me anymore!'" Bryce got his wish, and when he left the hospital in a wheelchair, a large museum bottle went with him.

The despised leg, however, had the last laugh. Bryce suffered from phantom limb pain in the extreme. The wound healed, but in his mind the leg lived on, hurting him as much as ever. He could feel the phantom calf muscles go into ischemic cramp, and now he had no prospect of relief.

Dr. Godder explained to us students that the leg, which should have been amputated two years before, had achieved an independent existence in Bryce's tormented mind. Even people born without limbs may have a felt image of the limb in the mind, and may experience phantom pain. Bryce had a richly developed felt image reinforced by feedback from the cut nerves in the stump. He hated that leg with such ferocity that the pain, which began as a signal reporting in from the periphery, had etched a permanent pattern in his brain. The pain existed at stage three only, in his mind, but that was sufficiently torturous. Though he could glare at the leg on the mantle shelf, it leered back at him inside his skull.

Unmaking the World

Phantom limb pain teaches me an unforgettable lesson about pain: the human body values it supremely. Years ago, Walter Cannon introduced the wonderful word "homeostasis" to describe the body's strong drive to get things back to normal. Step from a sauna into a snow-covered backyard in Alaska, and your body will valiantly strive to keep your temperature steady. The body automatically corrects imbalances in fluids and salts, regulates temperature and blood pressure, monitors glandular secretions, and mobilizes to repair itself. Working together in community, the body's cells seek out the most favorable conditions for the whole.

Phantom limb syndrome demonstrates a kind of homeostasis of pain. At an amputation site the cut nerves will branch out and try to connect with the stump of their own axon; unable to find it, they form knots of futile nerve twigs (often surgeons have to go back in and cut these neuromas). Failing that, the spinal cord may fabricate sensory messages on its own. And if all else fails, the brain endeavors to keep alive a memory pattern of the missing limb, as it did so convincingly for Mr. Bryce. In such cases, the pain network almost seems to take on a life of its own, frantically seeking new routes to reestablish the pain.

I have often thought about the paradox of pain illustrated by the unfortunate Mr. Bryce. On the one hand, pain from his leg went to great lengths to stay alive: nerves, spinal cord, and brain conspired to resurrect silenced pain signals. At the same time, Mr. Bryce himself was trying desperately to kill off those very signals. His mind and body were fighting a civil war, a dramatized version of the conflict all of us experience in pain. We feel the pain, urgently, and above all else we want to stop feeling it. We are divided. This most obvious fact about pain raises an important question: Why must pain so be distasteful as to produce a bodily state of civil war?

Human beings have an efficient reflex system that forcibly withdraws a hand from a sharp or hot object even before nerve messages reach the brain.* Why, then, must pain include the toxin of *unpleasantness?* My "substitute pain" project answered the question on one level: pain supplies the compulsion to respond to warnings of danger. But could not such warnings be handled as a reflex, without involving the conscious brain? In other words, why does there need to be a third stage of pain at all?

Nobel Laureate Sir John Eccles worried over this issue, and even performed experiments on decerebrated animals to see how they would respond to pain. He found that a brainless frog still pulls its foot from an acid solution and a decerebrated dog still scratches flea bites. After much study Eccles concluded that, although the reflex system does provide a layer of protection, the higher brain becomes involved for two reasons.

First, the hurt of pain forces the entire being to attend to the danger. Once aware of the cut on my finger, I forget all about my

---

*The higher brain actually plays a trick of perception. If I touch a pot on the stove with my hand and quickly withdraw it, it feels as if I am consciously reacting to the heat. But the act of pulling back my hand was actually a reflex response organized by the spinal cord, which did not even consult the conscious brain about the proper course of action—there was not time for delay. It takes fully half a second for my consciousness to sort through and interpret a pain message, while the spinal cord can order a reflex in a tenth of a second. My brain "backfills" my perception to the reflex so that it seems as if I made the choice consciously.

crowded schedule and the long line of patients outside—I run for a bandage. Pain ignores, even mocks all other priorities.

It astounds me that a coded bit of datum in the brain can induce such a feeling of compulsion. The tiniest object—a hair down the trachea, a speck in the eye—can commandeer the whole of a human being's consciousness. A distinguished poet who has just received a literary award returns to her seat, bows demurely to acknowledge the applause, gracefully arranges her skirt, bends to sit, and then gracelessly shoots up with a howl. She has landed on a jagged edge of the chair and her brain, flouting all decorum, attends solely to the distress signals emanating from the lowly lamina of her bottom. An operatic tenor whose career depends upon critical reception of this evening's performance rushes from the stage for a glass of water to calm the tickle in his throat. A basketball player writhes on the floor in front of a television audience of 20 million; the pain system cares not at all about the trivia of decorum and shame. By involving the higher brain so prominently, the response of self-protection overwhelms all others.

The second advantage of higher brain involvement, Eccles said, is that unpleasantness sears into memory, thus protecting us in the future. When I burn myself handling a hot pot, I determine from then on to use a glove or hot pad. The very unpleasantness of pain—the part we detest—makes it effective across time.

Pain is unique among sensations. Other senses tend to habituate, or lessen over time: the strongest cheeses seem virtually odorless after eight minutes; touch sensors adjust quickly to coarse clothing; an absent-minded professor searches in vain for his glasses, no longer feeling their weight on his head. In contrast, pain sensors do not habituate, but report incessantly to the conscious brain as long as danger remains. A bullet penetrates for a second and exits; the resulting pain may linger a year or more.

Oddly, though, this sensation that eclipses all others is hardest to remember once it fades. How many women have sworn after a difficult childbirth, "Never again will I go through that"? How many receive the news of another pregnancy with joy? I can close my eyes and summon up a constellation of scenes and faces from the past. Through sheer mental effort I can nearly replicate the smell of an Indian village or the taste of chicken curry. I can mentally replay familiar motifs from hymns, symphonies, and popular songs. But only weakly can I recall excruciating pain. Gallbladder attacks, agony from a ruptured disc, an airplane crash—my memories come to me stripped of the unpleasantness.

All these characteristics of pain serve its ultimate end: to galvanize the entire body. Pain shrinks time to the present moment. There is no need for the sensation to linger once the danger has passed, and it dare not habituate while danger remains. What matters to the pain system is that you feel miserable enough to stop whatever you're doing and pay attention *right now*.

In the words of Elaine Scarry, pain "unmakes a person's world." Try carrying on a casual conversation with a woman in the final stages of childbirth, she suggests. Pain can overrule the values we cherish most, a fact which torturers know all too well: they use physical pain to wrench from a person information which a moment before he had held precious or even sacred. Few can transcend the urgency of physical pain—and that is its intent, precisely.

15
Weaving the Parachute

———◆———

The mind is its own place, and in itself
Can make a heav'n of hell, a hell of heav'n.
John Milton, *Paradise Lost*

If I held in my hands the power to eliminate physical pain from the world, I would not exercise it. My work with pain-deprived patients has proved to me that pain protects us from destroying ourselves. Yet I also know that pain itself can destroy, as any visit to a chronic pain center will show. Unchecked pain saps physical strength and mental energy, and can come to dominate a person's entire life. Somewhere between the two extremes, painlessness and incessant chronic pain, most of us live out our days.

The good news about the third stage of pain, the mental response, is that it allows us to prepare for pain in advance. Hypnotism and the placebo effect prove that the mind already has within it powers to control pain. We need only learn to tap those resources. The varied responses I have seen as a physician—some patients face pain heroically, some stoically endure, and some cringe in abject terror—have shown me the advantages of making the proper preparations.

I like the concept of "pain insurance": we can pay up premiums ahead of time, long before pain strikes. As one doctor said in Bill Moyers's television series *Healing and the Mind*, "You don't want to start weaving the parachute when you're about to jump out of the plane. You want to have been weaving the parachute morning, noon, and night, day in, day out. And then when you need it, it might actually hold you." The worst time to think about pain, in fact, is when you are feeling its assaults, because pain demolishes objectivity. I have made most of my own preparations for pain while healthy, and the insights I gained helped prepare me for later ambushes.

It was while treating leprosy patients in India that I first recognized the value of the gift of pain, and afterward I tried to convey that sense to my six children. Is it possible to teach appreciation for pain to a child? I wondered. After a few bungled attempts, I concluded that a five-year-old screaming in panic at the sight of his own blood is not receptive to such a message. My children seemed much more open to an object lesson when *I* was the victim of cuts and scrapes.

"Does it hurt, Daddy?" the children would ask as I rinsed out a cut on my hand and scrubbed it with soap. I would explain that yes, it hurt, but that was a good thing. The tenderness would make me take extra care. I would skip my weeding chores in the garden for a few days in order to give my injured hand a rest. Pain, I pointed out, gave me a great advantage over our friends Namo, Sadan, and the other leprosy patients. My wound would likely heal faster, with less danger of complications, because I felt pain.

If I asked my grown children today to recall their most vivid lesson about pain, probably they would all mention the same scene from India. Each summer our entire family piled into a car and drove 280 miles to a magnificent site high in the Nilgiri Hills, an area of virgin jungle still patrolled by tigers and panthers. Our summer bungalow, lent to us by the manager of a tea estate whose staff we had treated as patients, sat in a clearing amid mountain lakes and grasslands some thirty miles from the nearest town. The Webbs, another Vellore staff family, often shared our summer bungalow, and it was John Webb, a pediatrician, who prompted the memorable lesson about pain.

Riding his motorcycle on the curvy, unpaved mountain road one day, John had to swerve so sharply to avoid a dog that his wheel caught a rock and flew out from under him. He fell clear of the motorcycle, but momentum sent him skidding chin-first along the gravelly path. Although his wounds were no more serious than scrapes and bruises, tiny pieces of dirt and gravel had ground into the flesh.

Knowing my views on pain, John was happy to let me use him as an object lesson for the children. "Paul, you know what you have to do," John said. "And I don't mind if the children watch." He lay down on the couch, the children encircling him, and I fetched a basin, plain soap, and a stiff nail brush. I had no anesthetics to offer.

During World War II John had served as a medical officer in the army that invaded Italy. He had drilled medics about the importance of getting every speck of dirt and grime out of wounds in order to prevent infection. Now that it was his turn, he gritted his teeth and grimaced. I scrubbed the raw flesh with my frothy brush, and our children furnished the sound effects. "Ooh! Yuk!" "I can't watch." "Doesn't it *hurt?*"

"Go on, Paul, go on," John said through clenched teeth if he sensed I was letting up. I scrubbed until I saw nothing but clean pink skin and deeper bleeding dermis, and then applied a soothing antiseptic ointment.

Over the next few days the children got a short course in physiology as John and I expounded on the magic of blood and skin and their remarkable agents of repair. He took no aspirin or other painkiller, and my children learned that pain can be borne. Perhaps more important, they saw John accepting pain as a valuable part of the recovery process. Daily, he would peel back the dressings to check the progress of healing and then give us a tenderness report. His body spoke to him in the language of pain, forcing him to take extra precautions. He chewed food slowly and deliberately. He slept on his back, or on his other side. And for the rest of our vacation he stayed off motorcycles.

My children got the message only too well. Hanging a picture on the wall back in Vellore soon after our vacation, I pounded my thumb with a hammer. I dropped the hammer and began hopping up and down, squeezing the offended thumb. "Thank God for pain, Daddy!" my son Christopher cried. "Thank God for pain!"

Gratitude

The notion that what we think and feel in the mind affects the health of our bodies has gradually seeped into medical consciousness. Every young doctor learns about the placebo effect. And thanks to popular authors like Bill Moyers, Norman Cousins, and Dr. Bernie Siegel, the general population too has become aware of the role emotions can play in healing. As one wry observer commented, "Sometimes it is more important to know what kind of fellah has a germ than what kind of germ has a fellah."

Dr. Hans Selye was the true pioneer in discovering the impact of emotions on health, and partly because of his influence I begin with gratitude as my first suggestion in making preparations for pain. In his Montreal laboratory Selye spent years conducting experiments on rats to find out what damages the body. He wrote thirty books on the subject himself, and well over a hundred thousand articles have been published about the "stress syndrome" which he first described in 1936. Selye observed that mental stress causes the body to produce extra supplies of adrenaline (epinephrine), which accelerates heart rate and breathing. Muscles also tense up, and the tension may lead to headaches or backaches. In searching for the root cause of stress, Selye found that such factors as anxiety and depression can trigger attacks of pain or intensify pain already present. (According to the American Academy of Family Physicians, two-thirds of office visits to family doctors are prompted by stress-related symptoms.)

As Selye summarized his research toward the end of his life, he named vengeance and bitterness as the emotional responses most likely to produce high stress levels in human beings. Conversely, he concluded, *gratitude* is the single response most nourishing to health. I find myself agreeing with Selye, in part because a grateful appreciation for pain's many benefits has so transformed my own outlook.

People who view pain as the enemy, I have noted, instinctively respond with vengeance or bitterness—*Why me? I don't deserve this! It's not fair!*—which has the vicious-circle effect of making their pain even worse. "Think of pain as a speech your body is delivering about a subject of vital importance to you," I tell my patients. "From the very first twinge, pause and listen to the pain and, yes, try to be grateful. The body is using the language of pain because that's the most effective way to get your attention." I call this approach "befriending" pain: to take what is ordinarily seen as an enemy and to disarm and then welcome it.

A radical change in outlook took place among the group of scientists and health workers at Carville as they saw daily proof of pain's benefits, both in patient wards and in the laboratory. Beyond all doubt, they learned to value the gift of pain with gratitude. Today, if any of our group should suffer from intractable pain, we may become afraid and depressed. We may plead for relief. But I doubt anything will shake our bedrock belief that the *system* of pain is good and wise.

I find it ironic that as a doctor (except in dealing with pain-deprived patients) I must rely so strongly on my patients' complaints about pain, for the very pain they grumble about is my main guide in determining the diagnosis and course of treatment. One reason some cancers are more fatal than others is that they affect parts of the body less sensitive to pain. Cancer in an organ like the lung or the deeper part of the breast may not be noticed by the patient, and the physician may have no clue until it has spread to a sensitive organ like the pleura, the membrane of the lung. By that time cancer may have entered the bloodstream and metastasized beyond the reach of local treatment.

I like to remind myself, and others, that even in bodily processes normally regarded as enemies, we can find a reason to be grateful. Most discomforts derive from the body's loyal defenses, not the illness. When an infected wound reddens and produces pus, for example, the redness and swelling come from an emergency surge of blood to the scene, and the pus, composed of lymph fluids and dead cells, gives proof of cellular battles fought on the body's behalf. Increased local heat results from the body's effort to move more blood to the affected part. A more generalized fever circulates blood more quickly and, conveniently, happens to create a more hostile environment for many bacteria and viruses.

Indeed, virtually every bodily activity that we view with irritation or disgust—blister, callus, fever, sneeze, cough, vomiting, and, of course, pain—is an emblem of the body's self-protection. While president, George Bush was embarrassed by an episode of vomiting at a state dinner in Japan. Perhaps he should have been grateful. I marvel at the physiological mechanism involved in vomiting, which recruits scores of muscles to reverse their normal processes violently: designed to coax food down through the digestive tract, they now regroup in order to expel unwelcome invaders. As President Bush learned, the reflex works on our behalf whenever it senses danger, regardless of the circumstances. Likewise a sneeze, abrupt and unpreventable, will evict foreign objects and germs from the nasal mucosa with near-hurricane force. Even the most unpleasant aspects of the body are signs of its struggle toward health.

Gratitude has become my reflex response to pain, especially, and I can testify that this fundamental shift in attitude has truly changed pain's effect on me. I no longer feel annoyance as I become reacquainted with my chronically sore back in the morning. I may wince and groan when I attempt to get dressed, but I also tune in to the message of pain. It reminds me that I do much better if I do not bend, but put my feet, one at a time, up on a chair to pull on my socks or tie shoelaces. It also gives veiled hints that I should rearrange my schedule and get extra rest, or do exercises to limber up stiff joints. Whenever possible, I try to follow its advice, for I know that my body has no more loyal advocate than pain.

Not long ago, after carrying a suitcase on a long overseas trip, I had a particularly painful bout with the pinched nerve in my back. At first, gratitude was the furthest response from my mind. I felt irritated and discouraged. When I sensed that the pain would not readily go away, however, I decided to apply consciously what I believed about gratitude. I began to focus my mind on various parts of my body, in a kind of litany of gratitude.

I flexed my fingers and thought of the synchronized activity of fifty muscles, scores of stringy tendons, and millions of obedient nerve cells that made such motion possible. I rotated my joints and reflected on the marvelous engineering built into ankles, shoulders, and hips. An automobile bearing lasts seven or eight years with proper lubrication; mine had exceeded seventy years, their lubrication self-renewing, with no time off for maintenance.

I breathed deeply and imagined the pockets in my lungs trapping tiny bubbles of oxygen and busily stowing them aboard a blood cell for transport to the brain. A hundred thousand times a day my heart muscles beat, propelling that fuel to its destination. I took breath after breath, renewing all the functions of my body with fresh, clean air. After ten deep breaths I felt slightly dizzy.

My stomach, spleen, liver, pancreas, and kidneys were working so efficiently that I had no way of perceiving their existence. Yet I knew that in an emergency they would find a way to alert me, even if they had to resort to the trick of borrowing pain cells from neighboring tissue.

I closed my eyes and experienced, for a moment, a world without sight. I reached out and touched the leaves and bark and grass around me, absorbing their texture with my fingertips. I thought of my family, and as their images came to mind, one by one, I marveled at my brain's extraordinary ability to summon them into consciousness. Then I opened my eyes and a sudden rush of light waves spilled in.

Even at its worst, seven decades old and achy, my body gave compelling reasons for gratitude and even praise. It did not occur to me to rail against God for the discomfort I was experiencing; I knew too well the dire alternative of a life without pain.

In the final stage of my litany, I turned my attention to the region of pain itself. I thought of the vertebrae, so well designed that the same basic structure can support the eight-foot neck of a giraffe. I recalled my most complex surgical procedures, when I had dissected out tiny strands from the web of nerves in the spinal cord. Such intricacy—a slip of the knife, and my patient would never walk again. One of those tiny nerves in my own back had already forced me to make major adjustments: corrections in my posture and walking stride, a choice of different pillows and sleeping positions, a reluctant decision to have porters carry my suitcase.

The pain did not go away that night. I still felt a dull, persistent throb as I lowered myself into bed. But somehow the sense of gratitude had worked a calming transformation in me. My muscles were less tense. Pain no longer dominated in quite the same way. What had seemed my enemy had become my friend.

A cynic might say, "These are tricks of the mind. You have lowered the threshold of fear and anxiety, nothing more." That, of course, is the point: Pain takes place in the mind, and what calms the mind will enhance my ability to cope with pain.

Listening

The reason I encourage gratitude is that one's underlying attitude (a product of the mind) toward the body can have a major impact on health. If I regard the body with respect, wonder, and appreciation, I will be far more inclined to behave in a way that sustains its health. In my work with leprosy patients, I could make repairs to hands and feet, but these improvements, I soon learned, amounted to nothing unless the patients themselves assumed responsibility for their limbs. The essence of rehabilitation— indeed, the essence of health—was to restore to my patients a sense of personal destiny over their own bodies.

When I moved to the United States, I expected to find that a society with such high standards of education and medical sophistication would foster a strong sense of personal responsibility in health. I have found exactly the opposite. In Western countries, an astounding proportion of the health problems stem from behavior choices that show disregard for the body's clear signals.

We doctors know this truth, but we shy away from interfering in our patients' lives. If we were fully honest, we might say something like this: "Listen to your body, and above all listen to your pain. It may be trying to tell you that you are violating your brain with tension, your ears with loudness, your eyes with constant television, your stomach with unhealthy food, your lungs with cancer-producing pollutants. Listen carefully to the message of pain before I give you something to relieve those symptoms. I can help with the symptoms, but *you* must address the cause."*

Albert Schweitzer once remarked that disease left him rapidly because it found little hospitality in his body. That would be a worthy goal for all of us, but it appears society is heading increasingly in the opposite direction. Each year representatives from the Public Health Service, including the Centers for Disease Control and the Food and Drug Administration, meet to discuss health trends and to set priorities for new programs. In the 1980s, in the midst of one such week-long conference, I started making a list of all the behavior-related problems on the agenda and the time devoted to each: heart disease and hypertension exacerbated by stress, stomach ulcers, cancers associated with a toxic environment, AIDS, sexually transmitted diseases, emphysema and lung cancer caused by cigarette smoking, fetal damage stemming from

---

*I readily admit that the medical establishment bears a large part of the blame. Imagine the ethical dilemma of a young surgeon, burdened with debt from medical school, who weighs a patient's options. The more conservative approach would ask the patient to assume responsibility for her own health: to exercise, undergo physical therapy, change diets, make life-style adjustments, learn to live with a little pain. In return for such sound advice, the surgeon gets a fifty-dollar office visit fee. The radical approach involves outside surgical intervention, requiring admission to the hospital, and fees to the surgeon of perhaps five thousand dollars.

A study by William Kane in 1980 showed that American doctors were seven times more likely than their counterparts in Sweden and Great Britain to perform lumbar laminectomies for back problems. In the previous decade the total number of disc operations in the United States had increased from 40,000 to 450,000.

maternal alcohol and drug abuse, diabetes and other diet-related disorders, violent crime, automobile accidents involving alcohol. These were the endemic, even epidemic concerns for health experts in the United States.

A comparable gathering of experts in India, I knew, would have dealt instead with malaria, polio, dysentery, tuberculosis, typhoid, and leprosy. After valiantly conquering most of those infectious diseases, the United States has now substituted new health problems for old.

We were meeting in Scottsdale, Arizona. That state's neighbor to the west, Nevada, ranks near the high end on most mortality tables, while its northern neighbor, Utah, ranks near the bottom. Both states are relatively wealthy and well educated, and they share a similar climate. The difference, various studies suggest, is probably best explained by life-style factors. Utah is the seat of Mormonism, which frowns on alcohol and tobacco. Family ties remain strong in Utah and marriages tend to endure (mortality tables show that divorce strongly increases the likelihood of early death from strokes, hypertension, respiratory cancer, and intestinal cancer). Nevada, in contrast, has twice the incidence of divorce and a far higher rate of alcohol and tobacco consumption, not to mention the unique stress associated with gambling.

I write as a physician, not a moralist, but any physician working in modern civilization cannot help noticing our cultural deafness to the wisdom of the body. The path to health, for an individual or a society, must begin by taking pain into account. Instead, we silence pain when we should be straining our ears to hear it; we eat too fast and too much and take a seltzer; we work too long and too hard and take a tranquilizer. The three best-selling drugs in the United States are a hypertension drug, a medication for ulcers, and a tranquilizer. These pain-mufflers are readily available because even the medical profession seems to look upon pain as the illness rather than the symptom.

Before heading for the medicine cabinet to silence pain, I try to sharpen my hearing. Listening to pain has become a ritual for me, the flip side of my litany of gratitude. Is there a pattern to the pain? I ask myself. Does it tend to occur at a regular time of day or night or month? Does it seem to relate to my job, or to relationships with people? How does eating affect it? Do I feel the pain before, during, or after meals? Does it correspond with bowel movements? Urination?* Does a change in posture, or abnormal exertion, seem to affect it? Am I anxious about something in the future, or do I tend to dwell on some memory of a past event? Am I having financial worries? Am I bitter or angry at someone—perhaps because he was partly responsible for my pain? Am I angry at God?

I may try experiments to attune myself better to my pain. What if I sleep with a different pillow, or sit on a chair instead of a couch? How about an hour of extra sleep a night? How do I respond to certain foods—fats, sweets, vegetables? What seems appealing? What seems revolting? I take notes of any correlations that come to mind.

I could not guess how many trips to the doctor this exercise has saved me over the years (physicians, you may be surprised to learn, are usually very reluctant to visit a doctor). I rarely feel grateful for the fact of pain, but I almost always feel grateful for the message that it brings. I can count on pain to represent my best interests in the most urgent way available. It is then up to me to act on those recommendations.

Activity

When listened to carefully, pain not only teaches what abuses to avoid, but also hints at the positive qualities the body needs. As a rule, body tissue flourishes with activity and atrophies with dis-

---

*"Civilization" often calls on us to overrule simple signals of pain. I remember a comment from student days in *Textbook on Surgery* by Hamilton Bailey. Wild dogs, he said, do not suffer from enlargement of the prostate gland, but house-trained dogs tend to have the same problems as their masters. When dogs (and humans) learn to overrule signals from the bladder and wait for more "appropriate" times to seek relief, our bodies pay the consequences.

Similarly, civilization makes it socially difficult for us to respond as we should to the need for a bowel movement. We ask for the "rest room," and the hostess averts her eyes and points down the corridor, while we apologize and sneak away. Or, more seriously, we may postpone until later what our bodies are telling us we should do now. By the time we get home the rectum, its message ignored, may not cooperate. The resulting strain can easily lead to hemorrhoids. Most of the constipation that people suffer in later life is due to (1) the lack of respect for normal reflexes, postponing action for social reasons, or (2) a diet dependent on refined foods and deficient in bulk and fiber.

use. I have seen this principle demonstrated most pathetically in stroke victims. As muscles in their hands remain in constant spasm, the fingers curl into a rigid claw position from lack of use. When I pry these fingers apart, in between them I find damp skin that has the texture of blotting paper and rips just as easily. The skin on the hand has lost its elements of strength because it has not been called upon to confront the real world it was designed for. "Use it or lose it" is the stern motto of physiology.

Early astronauts learned this principle the hard way. After the first space missions, medical researchers discovered that the astronauts had lost calcium in their bones and were in danger of severe osteoporosis. NASA added calcium supplements to the astronauts' diets, but subsequent missions showed the same results. Weightlessness, not diet, was the problem. If bones do not get exercise, the economical body judges that the bones must have more calcium than they need; it redistributes the calcium or excretes it in urine. The astronauts' bodies had simply been adapting to the less demanding rigors of weightlessness. To compensate, astronauts now do isometric-type exercises that imitate real work. Pushing one hand against another, even in weightless conditions, puts a strain on the arm bones that feels to them like work. The bones retain their calcium for reentry into the gravity of earth, where it will be needed.

In India I saw a vivid illustration of the body's need for activity. It struck me that Indian people rarely complained about osteoarthritis of the hip, a common malady of old age in the West. Osteoarthritis occurs when the cartilage cushion separating the femur and hip socket wears down, narrowing until the bones almost touch. Sometimes they rub together, resulting in friction and severe pain. The pattern shows up readily in X rays. Searching for clues, I compared the hip X rays of Indian and Western patients and found that the cartilage gap closes at the same rate in the elderly of both cultures. Uneven wear is what causes such difficulty in Western hips.

The ball of the femur starts out as a smooth sphere. Westerners tend to move their legs in only one direction, straight ahead and back, as they walk or run or sit in chairs. The bone scores along a single plane, resulting in some longitudinal grooving and the formation of tiny bumps and projections in the cartilage—the eventual source of arthritic pain. In contrast, Indians customarily sit with crossed legs, yoga style, rotating their hips in full abduction and complete rotation dozens of times a day. The ball of the femur wears evenly, not asymmetrically, and even though the aging cartilage of the joint shrinks, elderly Indians walk on a perfect sphere without grooves and projections. Sitting cross-legged is good insurance against old-age hip pain.

Artificial hip replacement is now a huge, profitable business in the West. It staggers me to realize how much expense and suffering could be avoided if we simply became more adept at listening to the body's message that we ought to give every joint a full range of activity every day. The average middle-aged person finds it painful to sit fully cross-legged, because he hasn't used the rotation of his hips for years. In contrast, someone who swims and climbs mountains, or walks on rough uneven ground as our ancestors did, uses every available movement and forestalls future pain. I toy with the idea of placing an ad in health journals offering "A Guaranteed Method to Avoid Hip Replacement" and charging $100 or so for the secret formula: Adopt the practice in youth of sitting cross-legged ten times a day on the floor or on a sofa.

Just as vigorous exercise causes muscles to develop and bones to harden, I believe there is even a sense in which nerve cells thrive when they are exposed to sensation. My leprosy patients taught me that the freedom to explore life is one of pain's greatest gifts. Unlike them, I am free to walk barefoot across rock-strewn ground, to drink coffee out of a tin cup, and to turn a screwdriver with all my strength, because I can trust my pain signals to alert me whenever I approach the danger point. I encourage healthy people to engage in strenuous physical activity and test their sensations to the limits for this reason: it may help prepare them to cope with later, unexpected pains.

Athletes are the one group of people in our society who study pain and who intentionally impose physical strain upon themselves. The marathon runner and the weightlifter listen intently to feedback from tendons and muscles and from heart and lungs as they labor to coax more effort from their bodies. The rock climber, wedging his fingers in the crack of a granite cliff, knows that his success, perhaps even his life, depends on his willingness to tolerate real pain in his fingertips and knuckles. He must sense the point of breakdown just in time, and then bring up reinforcements in the form of another hand or toe hold, or otherwise retreat.

Skilled athletes listen to their bodies with finely tuned equipment, pressing right to the edge of pain without falling off. For them, pain is an old friend. I saw a television interview with Joan Benoit just after she had won the Boston Marathon. "Was it a terrible ordeal?" the interviewer asked. "No, not really," Benoit replied. "I enjoyed it. I was listening to my body. From the start, my body was talking to me, telling me the limits it could stand. It was a kind of ecstasy." No doubt Joan Benoit would have known if the tendons in her legs or the organs of her cardiovascular system were in actual danger. Having learned to attend to her pain, she knew the difference between normal stress and urgent warning signals.

I applaud efforts to involve children in organized sports mainly because a comfort-oriented society offers few other places to learn the language of pain that Joan Benoit describes. I admit to holding rather unorthodox views of childrearing, developed partly as a reaction to this deficiency in modern society. For instance, I heartily advocate bare feet for young children. Living tissue adapts to the surfaces it is exposed to, and running barefoot is a fine way to stimulate nerves and skin. It trains a child to listen to the varied messages that come from running across grass, sand, and asphalt. An occasional stone might bruise the skin, but skin adapts, and the mixed messages from bare feet provide much more knowledge about the world than do neutral messages from shoe leather. (An added benefit is that bare toes spread out to distribute stress, whereas many shoes cramp toes and deform feet.)

To me, it seems that modern child-rearing techniques communicate how *not* to handle pain. Parents wrap babies in down comforters and clothing of soft texture, but this planet includes many rough textures as well. I wonder whether, when children begin to be more mobile, we would do better to replace baby blankets and mattress pads with a coarser material like coconut matting. Just when growing children need tactile stimulation for normal development, we surround them instead with neutral sensations. To complicate matters, modern parents lavish sympathy every time their son or daughter suffers any slight discomfort. Subliminally or overtly, they convey the message "Pain is bad." Should it surprise us that these children become adults who flee all pain in fear, or allow themselves to become dominated by it, or, at the least, share the intimate details of every ache and pain with anyone in range?

As I mentioned earlier, studies of various ethnic groups indicate that response to pain is in large degree learned. Ancient Sparta trained its children to prepare for pain. Modern society may have gone to the other extreme: our skill at silencing pain has brought about a kind of cultural atrophy in our overall ability to cope with it. I find some encouraging signs in the younger generation's fondness for aerobics and triathlon competitions, and in the emergence of programs such as Outward Bound. An active body, one that seeks challenges and pushes the limits of endurance, is best equipped to handle unexpected pain when it does occur—and it always will. The only way to conquer pain is to teach individuals to prepare for it in advance.

Self-Mastery

I remember my very first aspirin. I never took pain relievers as a child because my mother, a dedicated homeopath, opposed treating symptoms, preferring to trust the body's ability to heal itself. When I moved to England for schooling at the age of nine, I stayed with my grandmother and two unmarried aunts who shared my mother's homeopathic beliefs.

At twelve, still in England, I fell victim to influenza. My fever soared, and I felt as if someone had pummeled my entire body. I could hardly sleep for the headache pain, and I needed rest. My moans and groans must have alarmed my aunts because they called in a doctor, my first cousin, Vincent.

Even in my febrile state I could hear snatches of the debate whispered in the hallway outside my room.

"The fever's a normal part of the influenza. It will run its course. Why don't you give him some aspirin?"

"Aspirin? Well, I just don't know. He's never had anything like that!"

"Yes, but it will make him so much more comfortable. And it will help him sleep."

"You're sure it won't hurt him?"

At the end of the discussion my aunt came in with a single large white pill and a glass of water. "The doctor says you may take this, Paul. It will help your headache."

From my mother I had inherited a suspicion of all medicines, and the hushed discussion in the hallway had only confirmed that suspicion. I determined to try to handle the pain without the aspirin. I repeated to myself over and over, "I can handle it. I'm strong. I can handle it." All that night the white pill sat on my bedside table, unswallowed, looming, a magic potion with vast but not-quite-trustworthy powers. I slept undrugged.

Let me quickly add that in the years since I have taken drugs and have administered many others, both to my patients and to my own children. Nevertheless, I look back with gratitude on an upbringing that taught me a lasting lesson: *my sensations are my servants, not my masters.* I remember the next morning feeling a certain pride as my aunt came into the room and found the pill sitting on the table. I had mastered pain, for one night at least.

The aspirin incident gave me confidence that "I can handle it"—the same lesson John Webb would later try to convey to our children after his motorcycle accident. Hence a small victory helped prepare me for more intense pain to come, such as what I would feel in my spinal cord, gallbladder, and prostate gland. Early on I learned a pattern of self-mastery that has since served me well in circumstances when I could not readily find relief.

Once, during World War II, when army conscription had brought about an acute shortage of dentists, I decided to drill my own teeth and fill some bothersome cavities. Using a complex of mirrors, and twirling dental drill bits between my finger and thumb, I managed to clean out the decay and insert a filling. To my surprise, it seemed easier than having a dentist do the work. I felt in control. I could sense the tender spots and guide the drill bits around the edges of pain; a dentist would have had to interpret my grunts and groans. I thought back with gratitude on the discipline I had learned in mastering pain years before.

Nearly all of us, even in a comfort-oriented society, voluntarily endure some pain. Fashion-conscious women pluck their eyebrows, jam their feet into too-small shoes, wear thin stockings on winter days, and even undergo major surgery to change details of the face or figure. Athletes condition themselves to face the blows awaiting them on the basketball floor, hockey rink, or football field. A major manufacturer of exercise machines invites its users, "Feel the burn." What often happens, though, is that people who willingly undergo pain for some desirable end find involuntary pain shocking and unmanageable. Pain from illness or injury seems an intrusion in a culture that gives the illusion that all discomfort can be controlled.

My time in India exposed me to a society that has no illusions about controlling discomfort. In a country where the climate is

234 THE GIFT NOBODY WANTS

harsh, tropical diseases abound, and natural disasters roll in with each typhoon, no one can pretend to "solve" pain. Nonetheless, over the centuries the culture has discovered ways to help its people cope. A society that lacked many physical resources was forced to turn to mental and spiritual resources.

First as a child, then later as a physician in India, I was fascinated by the fakirs and *sadhus* who had exquisite command of their bodily functions. They could walk on nails, hold a difficult posture for hours, or fast for weeks. The more advanced practitioners even managed to control heart rate and blood pressure. Hindu "holy men" were known for their asceticism, and esteem for that high cultural value percolated down to the society at large. From an early age, the Indian people learned to respect discipline and self-control, qualities which helped equip them to cope with suffering.

Buddhism, a philosophy specifically designed to come to terms with human suffering, grew out of Indian soil. Shocked by the Four Distressing Sights (sickness, a dead body, old age, and a beggar), Gautama Buddha renounced his princedom and set out to find a riddle to the world's suffering. The solution he arrived at could not be more opposed to the Western philosophy of consumerism and the pursuit of pleasure. "The whole truth concerning the conquest of suffering lies in the self-conquest which leaves no passion remaining," concluded the Buddha. If life consists of suffering, and suffering is caused by desire, then the only solution to suffering is to end desire.

I am neither Hindu nor Buddhist, but it impresses me that both beliefs approach pain in the same way. According to Eastern thought, human suffering consists of "outer" conditions (the painful stimuli) and "inner" responses that take place in the mind. Although we cannot always control the outer conditions, we can learn ways to control our inner responses. As I became acquainted with these philosophies, I could not help noting the parallel to the signal-message-response stages of pain I had learned in medical school. In effect, Eastern philosophy affirms that stage-three pain, the response in the mind, is the dominant factor in the experience of suffering, and also the one we have most control over.

"The greatest discovery of my generation," wrote William James at the dawn of this century, "is that human beings, by changing the inner attitudes of their minds, can change the outer aspects of their lives." I smile when I read that statement, because Williams James's "discovery" has been taught by the major religions for several thousand years. After exposure to such teaching in the East, I began to pay more attention to the rich tradition of self-mastery in my own faith, Christianity.

During the Middle Ages, for example—significantly, a time of chaos and great suffering—religious orders devised a series of contemplative exercises. Most of them included prayer, meditation, and fasting, all disciplines directed toward the inner life. Consider these instructions for the "Prayer of the Heart" from Gregory of Sinai in the fourteenth century:

> Sit down alone and in silence. Lower your head, shut your eyes, breathe out gently and imagine yourself looking into your own heart. Carry your mind, that is, your thoughts, from your head to your heart. As you breathe out, say "Lord Jesus Christ, have mercy on me." Say it moving your lips gently, or simply say it in your mind. Try to put all other thoughts aside. Be calm, be patient and repeat the process very frequently.

Although intended primarily as worship aids, these disciplines have the added benefit of teaching self-mastery, a form of "pain insurance" that pays good dividends in times of crisis. Dr. Herbert Benson, a cardiologist at the Harvard Medical School, has proved conclusively that spiritual disciplines aid in what he calls "the relaxation response," which has a direct effect on perceived pain. Meditation (an act of mind) triggers physiological changes in the body: a gradual lowering of the heart and respiratory rates, changes in brain wave patterns, a general decrease in sympathetic nervous system activity. Tense muscles relax, and a state of inner stress gives way to calmness. In one study the majority of patients who had failed to find relief for chronic pain in conventional ways reported at least a 50 percent reduction in their pain after training in the relaxation response; in another, three-fourths of the patients reported moderate to great improvement. For this reason, most chronic pain centers now include programs of relaxation and meditation.

In modern times we have turned away from such practices, so that spiritual disciplines are often regarded as quaint and burdensome. But I have found that disciplines of the spirit can have an extraordinary effect on the body, and especially on pain. Prayer helps me cope with pain, by moving my mental focus away from a fixation on my body's complaints. As I pray, nourishing the life of the spirit, my tension level goes down and my consciousness of pain tends to recede. It did not surprise me at all to learn recently from a medical researcher that people who have strong religious faith have a lower incidence of heart attack, arteriosclerosis, high blood pressure, and hypertension than those who do not.

Community

My final suggestion for pain preparations, unlike the others, does not depend primarily on the individual. Just the opposite. The best single thing I can do to prepare for pain is to surround myself with a loving community who will stand beside me when tragedy strikes. This factor, I concluded, accounts in large measure for the Indians' ability to handle suffering.

Because of the tight extended family system, an Indian rarely faces suffering alone. When I was at Vellore, I saw many remarkable examples of community in action. A man with tuberculosis of the spine would travel seven hundred miles from Bombay for treatment, accompanied by his wife. If the second cousin of his wife's great-uncle lived anywhere nearby, that man had nothing to worry about. The cousin's family visited the hospital every day and supplied hot meals; the patient's wife slept under the bed on a mat and stayed close by to serve him. Nearly always, patients in great pain had a family member nearby to hold a hand, moisten dry lips, speak gentle words into the ear.

I had no way to measure the impact of community on the relief of pain, but I do know that in a land where pain-relieving drugs were in short supply and there was no universal health care, patients learned to depend on their families with confidence and trust. I certainly saw more pain, but less fear of pain and suffering, in India than I have seen in the West. In general, patients had less anxiety about the future. For example, when time came for release and home care, the man with tuberculosis of the spine naturally moved into the second cousin's house. As a matter of course, the host family would clear out the best room in the house, assume all responsibilities for daily care, and provide full board. They would not think of asking for payment, even if the period of recuperation lasted several months.

The sense of community extended to important medical decisions as well. I often found myself dealing with the patient's entire family, or with an informal council appointed by the family to oversee care. This council would send a representative to discuss with me all the relevant issues: What dangers does the patient face? Is permanent relief possible? Will the cancer likely return even after surgery? How will old age affect the risks? After quizzing me, the representative would return to the family council to ponder these issues. Sometimes the councils called upon other members of the family to share the expense and the demands of post-hospital care. Other times, they overruled my advice: "Thank you for your help, Dr. Brand, but we have decided against the surgery. It seems clear our aunt will die before long, and we will spare her this strain. She has lived a long time, and these treatments would put a financial hardship on the family. We will take her home where we can care for her until she dies."

I did not resent these family councils, time-consuming though they were. As a rule, they made wise decisions. The elder members, who had seen many people die in their villages, worked through the difficult issues with compassion and good sense. I also observed the impact of this system on the patients themselves, who placed complete trust in the family council and looked to the family, rather than to technology or drugs, as their main reservoir of strength. When we told a patient that her condition was terminal, she would have no desire to stay in the high-tech hospital, doped up with morphine. Rather, she wanted to go home where the family could surround her during her last days of life.

I contrast this approach to situations I have seen in the West, where elderly parents must often face their last days alone. Grown children, scattered all over the country, suddenly get word that their mother faces a difficult medical choice. They catch the next flight to the hospital. "Oh, Doctor, you must do everything possible to keep Mother alive," they tell the physician in a flurry of concern. "Spare no expense at all. Use feeding tubes, breathing tubes, whatever is necessary. And make sure she has plenty of pain medication." Then they fly back to their hometowns. If Mother survives, she'll probably be sent to a nursing home, alone.

India is fortunate to have community built into the family structure, a system that cannot, and probably should not, be imposed on a very different society in the West. Yet we have much to learn from their example of a wider community absorbing the impact of pain. I saw something comparable happen in London during the Blitz, when an entire city rallied around the common purpose of helping people who were in pain. A volunteer corps of nurses' aides sprang up spontaneously. People started checking regularly on their neighbors. The injured were not hidden away, but rather honored. Why, though, must we wait for times of emergency before forming a sense of community?

Perhaps because of the Indian influence, I tend to rely on my own family as a support community for pain. I am now approaching the last phase of my life. Rather than waiting passively for some disaster, I am trying to involve my family in what may lie ahead. The process begins with my wife, my companion for five decades. Margaret is teaching me some of the intricacies of caring for the house that I have never mastered. I am teaching her how I keep accounts, so that if I die just before income tax time, she will not feel stranded. I admit, we both worry about the possibility of having to depend too heavily on the other. What if one of us becomes incontinent? Or has a stroke and loses mental functioning? Margaret once suffered a temporary but almost total loss of memory after a bad fall, giving me a foretaste of what might lie around the corner. Together, we are trying to overcome any sense of shame over having to be dependent.

A support group can become a community of shared pain. So can a church or synagogue. Margaret and I may need help in coping with some emergencies, and know we can count on the church community to help shoulder the burden. Wherever we have lived we have sought out and have had the good fortune of finding a caring church. In fact, our present church has taken the far-sighted step of initiating a home hospice plan. Thirty-two volunteers, have taken a course of training offered by a local hospital-based program. As long as we are able, we will each help the others. When we have needs, they will help us.

The home hospice program relieves some of our anxiety in preparing for death. We have also worked out and signed a "living will" that sets strict limits on the artificial prolonging of life. Death is the one sure fact of life, of course. I trust the words of the Psalmist, "Yea, though I walk through the valley of the shadow of death, I will fear no evil, for You are with me." I have learned the best way to disarm my fears about terminal illness, and about the possibility of great pain, is to face them in advance, before God, and within a community that will share them.

16
Managing Pain

—◆—

It is a distortion to picture the human being as a teetering, fallible contraption, always needing watching and patching, always on the verge of flapping to pieces; this is the doctrine that people hear most often, and most eloquently, on all our information media. . . . The great secret of medicine, known to doctors but still hidden from the public, is that most things get better by themselves.
Lewis Thomas

No matter how well we prepare, pain almost always comes as a surprise. I bend over to pick up a pencil and suddenly it feels as if a spike has been driven into my back. Instantly my concern changes from pain preparation to pain management—and the difference between the two is the difference between a San Francisco practice drill and an actual earthquake. No amount of planning can fully equip us for the time when, without warning, the ground shifts.

I have expressed my suspicion that, in Western countries at least, people have grown increasingly less competent at handling pain and suffering. When pain's emergency sirens sound, the average person trusts his or her own resources less and the "experts" more. I believe the most important step in pain management is to reverse that process. We in medicine need to restore our patients' confidence in the most powerful healer in the world: the human body.

Doctors tend to exaggerate their own significance in the scheme of things, and for this reason I love the revisionist scene described in *The Healing Heart*. In the emergency room of a hospital, the Dean of the UCLA School of Medicine stands alongside the school's top cardiologists to await the arrival of a VIP patient suffering from heart failure. Suddenly the doors swing open and a stretcher rolls through. The patient—Norman Cousins—sits up,

grins, and says, "Gentlemen, I want you to know that you're looking at the darnedest healing machine that's ever been wheeled into
this hospital."

I know of no doctor who would seriously disagree with
Cousins's statement.* Franz Ingelfinger, the distinguished editor
of the *New England Journal of Medicine* for many years, estimated
that 85 percent of patients who visit a doctor have "self-limiting
illnesses." The doctor's role, he said, is to discern the 15 percent
who really need help as opposed to the 85 percent whose ailments
the body can handle on its own.

When I first studied medicine, in the days before penicillin,
we had limited resources to offer and by necessity a doctor func-
tioned more as an adviser or counselor. Without question the most
important person in the transaction was the patient, whose willing
participation in the plan for recovery would largely determine the
outcome. Now, in the patient's view at least, the tables have
turned: the patient tends to regard the doctor as the important
party.

Medicine has become so complex and elitist that patients feel
helpless, and doubt whether they have much contribution to make
in the struggle against pain and suffering. Too often the patient
sees himself or herself as a victim, a sacrificial lamb for the experts
to pick over, not a partner in recovery and health. In the United
States advertising further feeds the victim mentality by condition-
ing us to believe that staying healthy is a complicated matter far
beyond the grasp of the average person. We get the impression
that, were it not for vitamin supplements, antiseptics, painkillers,
and a trillion-dollar annual investment in medical expertise, our
fragile existence would soon come to an end.

The Doctor Within

Many patients view their own bodies with a sense of detachment or even hostility. Once pain has announced that a part of the

*To take just one example, if through some strange fiat we doctors
were forced to choose for our own selves either (1) the human immune system alone or (2) all the resources and technology of science but with the loss
of our immune system, we would without a moment's hesitation choose the
former. The disease AIDS exposes the helplessness of all modern technology when a person's immune system shuts down: pneumonia, cold sores, or
even diarrhea can pose a mortal danger.

body has broken down, the affected person, feeling helpless and irritated, seeks out a mechanic-doctor to repair the broken part. A young man who came to me with a very minor ailment illustrates the modern attitude. A beginning guitar player, he complained to me about tender spots on his fingertips. "Can't you do something about these sore spots?" he asked. "I can only play for half an hour before I have to quit. At this rate I'll never learn to play the guitar."

As it happened, I had personal experience with that very problem. One year in medical school I spent the summer sailing on a schooner on the North Sea. The first week, as I pulled on heavy ropes to hoist the sail, my fingertips became so sore that they bled and kept me awake at night with the pain. During the second week calluses were forming, and soon afterward thick calluses covered my fingers. I had no more trouble with tenderness that summer, but when I returned to medical school two months later I found to my chagrin that I had lost my finer skills in dissection. The calluses made my fingers less sensitive and I could scarcely feel the instruments. For a few weeks I worried that I had ruined my career as a surgeon. Gradually, though, the calluses disappeared with my sedentary life, and sensitivity returned.

"Your body is in the process of adapting," I told the young guitarist. "The calluses show that your fingers are getting used to the new stress of being drawn across steel strings. Your body is doing you a favor by building up extra layers of protection. As for the tenderness, it's only a temporary phase, and you should be grateful for it." I told him of insensitive leprosy patients who had badly damaged their hands trying to learn the guitar or violin because they had no pain warnings to prevent them from over-practicing. Others adhered to a restricted timetable of practice so as to allow their tissues a chance to build up callus. (Skin tissue responds to the stimulus at a local level even though the brain never receives the pain sensations.)

I failed to sway the guitarist, who left my office disappointed that I had not "fixed" his hand. In an odd way, vaguely reminiscent of my leprosy patients, he seemed estranged from his own body. His hand was an object—almost a nuisance, really—that he had brought to me, the body specialist, for repairs. Such an attitude has become almost typical of modern patients.

Sadly, medical professionals sometimes foster such an attitude. I frequently meet with groups of students in medical school and ask about their frustrations in the field. The most common response I hear centers on the clumsy word *depersonalization*. As one bright young woman told me, "I chose medicine out of a sense of compassion and a desire to relieve suffering. But more and more I find I have to fight off cynicism. We don't talk much about patients here; we talk about 'syndromes' and 'enzyme failure.' They encourage us to use the word 'client' rather than 'patient,' which implies that we're selling services rather than ministering to persons. Some of the younger teachers speak of patients almost as if they were adversaries. They say, 'Watch out for older patients—they're chronic complainers, and will eat up too much of your time.' And we spend hours studying the latest MRI and CAT scan diagnostic techniques, but I haven't had a single class session on bedside manner. After a while, it's easy to forget that the 'product' we're dealing with is a human being."

I cringe when I hear such words, and think back with gratitude on my old-fashioned professors: H. H. Woolard, who treated even cadavers with reverence, and Gwynne Williams, who would kneel by a patient's bedside so that, at eye level, he would appear less intimidating and thus help the patient relax. The current biomedical approach, which narrows the focus from the patient to the disease itself, has taught us much about hostile organisms, but at the risk of devaluing the patient's own contributions. We dare not let technology distance us from patients, because certain things technology cannot do. It cannot hold your hand, inspire confidence, make you a partner in the recovery process. Used wisely, technology should be a servant of the human side of medicine: by handling facts and data, it can free the physician to spend more time with the patient so that he or she can apply the compassionate, humane wisdom that can only come from a human mind.

On the surface a doctor's task may resemble an engineer's—they both repair mechanical parts—but only on the surface. We treat a person, not a collection of parts, and a person is far more than a broken body in need of repair. A human being, unlike any machine, contains what Schweitzer called "the doctor within," the ability to repair itself and to affect consciously the healing process. The best physicians are the humblest ones, those who listen closely to the body and work to assist it in what it is already instinctively doing for itself. Indeed, in pain management I have no choice but to work in partnership: pain occurs "inside" the patient, and the patient alone can guide me.

I have learned about pain management primarily through

hand surgery, in which all parties involved must tune in to pain. If you injured your hand and came to me for surgery, we would both look to pain to help steer the recovery process. I could artificially dull the pain before therapy sessions to make you more comfortable, but if I did so you might well (like my leprosy patients) exercise too vigorously and tear out the transplanted tendons. On the other hand, if you avoided any movement that caused even a little pain, your hand would become stiff, for scar tissue would fill in the spaces and immobilize the hand. Together, we must seek the boundary of pain and then push through it and just beyond it.

The best rehabilitation takes place, I have found, if I can convince you of the truth that you are doing it all yourself. I have done my job by rearranging the muscles and tendons. Everything else depends on you. Your body will have to reunite the nerves and blood vessels I have cut, and deal with scar tissue and collagen. I attached the tendons to their new sites with flimsy stitches; your fibroblasts will provide strong, permanent attachments. Your muscles will gauge the new tensions and add or subtract tiny units called sarcomeres, covering the mistakes of the surgeon. Your brain will have to learn new programs to order movement. As the wound heals, it is you who must start to move the hand. The hand belongs to you, and only you can make it work again.

At the Carville clinic we make available instruments that patients can use as a kind of biofeedback of the healing process. By using a thermistor probe, for example, they can monitor the changing temperature of joints: the temperature goes up with activity and then down after rest, but stays up if the patient exercises too strenuously. We tell patients how much swelling to expect, then give them a measuring jar to dip the hand into. The rise in water level will show whether the patient has done something to cause excessive swelling, even something as simple as letting the injured hand hang below the waist. In these ways we teach patients to take personal responsibility for their own healing even when they have lost the internal monitor of pain.

No instrument, however, can measure what is beyond doubt the most important factor in hand therapy: the patient's will to recover. The mind, not the cells of the injured hand, will determine the final extent of rehabilitation, because without strong motivation the patient simply will not endure the disciplines of recovery.

My least favorite hand surgery patients are those involved in litigation as a result of injury on the job. These men and women have a powerful incentive *not* to gain full recovery of the hand, because a permanent disability means a larger financial settlement. Their pain threshold often seems to get lower and lower until at the first twinge of pain they pull back from the physical therapy exercises. If they successfully avoid all pain, they will likely have a permanent disability. (One 1980 study showed that people in Great Britain injured through industrial accidents returned to work at a rate 25 percent slower than those who sustained comparable injuries through road accidents. The suspected reason: in that country, injuries from industrial accidents are compensated better, giving the patient less incentive to recover.)

In contrast, one of my best patients was an inmate of the state penitentiary in Louisiana whose hand had been so damaged by a bullet that I had to devise some new tendon transfer techniques during the surgery. I assumed the patient would have to undergo extensive therapy, with no guarantee of success. But, as we later learned, this prisoner had a powerful incentive to recuperate quickly. During the period of postoperative hospitalization he removed the plaster cast, filed off his shackles, and escaped. Three years later I saw him at another hospital, still on the loose. The damaged hand had healed perfectly: his urgent need to regain active use, moderated only by pain, had provided the perfect environment for full recovery.

The reason subjective issues like "incentive to recover" carry such weight in pain management traces back to the three stages of pain: signal, message, and response. After surgery, a hand patient has the overpowering sensation "My hand hurts." But as we have seen, that sensation is a clever invention of the mind: what really hurts is the felt image of the hand stored away in the spinal cord and brain. Since pain involves all three stages of perception, effective pain management must take into account each of these stages.

Signal

Most of us attack pain first at stage one: we open the bathroom cabinet and select a medication designed to block pain signals at the site of damaged tissue. Aspirin, the most widely used drug in the world, works at this stage. Although an aspirinlike substance was extracted from the willow in 1763 and used for treatment of rheumatism and fever, it took two hundred years for scientists to figure out what makes aspirin so effective: it prevents the production of something called prostaglandin in damaged tissue, hence suppressing the normal responses of swelling and hypersensitivity.

Other common drugs work directly on the nerve endings, interfering with their ability to send pain signals. Sunburn sprays and topical treatments for cuts, wounds, and mouth sores often contain these chemicals, as do the more powerful local anesthetics used by dentists and doctors in minor surgeries.

I am slow to interfere with pain signals from the periphery. Having spent my life among people who destroy themselves for lack of pain, I treasure these signals. A harried executive who swallows a handful of aspirin and tranquilizers after a hard day's work, much like the athlete who accepts a painkiller injection before an important game, is overriding a fundamental principle of the pain system. Pain signals at stage one report in loudly and insistently so that their message will seize consciousness and bring about a change in behavior. To silence the signals without changing behavior is to invite the risk of far greater damage: the body will feel better while getting worse. Certainly painkillers like aspirin offer benefits, such as a good night's sleep and a reduction in inflammation, but in every case I believe we must first consider the positive use of pain, and then act in a way that achieves the proper balance.

Once again, my experience in hand therapy comes to mind. Unless we can persuade our patients to accept a little pain as part of their rehabilitation, the joints will freeze up and the hand go rigid. "Just give me some drugs to keep it from hurting, and I'll do my exercises gladly," some patients say. They are quite right. Modern surgeons, before closing up the hand, may leave a tiny catheter next to the nerve so that a local anesthetic can be dripped into the wound; their patients then do exercises they might otherwise balk at, speeding recovery. I do not oppose this practice, but I have learned to reserve it for my most careful and cooperative patients. Most patients need pain's boundary of inhibition; without it, they tend to move too strongly and break the wound open. The key in pain management is to recognize the links between the stages of pain. I will block pain signals at stage one only if I have confidence that my patients will take responsibility at stage three, conscious response. Will they follow the precise instructions of the therapist even in the absence of pain?

When I confront pain personally I prefer to counteract all

three stages at once. It seems appropriate to give a unified response to a sensation that involves my body so inclusively. A few years ago I had a problem with my gallbladder. When I first felt the urgent pain signals (stage one) from my upper abdomen, I had no idea what danger they were trying to alert me to. It was an intense and cramping pain, far too severe for indigestion. Antacids had no effect. Its location made the gallbladder or pancreas the possible site. My age was about right for cancer to appear, and by the time I visited the doctor I had worked myself into a churning state of fear and foreboding.

An X ray revealed that I had gallstones, not cancer, a painful condition to be sure but one easily treatable with surgery. I felt foolish about my panicky reaction. The abdominal attacks kept occurring, but right away they seemed less painful. Although the pain signals themselves did not diminish, my perception of them (stage three) surely changed as my anxiety lessened.

Because of scheduling difficulties I had to delay the gallbladder surgery for a few months. Pain from gallstones and kidney stones ranks very high on the intensity charts, and I now understand why. I had many opportunities to practice my mastery over pain (and many opportunities to reconsider my "Thank God for pain" philosophy!). I suppose I have never outgrown the boyhood spirit that made me resist the temptation of an aspirin, because I consistently tried to avoid running to the medicine cabinet for Demerol.

Night attacks were the worst. I remember one especially difficult night when I got out of bed, slipped on a robe, and walked around the paths of the leprosarium in my bare feet. The Louisiana night was steamy, and alive with sound. Frogs bellowed out their choruses in the pond, with crickets and other insects filling in the notes they missed. Nell, our frisky mongrel dog, ran ahead of me, delighted by the unscheduled walk at such a strange hour.

I deliberately chose to walk on the paths made of shell gravel dredged from southern beaches. These shells are very sharp, and painful to bare feet. I had to select my steps with care and ease my feet down gingerly, and I alternated by walking on the wet grass. As I walked along, I also picked up small tree limbs and stones and fingered them. All these minor acts helped to combat the pain: the flood of sensations from shells on my bare feet competed with and partially drowned out the pain signals from my gallbladder. The pain I felt now was quite different—and much more tolerable—than what I had felt in a dark, quiet bedroom.

I'm not sure when the singing began. I think I spoke at first, expressing aloud to God my wonder and appreciation for the good earth around me and the stars blazing overhead. Then I found myself singing a few bars of a favorite hymn. Birds started and flew away in disorder. Nell cocked her ears and looked quizzical. I glanced around, self-conscious, suddenly aware how it would look if a night watchman caught the senior staff surgeon outdoors at 2:00 A.M., barefoot, wearing pajamas, and singing a hymn.

That bayou evening still shines in my mind. At other times, especially when I needed a full night's sleep, I did take some painkiller to quiet the pain I felt in the dark and stillness of my bedroom. But that night I marshalled my whole body in a counterattack on the pain that had rudely got me out of bed. By walking on the shell path, I generated new, more tolerable stage-one signals of pain which had flooded the spinal gate, affecting stage two. And attentiveness to the world around me influenced stage three, bringing about a state of calmness and serenity. The muscle spasm and with it the colic finally subsided and I climbed back into bed a new man, and slept through the night.

Message

If I had been willing to invest several hundred dollars in a Transcutaneous Electrical Nerve Stimulator (TENS), I might have stayed in bed. The TENS represents a quintessentially modern approach to pain management. A battery-powered device about the size of a Walkman radio, it generates a small electrical current that passes between two carbon-rubber electrodes. Strapped to the skin and positioned directly over a nerve, the TENS produces a slight tingling sensation, which the wearer can adjust up or down depending on the intensity of the pain. (Other devices deliver electrical current directly to platinum electrodes implanted beside nerves or even in the spinal cord, but the skin-stimulating models usually win out because they avoid the complications of surgery.)

Is it due to sheer old-fashionedness that I prefer bayou sounds and the feel of shell gravel to a tingling electrical sensation? Both techniques work partly by generating new nerve signals that overwhelm the spinal "gate." As the spinal gate-control theory explains it, nerves from the spinal cord pass through a relatively narrow channel just below the medulla oblongata of the brain, and when that bottleneck becomes clogged with extraneous sensations, pain messages tend to diminish. Drowned out by the competition, fewer pain signals are converted into messages and forwarded to the brain.

The effectiveness of TENS varies from patient to patient, but I have noticed one positive benefit. When a chronic pain patient learns that he or she has a measure of control over pain just by turning a dial on a machine, the pain suddenly seems less threatening, more tolerable. In this way TENS, a pain treatment directed at stage two, also has an impact on pain perception at stage three. It reduces fear and anxiety, two common intensifiers of pain. Over time, the patient may stop using the machine entirely. The patient has, if not befriended the pain, at least learned to live with it. I wholeheartedly approve of this training exercise in pain mastery, though I admit to a bias toward midnight walks, hairbrushes, and hot baths as means to achieve the same end.

The field of dentistry is also experimenting with TENS. Since most patients regard the needle as the most unpleasant part of dental care, researchers keep looking for ways to provide anesthesia without needles. In one technique, a dentist using TENS places a thin electrode on a patient's hand, another behind the ear, and a third wrapped in cotton beside the tooth requiring dental work. For a majority of test subjects, a mild current at 15,000 cycles per second can provide pain relief equivalent to novocaine.

Many prescription drugs likewise address pain at the message stage. The painkilling properties of opium have been recognized for most of recorded history, and varieties of the poppy plant grow all over the world. Only recently, however, was it discovered that the drug works directly on the spinal cord as well as on the brain. Opium-type molecules (the opium family includes the powerful drugs codeine, morphine, and heroin) lock on to opiate receptor sites in the spinal cord, slowing the rate at which cells fire and reducing the number of messages conveyed to the brain. New epidural techniques drip the narcotic directly into the spinal canal, affecting the sensory nerve roots on the way into the spinal cord, a precise anesthesia that can provide relief for such excruciating conditions as pancreatic cancer.*

The most radical pain management technique is invasive surgery, and surgical procedures aimed at stage two seem the most promising, albeit not foolproof. Surgery for pain at stage three, within the brain itself, involves much risk, and frequently fails to solve the problem: after a short relapse, the pain reappears. Cutting the peripheral nerves that produce the pain signals at stage one may relieve some chronic pains, especially facial neuralgia, but there is no guarantee that blocking pain at the site of its origin will end it.

The complex phenomenon of pain cannot easily be "fixed," not by the best surgeon in the world. I have read one report of a race car driver who lost his left forearm in a racing accident. The man suffered phantom limb pain, and, after electrical implants on the local nerves did nothing to relieve it, his surgeon opened up the spinal cord. To his great surprise, he found that the nerves running from the arm to the spinal cord had already been severed by the accident. Pain signals could not possibly be coming from the periphery; the spinal cord itself was generating a message that the brain interpreted as "My left arm is hurting."

Not even surgery on the spinal cord itself, however, gives a permanent guarantee against pain. As an act of mercy, surgeons may remove a section of the spinal cord from a cancer patient who has a short life expectancy, but if the patient lives more than eighteen months the pain sometimes returns. Either the brain or another part of the spinal cord mysteriously finds a way to resurrect the pain messages.

I am not a neurosurgeon, and I can only recall a few times when I agreed to treat pain surgically. The most memorable involved an Indian woman named Rajamma, who suffered from

---

*A drug like opium or morphine does not usually produce hallucinatory effects if taken for the relief of pain. And, for reasons not fully understood, narcotics given for pain treatment do not normally result in addiction. A study published in 1982 reported on twelve thousand Boston hospital patients who had received narcotic painkillers: only four became addicted to the drugs they had received as patients. Studies also show that patients who control their own access to injected narcotics use less than the hospital staff would have administered.

the bedeviling condition of tic douloureux, a severe neuralgia of the face. Unpredictably, spasmodically, she would be jolted by a fiery shot of pain to one side of her face. She came to me in desperation after trying many alternative treatments.

"I had all the teeth removed from one side of my face, but the pain did not go away," Rajamma said. "Then I let a local medicine man scar me with burns." She pointed to the scar marks on her left cheek. "The pain got worse. Now, any small movement or sound may bring on an attack. My children cannot play near the house. We keep the chickens penned so they will not fly up and startle me."

I knew that the procedure for treating tic douloureux involved a delicate exploration of the gasserian ganglion, located where the fifth cranial nerve enters the brain, and should only be attempted by a trained neurosurgeon (if the nerve twig to the eye were cut accidentally, the loss of eye sensation could lead to the loss of the eye). But I was in South India, where no neurosurgeon was available. First I tried deadening the site with an anesthetic, which failed. Rajamma and her husband begged for me to attempt the surgery, even if it meant blindness, even if it meant death. "What kind of life do I lead now?" Rajamma asked. "Look at me." She was already dangerously thin. "I dare not chew," she explained. "I live on fluids."

Finally, I did attempt the surgery, and located two tiny nerves, fine as cotton threads, that seemed the most likely carriers of her pain. I held them in my forceps for a few seconds before cutting them. Could these thin wires be the source of the tyranny? What if I had the wrong nerves? I snipped them, and closed the wound.

I am sure that my tension was as great as Rajamma's as I sat with her in the ward and mapped the area of her cheek that now had no sensation. Haltingly, she began to attempt the movements that had previously triggered spasms of pain. She tried a slight smile, her first intentional smile in years, and no attack came. Her husband beamed back at her.

The surgery proved a success and, little by little, Rajamma's world fell into place. When she returned home, chickens were welcomed into the house again. The children began to play without fear of hurting their mother. In ever-widening circles, the family's life returned to normal. Pain, gone wild, had at last been tamed.

Response

Transcutaneous stimulators, epidural blocks, spinal cordotomies—these techniques may help persistent, long-term pain, but in many cases the body finds a new avenue and the pain returns. For this reason, chronic pain centers have learned to attack pain on all three fronts: signals from the injury site, messages along the transmission routes, and response in the mind. Actually, attending to a patient's psychological health and family environment may have as much effect on the pain as prescribing analgesic drugs or a TENS device. As one Boston psychiatrist puts it, "Half the people who go to clinics with physical complaints are really saying, 'My life hurts.' Pain is really an existential expression."

In my own approach to pain, I give highest priority to the third stage. That may seem odd, since I have spent so much of my career working with leprosy patients, who suffer from the lack of pain signals in the periphery (stage one). But the very fact that they do "suffer" proves the importance of the mind in the pain experience. Leprosy patients helped me understand the difference between *pain* and *suffering*. "I'm suffering in my mind because I can't suffer in my body," is how my patient Namo had put it.

In more advanced cases of leprosy, my patients felt no "pain" at all: no negative sensations reached their brains when they touched a hot stove or stepped on a nail. Yet all of them suffered, as greatly as any people I have ever known. They lost the freedom that pain provides, they lost the sense of touch and sometimes sight, they lost their physical attractiveness, and because of the stigma of the disease they lost the feeling of acceptance by fellow human beings. The mind responded to these effects of painlessness with a feeling that could only be called suffering.

For the rest of us, pain and suffering often arrive in the same package. My goal in pain management is to seek ways to employ the human mind as an ally, not an adversary. In other words, can I prevent "pain" from becoming undue "suffering"? The mind offers wonderful resources to accomplish just that.

In my days of medical training, I was mystified by some of the puzzles of pain: the "Anzio effect" response to battlefield wounds and the mysterious powers of placebo, hypnosis, and lobotomy. At the time, science had no explanation for these phenomena; like the Hindu fakir's mastery over pain, they belonged more to the field of magic than of medicine. In more recent years, researchers have unlocked some of the secrets of the brain's alchemy. It seems the body manufactures its own narcotics, which it can release upon command to block out pain.

The brain is a master pharmacologist. Its tiny opiate etorphin has ounce for ounce ten thousand times the painkilling power of morphine. Neurotransmitters such as these modify the synapses of the brain's neurons, literally changing the perception of pain as it is being sorted and processed. The soldier who reacts spontaneously to the excitement of battle and the fakir who exercises an acquired discipline have probably found ways of tapping into the brain's natural painkilling forces. The peripheral nerves are sending signals, the spinal cord is transmitting messages, but brain cells alter that message before it becomes pain.

Once discovered (in the 1970s), brain neurotransmitters opened up the possibility of intriguing new approaches to pain management: (1) perhaps the brain's neurotransmitters could be artificially produced, allowing us to manage pain better by outside intervention; (2) perhaps we could teach the brain to dispense its elixirs on demand, whenever we want them.

The first line of inquiry is still in its infancy. Researchers have synthesized several powerful enkephalins, but major barriers remain. For one thing, protective enzymes intercept most foreign chemicals as they try to pass from the bloodstream into the brain, and a painkiller that must be injected directly into the brain has obvious drawbacks. Also, the synthetics tend to be addictive: the brain stops producing its own enkephalins in the presence of the artificial ones, leaving the user with a choice of permanent addiction or an agonizing withdrawal.

The opposite approach, to stimulate the brain's own painkillers, has nearly unlimited potential. Inside the ivory box of skull, psychology and physiology come together. We know that a person's response to pain depends to a very large degree on "subjective" factors, such as emotional preparedness and cultural expectations, which in turn affect the brain's chemistry. By altering these subjective factors, we can directly influence the perception of pain.

Pain accompanying childbirth provides an excellent example. Societies that practice *couvade* give dramatic proof that culture plays an important part in determining how much pain the delivering mother perceives. To all appearances—and the appearances defy comprehension for women who have gone through painful deliveries themselves—the mothers in *couvade* societies do not experience much pain. In Western culture, however, childbirth ranks as one of the highest pains. Using the McGill Pain Questionnaire, Ronald Melzack interviewed hundreds of patients and determined that mothers rated labor pain during childbirth higher than pain from back injury, cancer, shingles, toothache, or arthritis.

Yet Melzack also found that second-time mothers rated their labor pains lower. Their prior experience helped to lower the threshold of fear and anxiety, and subsequently the perception of pain. First-time mothers who had prenatal training, such as classes in the Lamaze method, also rated their pains lower. The Lamaze method can in fact be viewed as a wide-scale attempt to change the perception of childbirth pain. Lamaze teachers stress that childbirth entails hard work, but not necessarily pain. They reduce fear and anxiety (stage three) by educating pregnant women about what to expect. And they teach concrete, practical ways of coping with pain at stages one and two: the breathing exercises and the father's assistance in pressing on the back during labor contractions all help counteract pain at the spinal gate.

The Lamaze course employs one simple exercise that any of us can do at any time to modify pain at stage three: conscious distraction. I first learned of the effect of distraction from Tommy Lewis's research. When bells were rung and adventure stories read aloud, the laboratory volunteers had much greater tolerance for pain. Lab assistants using radiant heat machines were surprised to see blisters swell up unnoticed on volunteers' arms as those subjects concentrated on counting backward from fifty to one.

A few years ago, American dentists had high hopes about the potential of audio techniques in controlling pain. Patients who wore earphones and listened to loud stereo music, or even artificial "white noise," sat contentedly without painkiller while dentists probed and drilled. Stereo equipment would replace the hypodermic needle, some predicted. At dental conferences, dentists cited Melzack's spinal gate-control theory as a way to explain the phenomenon. But when Ronald Melzack himself tested the findings against those for a placebo stimulus—a worthless sixty-cycle hum that should have had no effect on the patients—to his surprise even the placebo noise diminished pain. Melzack concluded that the key element in the audio machine's success was the value of conscious distraction. As long as the subjects concentrated on the music or noise, and as long as they had knobs and levers to operate, they felt less pain. They were attending to something else.

In the book *Living with Pain*, Barbara Wolf tells of her long struggle against chronic pain, an odyssey which included having subcutaneous neural transmitters implanted in both hands. After trying a host of methods, she decided that distraction was the best and cheapest weapon available. She used to cancel activities when she felt pain, until she noticed that the only time she felt completely free of pain was during classroom hours when she taught English. Wolf recommends work, reading, humor, hobbies, pets, sports, volunteer work, or anything else that can divert the sufferer's mind from pain. When pain strikes with fury in the middle of the night, Wolf gets up, maps out the day ahead, works on a lecture, or completely plans a dinner party.

Pain need not necessarily dull the mind. Blaise Pascal, plagued with acute facial neuralgia, worked out some of his most complex geometry problems while tossing uncomfortably in bed. Composer Robert Schumann, suffering from a chronic illness, would get out of bed and correct his musical scores. Immanuel Kant, his toes burning from gout, would concentrate with all his might on one object—for example, on the Roman orator Cicero and everything that might relate to him. Kant claimed this technique succeeded so well that in the morning he sometimes wondered whether he had imagined the pain.

When I confront intense pain, I look for activities that will fully absorb me, either mentally or physically. I go out for a walk or work at my computer. I dredge up tasks that I have avoided out of busyness: I clear out a closet, write letters, go bird watching, weed the garden. I too have found that conscious distraction and the discipline of activity can be helpful tools in combating pain.

One specialist at a chronic pain center told me that many patients want to wait until the pain subsides before they resume normal functioning. But he has learned that coping with chronic pain depends on a patient's willingness to exercise and increase productive activity *despite* the feeling of pain. Chronic pain management succeeds when the patient accepts the possibility of living a useful life in the presence of pain.

We in the West, who rely on pills and technology to solve our health problems, tend to discount the role of the conscious mind. After meeting Dr. Clifford Snyder, I can never again underestimate our inherent power to alter pain perception. This gentle man, a respected plastic surgeon and former coeditor of the *Journal of Plastic Surgery*, has learned to harness the mind's amazing capacity for pain management. After several trips to China to investigate acupuncture, Snyder became convinced that much of the potency of acupuncture in relieving pain was due to a person's mental belief in it—a glorified placebo effect. A few years later, he had a chance to test his conviction about the mind's power.

Snyder needed surgery on his hand, a complicated procedure to strip away the synovial lining covering his wrist tendons. It involved deep cuts in an area of many nerve endings. Snyder had a busy schedule the next day, with a major address to deliver, and he did not want to risk general anesthesia, which could leave him groggy. He decided to *will* away pain, with no resource but the power of mind.

The attending surgeon, whom I also know well, agreed to honor his colleague's peculiar request. He allowed Dr. Snyder a few minutes to gather his thoughts, tied a tourniquet around the upper arm, and then without the application of any anesthesia proceeded to perform the surgery. Through sheer autosuggestion, Snyder concentrated on feeling no pain. He remained conscious throughout, and he insists that he felt absolutely no pain until about an hour after the surgery. The surgeon on the other end of the scalpel verifies his account.

Afterward, Dr. Snyder tried to incorporate what he had learned about pain management into his medical practice. "I always try to divert my patient's attention to something pleasant," he says. "I talk about football, or the president's recent news conference, and avoid expressing any alarm. I try to calm my patients. I touch and rub the site of injury, especially with children, and always tell them exactly what I'm going to do. I never lie to them. I want their complete trust."

Snyder reports remarkable results among some of his patients. One schoolteacher who came in for removal of a ganglion became so involved in a conversation with a medical student that Snyder removed the ganglion without even applying a local anesthetic. A teenage boy with severe acne came in to have his face "sandpapered" with an abrasive. "Doctor, I'll give you one hour," he said. "I don't want anything for the pain." He lay still for sixty minutes and showed no sign of pain. Then he held up his hand and said, "Now it's beginning to hurt. You'll have to stop."

Not everyone can master the skill of autosuggestion over pain. But the examples cited should encourage us to believe that, even if we cannot abolish a specific pain, we can probably make it hurt less and thus eliminate the need for drugs. They confirm the amazing capacity for pain management that all of us carry around atop our necks.

Worst Case

I once met with nuns, caregivers, and a few pain specialists from around the world at a conference in Dallas, Texas. In a televised interview afterward, I explained my personal philosophy of pain based on gratitude and appreciation for pain's benefits. "The system of pain is good," I said, "even though there will surely be times when individual pains are not good." I mentioned the pain that sometimes accompanies terminal cancer, a debilitating pain that serves no helpful purpose—the patient knows death is coming soon—and frustrates most of the pain management techniques I have described in this chapter.

"The challenge of medicine in such a case," I said, "is to give enough medication to quell the pain, but not so much as to cloud the patient's mind. Yet if the pain persists, as an act of mercy it may be necessary to give so much medication that the patient may not be conscious enough to communicate."

I heard a sudden eruption at the other end of the table and turned to face a slim, distinguished-looking Englishwoman. Dr. Therese Vanier had almost jumped out of her seat. "I'm sorry, Dr. Brand, but I must strongly disagree! I am a physician at the St. Christopher's Hospice in London, and this is not the philosophy of our hospice! We promise our patients that they will be free of severe pain but also will remain lucid. We can almost guarantee that."

The vigor of Dr. Vanier's response startled me, and after the interview I sought her out. She invited me to visit the hospice founded by Dame Cicely Saunders in 1967, in order to observe what they had learned about worst-case, terminal pain. Several years later I made the trip. St. Christopher's is, in essence, a place where people go to die. Forty percent of its admitted patients die within their first week.

"The majority of patients come to us in severe pain, in the final stages of their illness," Vanier explained during my visit. "Pain from a terminal disease is unique. Pain from a bone fracture, sore tooth, childbirth, or even postoperative recovery has meaning, and there is an end in sight. Pain from progressive cancer has no meaning except the constant reminder of approaching death. For many of the patients who come to us, pain fills the entire horizon. They can't eat, sleep, pray, think, or relate to people without being dominated by pain. Here at St. Christopher's we try to combat that particular kind of pain."

After visiting with Vanier, I met with Dr. Cicely Saunders, who told me the origin of the hospice movement. She had founded the first hospice, she said, after seeing how poorly the medical profession handled death. For the sake of a patient with some prospect of recovery, a modern hospital would go to any length. But a patient without hope was an embarrassment, a shameful emblem of medicine's failures. Doctors mostly avoided terminally ill patients, or spoke to them in platitudes and half-truths. Treatment for their pain tended to be grossly inadequate. In the midst of busy, crowded hospitals, terminal patients died afraid and very much alone.

The standard treatment of terminal patients offended Saunders's deep Christian sensibilities. A nurse at the time, she enrolled in medical school at the age of thirty-three for the express purpose of finding a better way to minister to the dying. After working at a home for the dying run by the Sisters of Charity she wrote, "Suffering is only intolerable when nobody cares. One continually sees that faith in God and his care is made infinitely easier by faith in someone who has shown kindness and sympathy." She went on to found St. Christopher's, and out of that sprang the worldwide hospice movement. Saunders notes that hospice actually resurrects a theme from the Middle Ages, when the church counted care for the dying as one of the seven cardinal virtues.

Working together, Saunders and Therese Vanier pioneered the "preventive" approach to pain from terminal disease. In many hospitals the standard order for pain medication says "PRN" (for *pro nata*, "as needed"). That order leaves medication to the discretion of the health worker, who has been sternly warned about the dangers of addiction. As a result, if the pain returns before expected, a patient in agony may have to plead for the next injection. Saunders tried a different approach. She carefully determined dosages in advance, then made them available to the patient at regular intervals so that the pain never returned at all. A steady blood level of medication, she found, helps to prevent both severe pain and oversedation. Saunders also tested patient-controlled dosages and discovered that terminal patients rarely overmedicate.

Under supervision, they usually come up with a program that controls pain around the clock without mental clouding.

The design of St. Christopher's reflects Saunders's wisdom about care for the dying. Most patients live in four-bed bays, not private rooms, with space enough for family members to stay overnight. Dividing curtains permit privacy as needed, but the presence of other human beings allows for a kind of community to develop, a community based on seeing others face death in an atmosphere of trust and not cringing fear. Rooms are filled with furniture purchased from a department store, not an institutional catalog. Front windows frame a park manicured in fine English tradition; rear windows overlook a flower garden and goldfish pond.

A visitor to the hospice sees signs of life everywhere: staff gathered around a bedside singing "Happy Birthday," artwork hanging from every blank wall space, a minijungle of potted plants, a patient's pet cocker spaniel frolicking on a visit. Every two weeks or so the staff organizes a concert, with a string quartet or harpist or children's handbell choir visiting the wards. Volunteers transport able patients to the local McDonald's or pub, depending on their preference. As much as possible, St. Christopher's functions at the convenience of patients, not staff.

My day at St. Christopher's convinced me that Therese Vanier's outburst on the panel in Dallas was fully justified. Even the worst pain imaginable, the severe pain that accompanies terminal illness, need not debilitate. It struck me that Dame Cicely, Dr. Vanier, and the others at St. Christopher's have incorporated nearly everything I have learned about pain management and more. They allow for diversion and conscious distraction. They help soothe the subjective factors (fear, anxiety) that contribute to pain. They work hard to make the patient feel like a partner, not a victim, one who retains control over his or her own body. They create a caring community.

In a word, the hospice movement has shifted the focus of medicine from *cure* to *care*. Daniel Callahan has criticized contemporary medicine for precisely this failure.

> The primary assurance we all require is that we will be cared for in our sickness regardless of the likelihood of cure. . . . The greatest failure of contemporary healthcare is that it has tended to overlook this point, has become dis-

tracted from it by the glamour of cure and the war against illness and death. At the center of caring should be a commitment never to avert its eyes from, or wash its hands of, someone who is in pain or is suffering, who is disabled or incompetent, who is retarded or demented; that is . . . the one commitment a healthcare system can almost always make to everyone, the one need that it can reasonably meet.

St. Christopher's, which grew out of one woman's deep Christian compassion, shows what can be done. Many church and community groups have followed Dame Cicely's model and now extend loving care to the terminally ill who have chosen against artificial methods of prolonging life. By definition, these patients are beyond the range of medical cure. Yet hospice has found a way to treat this most distressing human condition with dignity and compassion. Dame Cicely takes pride in the fact that fully 95 percent of the patients at St. Christopher's have been able to stay both alert and free of pain. She has demonstrated it is possible to disarm the last great fear most of us will face, the fear of death and the pain which accompanies it.

17
Intensifiers of Pain

❖

*One's own clothes are replaced by an anonymous white nightgown,
one's wrist is clasped by an identification bracelet with a number.
One becomes subject to institutional rules and regulations. One is
no longer a free agent; one no longer has rights; one is no longer
in the world-at-large. It is strictly analogous to becoming a
prisoner, and humiliatingly
reminiscent of one's first day at
school. One is no longer a person—one is now an inmate.*
Oliver Sacks, *A Leg to Stand On*

If the hospice movement is designed to help patients face the final challenge of pain, the typical modern hospital seems designed to render its patients helpless before all pain. Confined to a private, sterile room, entangled in a web of tubes and wires, the object of knowing glances and whispered conversations, the patient feels trapped and alone. In this alien atmosphere, pain thrives. I sometimes wonder if pharmaceutical companies have masterminded the scheme of modern hospitals in an attempt to promote the use of pain-relieving medications.

I got a dose of modern medicine in 1974 when I finally agreed to let a surgeon remove my troublesome gallbladder. After a lifetime of prowling hospital corridors, I should have known what to expect. But I soon learned a new perspective—the patient's. In surgery, I discovered, it is far more blessed to give than to receive.

All day long I lay in a spare white room void of any distractions except a television set and its irritating lineup of daytime programs. (Why doesn't someone decorate hospital ceilings since that's what most patients stare at?) A parade of technicians filed through my cell. I had not heard such brusque commands since my days in the Missionary Training Colony. "Roll up your sleeve."

"Pull down your pants." "Keep still." "Roll over." "Give me your arm." "Breathe deeply." "Cough."

The nurse who had ordered my pants down was holding a rubber catheter tube. I summoned up my courage to protest. "Why do I need a catheter?" I knew the danger of infection and, besides, who wants a rubber tube jammed up his private parts?

"You haven't passed any urine since your surgery" was his stern reply.

I felt a flicker of guilt. "That's because I haven't had much fluid input! It's my gallbladder that's missing, not my bladder. Give me a few minutes." He left the room, I staggered over to the pot, clutching my wounded abdominal wall, and with much effort triumphantly produced a few drops. It was my one proud moment in an otherwise grim day.

When a lab technician came for the second time within an hour to collect a specimen of blood from my vein, I timidly reminded her that she already had taken one. She frowned and said in a patronizing tone, "Yes, but it clotted. The sample was worthless." I nearly apologized for my defective blood.

My body was producing an impressive array of electronic read-outs for the laboratory, but all were hidden from my eyes. No doubt aware that doctors tend to be nosy patients, the hospital staff maintained an unbroken conspiracy of silence around me. The radiologist, for example, held up my X-ray film to the light, then looked at me, shook his head somberly, and departed to consult my surgeon.

Responsibility for my bowels belonged to one person, my blood to another, and my mind to yet another: the nurse in charge of my pain medication. I got to know her well, for I stayed in constant awareness of pain. I had no gravel walkways to tread, no research reports to pore over, no stereo systems to play soothing music. I was all alone with my pain. In the stillness, I could feel the sting from the most recent injection and even the pressure on my skin from the adhesive. I felt an irresistible temptation to hit the buzzer and call for more medication.

The word hospital comes from the Latin for "guest," but in some modern hospitals "victim" seems more apt. Despite my medical background I felt helpless, inadequate, and passive. I had the overwhelming impression of being reduced to a cog in a machine, and a malfunctioning cog at that. Every sound filtering in from the hallway somehow related to my predicament. A rolling cart—*they must be coming for me.* A groan from the hallway—*Oh no, they've found something.*

In a study conducted on the Isle of Wight off the southern coast of England, researchers determined that gallbladder patients who could see a cluster of trees outside their hospital windows had shorter postoperative stays and took fewer painkillers than patients who looked at a blank brick wall. Their report bore the title "View through a Window May Influence Recovery from Surgery." I came away from my own gallbladder surgery impressed that far more than a view influences recovery.

I use the term "pain intensifiers" for responses that heighten the perception of pain within the conscious mind. They are what I battled in my hospital room. These intensifiers—fear, anger, guilt, loneliness, helplessness—may have more impact on the overall experience of pain than any prescription drug I might take. Somehow we in medicine must find ways to nourish, and not starve, a patient's own contribution.

Fear

Dr. Diane Komp, an oncologist who works with children, started making house calls after she fully understood the importance of the environment to young patients. "I have visited children at home who experienced physical pain," she writes, "but I have never seen a child at home experience fear. In their homes, I was the guest and they were clearly the hosts. Children accurately reported their medical condition in this environment, since they were in control."

I better understood my feelings in the hospital when a friend showed me a book filled with drawings made by sick children. One boy had drawn a large army tank bearing down on a tiny stick figure—himself—holding up a red stop sign. In another drawing, an eight-year-old girl depicted herself lying in a hospital bed: "I'm lonely," the caption read. "I wish I was in my own bed. I don't like it in here. It smells funny."

My favorite drawing showed a boy cringing before an oversized hypodermic needle with one slight design modification: the end of the needle was a barbed fishhook. I share his point of view. Thanks to the homeopathic beliefs of my mother and aunts, I received few injections in childhood, and saw them as invasions of my person. An irrational fear of needles persists in my mind. To this day I have never succeeded in giving myself an injection. I drive the needle toward my skin and mysteriously, just before it reaches me, a barrier springs up and deflects it.

Research studies in the laboratory and in the hospital confirm that fear is the strongest intensifier of pain. Newcomers in laboratory tests report a lower pain threshold until they learn they can control the experiment and have nothing to fear. In measur-able physiological ways, fear increases pain. When an injured person is afraid, muscles tense and contract, increasing the pressure on damaged nerves and causing even more pain. Blood pressure and vasodilation change too, which is why a frightened person goes pale, or flushes red. Sometimes this product of the mind translates into actual bodily damage, as is the case with spastic colon, a by-product of human anxiety unknown in other animal species.

I think of my own experience with illness. One reason doctors and nurses have gained a reputation as ornery patients is that our medical knowledge makes us even more susceptible to fear. We have seen that the slightest symptoms can betray the presence of a life-threatening illness. John Donne said it well in his seventeenth-century diary of sickness: "Fear insinuates itself in every action or passion of the mind, and as gas in the body will counterfeit any disease, and seem the stone, and seem the gout, so fear will counterfeit any disease of the mind."

I had just taken an assignment as a medical resident in London when a nasty attack of fever and headache confined me to bed. I noticed that when I lifted my head off the pillow I felt pain in my neck and at the lower end of my spine. Panic set in. Not long before, I had studied the symptoms of cerebrospinal meningitis, a terrifying diagnosis in those preantibiotic days. I had the family order an ambulance, and a few hours later I was admitted to University Hospital under the care of the senior professor of medicine, Harold Himsworth. I reviewed my symptoms and told him of my provisional diagnosis of meningitis. There was, of course, the imminent possibility of brain damage. I indicated I was ready for the spinal tap that I assumed would be necessary.

Dr. Himsworth listened solemnly and examined me with much care. He assured me he would be able to forgo the spinal tap because careful examination had made him absolutely certain of his diagnosis and the appropriate treatment. No, he would not tell me the name of the drug he was prescribing; I must trust him. He looked so confident and wise that I obediently took the medicine and calmed down. The pain faded away and I promptly fell asleep.

Three days later, after I had made the fastest known recovery from cerebrospinal meningitis, Dr. Himsworth revealed to me the name of his mystery drug: aspirin. He smiled paternally as he told me he had quickly judged my symptoms to be 25 percent influenza and 75 percent fear of meningitis. I felt terribly ashamed of the fuss I had made, but Professor Himsworth suggested the experience could be a valuable part of my medical education. "When patients come to you complaining of a pain out of all proportion to its physical cause, perhaps you will be more understanding. They feel real pain. As a doctor, you will be treating their fears as well as their organic illness or injury."

Dr. Himsworth was right, of course. Almost every person in pain experiences fear, and no pill or injection will drive it away. The gentle and honest wisdom of health practitioners and the loving support of friends and relatives are the best remedies. I have found that the time I spend "disarming" fear for my patients has a major impact on their attitude toward recovery, and especially their attitude toward pain.

My initial consultations with hand surgery patients sometimes resemble counseling sessions because I have learned that pain cannot be treated as a purely physical phenomenon. Together, doctor and patient, we must face into the fear. What does the pain mean to the patient? Will the wage earner ever be able to support a family again? Will the hand ever look beautiful again? How much pain will be involved in the recovery process? Do painkillers or steroids pose a danger to health? I try to disarm fear by giving the patient honest, accurate information. In the end, though, the patient alone must make final choices about the course of treatment. My recommendations will not produce much benefit apart from the patient's own cooperation.

I once counseled a famous pianist, Eileen Joyce, who gave annual benefit concerts in London's Royal Albert Hall to support our hospital in India. She had stumbled and fallen on her hand while walking her dog, injuring her thumb. I saw her some time after the accident, and as she was telling me about it I manually rotated her thumb in all directions. The fall had damaged a joint, a bony projection at the base of thumb. Apparently it had healed back with a tiny roughness of bone, because when I moved it in one certain way she cried out, "Yes, that's it! That's the pain! Can you operate and fix it?"

I had to tell Eileen that I would not advise surgery. (Artificial thumb joints were not yet available.) The likelihood of solving her pain was small compared to the possibility of causing more damage with the surgery. "Is it possible you could learn to live with the pain?" I asked.

Eileen was crestfallen. "Of course, it isn't a frequent pain. I know that I can play for an hour or so without my thumb hurting, and some days I never feel it at all. But then I put it in the wrong position and suddenly I feel the pain. The fear of that happening takes over. How can I concentrate on Beethoven when I'm fearing the possibility of pain?"

As a hand surgeon, I had often marveled at how effortlessly concert pianists can draw upon the full capacity of the hand without really knowing the mechanics involved. They think about music, not about joints, muscles, and tendons. Now, though, awareness of a tiny speck of bone was dominating everything else in Eileen Joyce's mind. We discussed the various alternatives for dealing with the pain, and I heard later that Eileen decided to retire from the concert stage. She could not find a way to come to terms with the fear of a pain that just might rob her concentration during a concert, even though the pain itself was not severe.

I encourage patients to talk about their fear so that together we can relate the fear to the pain signal. Fear, like pain, can be good or bad. Good fear backs me away from cliffs and makes me duck when I hear a loud noise. It stops me from taking foolish risks when I drive a car or go downhill skiing. Problems only develop when fear (or pain) grows out of proportion to the danger, as happened with me and my fear of injections and perhaps happened with Eileen Joyce as well.

The only way I or any other doctor can disarm "bad" fear is to earn the patient's trust. I released my fear of meningitis into Harold Himsworth's hands because I trusted him and believed him when he told me I had nothing to fear. And that is why as a surgeon I must pay careful attention to my patients' fears. I want them to respect the "good" fear that keeps them from pushing too fast and redamaging what I have repaired. At the same time, I want them to overcome the "bad" fear of pain that tempts them away from rehabilitation exercises.

A friend of mine in California, Tim Hansel, taught me an important lesson about good fear and bad fear. An enthusiastic outdoorsman, Tim directed a program that led strenuous camping

trips in the Sierra Nevada mountains. On one of these trips he fell
headfirst into a crevasse, striking a rock at the bottom. The impact
compressed his spinal vertebrae together, rupturing discs in his
upper back, and soon arthritis settled in the bones. Hansel lived
with constant, intense pain. He consulted several specialists, and
each one told him the same thing. "You'll just have to live with the
pain. Surgery can't help."

As the months stretched into years, Hansel learned various
ways to cope with the pain. Afraid of causing further injury, he cut
back on many of his activities. In time, however, his spirits sank.
The sedentary life was making him depressed. Finally, Hansel
voiced his fears to his doctor. "I've been afraid of reinjuring
myself, but it's driving me crazy. I feel paralyzed by the fear. Tell
me specifically, what must I avoid? What might cause more
damage?"

His doctor thought for a moment and replied, "The damage
is irreversible. I suppose I would recommend against painting
eaves—that would put too great a strain on your neck. But as far as
I can tell, you can do whatever else the pain will allow you to do."
According to Hansel, that word from the doctor gave him a new
lease on life. For the first time, he realized that he was in control
of his pain, his future, his life. He determined to live the only way
he knew—with a sense of abandonment. He went back to climbing
mountains and leading expeditions.

Tim Hansel's pain did not go away. But his fear did. And
Hansel found that with the reduction in fear, his pain eventually
decreased as well. I have been with Tim, and believe him when he
says that pain no longer has any negative effect on the quality of
his life. He has learned to master it, because he no longer fears it.
"My pain is unavoidable," he says. "But my misery is optional."

Anger

Hand surgeons dread one condition above all others: "reflex
sympathetic dystrophy" (RSD), a particular manifestation of the
stiff hand phenomenon. After an injury or minor surgical procedure, severe pain may begin to spread throughout a limb. The
symptoms sometimes appear after a joint or tendon surgery that
initially seemed wholly successful. The patient's hand comes out of
a plaster cast looking fine but, day by day and inch by inch, a grad-

ual, inordinate pain creeps in. Muscles go into periodic spasm. The hand swells and the skin tightens. Inexplicably, over time the hand locks up and becomes as stiff as a mannequin's.

Many things may cause a stiff hand (a reaction to an infection, for example), but the RSD phenomenon can also develop from simple fear or anger. A person under poor medical supervision may be surprised by the amount of soreness in a hand just released from a cast. If he or she becomes bitter and resentful, and resists any movement that might cause pain, that combination of emotion and lack of understanding will begin to affect the hand.

Sheer anger provoked the most dramatic case of stiff hand I have seen. In India, I treated a woman patient who had lost the tip of her nose. Suspecting his wife of infidelity, her husband had taken revenge by biting her nose, thus spoiling her beauty. (India was probably the origin of the ironic proverb "Cut off your nose to spite your face.") Lakshmi came to me for treatment of her hand, however, not her nose. She had a beautiful face, even with the thickened skin around her surgically repaired nose, but as she told me the story of the stiff hand, her face contorted in rage— curiously, against the surgeon who repaired the nose and not the husband who bit it off.

The story tumbled out in a torrent of words, and since Lakshmi had no medical comprehension I could barely piece together a picture of what had happened. She had gone to a plastic surgeon in Madras, who agreed to fashion a new tip for her nose out of abdominal skin. After a perfectly acceptable procedure (which we had used on leprosy patients for a while), he transplanted the skin from her abdomen to her face in two stages. First he cut a strip of skin from the abdomen, leaving it attached to the belly at one end and lifting the other end free to form a bridge to the side of her wrist. In order to allow the graft time to develop a new blood supply in the wrist, he kept her hand strapped to the abdomen for three weeks.

Afterward, in a second operation, the surgeon snipped the bridge at the belly end so that the strip of skin hung free, nourished now by blood vessels in the wrist. He lifted Lakshmi's hand to her forehead, letting the tube of skin hang in front of her nose. After making a few cosmetic adjustments, the surgeon stitched the new skin in place and swathed her forehead, hand, and wrist in adhesive strapping. His plan was to come back at the end of three weeks and cut the hand free of the tube of skin, leaving a new tip of nose on the base of the old.

At this point in her story, Lakshmi trembled with rage. "He did not tell me!" she cried. "I wanted a nose and he ruined my hand. He made my shoulder hurt. For three weeks my shoulder did not stop hurting. And still it hurts!" I rarely heard a woman use profanity in India, but Lakshmi could not speak of her surgeon without cursing. Finally, she calmed down enough to finish the account.

She awoke from surgery feeling pain in her shoulder. The surgeon, probably assuming that a young woman would have a perfectly free joint, had never bothered to find out whether she had a full range of movement in her shoulder. In fact, Lakshmi had suffered from arthritis in her shoulder for some years and had never been able to lift her arm freely without pain. Now she found her arm strapped into a position that caused constant pain. She cried and sent messages to the surgeon, who informed her the pain was normal and would soon go away. Day after day she screamed at him, telling him she couldn't bear the pain in her shoulder. He made light of the problem. Others on the hospital staff joked about the hysterical woman with her hand fixed to her nose.

By the time the surgeon removed the strapping around her head and finished the nose, Lakshmi had an advanced case of reflex sympathetic dystrophy. Her entire arm, from shoulder to hand, was hypersensitive to pain and the hand absolutely immobile. Whenever she tried to move her hand the muscles went into a kind of spasm and the fingers refused to bend.

When Lakshmi came to me, several months later, her hand was stiff. As far as I could determine, her surgeon had not made any procedural errors; he simply had not communicated with his patient. If he had taken the time to discuss the procedure with this frightened woman, and to test out the posture required, he would have learned about the stiffness in her shoulder. Instead, he attached the arm to her forehead while she slept under general anesthesia. When she complained about intense discomfort, he casually dismissed her.

Lakshmi's hand was as useless as any claw-hand I had treated on a leprosy patient. The fingers stuck straight out, unbending. I divided some of the rigid structures that held her fingers straight, and cut and lengthened the tendons of the muscles that had become contracted. On the operating table, with Lakshmi under anesthesia, I could bend the fingers to some extent. I performed a second surgery on the hand, and my therapists tried to restore motion by splinting and massage. I even tried an injection into the sympathetic nerve ganglia at the root of her neck. But the hand behaved as though it was determined to be stiff. Each time, the muscle spasms returned. I concluded the woman had lost use of her hand because of anger and distress. I could find no other physiological cause. As far as I know, Lakshmi never used her hand again, and she certainly never overcame her bitterness against the surgeon.

The stiff hand syndrome caused by RSD makes obvious the link between psyche and soma. Sympathetic nerves control involuntary activities in the body such as blood pressure, digestion, and heart rate, and the entire sympathetic nervous system is highly responsive to emotional influences such as anger or embarrassment. ("Man is the only animal that blushes—or needs to," said Mark Twain, referring to one sign of the sympathetic nervous system at work.) In reflex sympathetic dystrophy the nerves overreact and produce a pain of their own, a pain slow in onset but relentless, and very difficult to treat. Because of the sympathetic nervous system's close ties to the emotions, a poor doctor-patient relationship, such as Lakshmi had experienced, can have a profound effect on the healing process.

Experts on RSD disorders have identified psychological traits that provide warning signs of these disorders: "fearful, suspicious, emotionally labile, chronic complainer, dependent personality, introspective, worrying, apprehensive, hysterical, defensive, hostile." When I meet a patient who shows evidence of these traits, I know that I must spend much more time in personal consultation before I operate. My effort to nurture mutual understanding and trust does not represent time lost, but rather time saved from postoperative complications.

Some patients who come to me for initial consultation remind me of the possums who lived near my home in Louisiana. When frightened, a possum goes into a rigid catatonic state, stiff from snout to tail. I have seen patients like that. Their eyes widen, and they follow all my movements. They are reluctant to be tested. Often their hands feel cold to the touch. I recognize that such patients need time to gain confidence. I hold the problem hand gently while I talk and explore the patient's history. Usually I stroke the hand. I ask about the family and the home. I stress that

I will not make decisions on my own: "It is your hand, after all, not mine," I tell them. Gradually, I find, the hand grows warmer and begins to relax, and early signs of confidence and hope appear.

Physiologically, we do not really understand why a hand may become stiff after a minor injury, but we do know that it is more likely to happen when anger and bitterness are present. Lakshmi in India may have been the most dramatic case of RSD I have witnessed, but I must say there are more cases proportionately in the United States. The pattern surprised me at first. I could not imagine a comparable scenario of doctor-patient misunderstanding being played out in the United States, with its high standards of medicine and education. I have since concluded that the litigiousness in the United States provides much more fertile ground for anger, resentment, and frustration, the very feelings that foster conditions like reflex sympathetic dystrophy.

Doctors involved with insurance settlements speak of the "compensation syndrome" in which patients who have something to gain from disability tend to experience more pain and heal at a slower rate. Some lawyers even coach their clients on grimaces and outward signs of pain that will elicit sympathy from the jury. One pain expert says bluntly, "There is almost a unanimous agreement among the directors of various pain control facilities in the United States and abroad that current laws in cases of injury compensation and the adversary legal process in itself are major operant factors in conditioning pain behaviours."

I have no bone to pick with lawyers or with legitimate grievances against negligence. I am retired from medical practice now, and have never had a malpractice suit against me. But I must observe that, strictly from a medical perspective, a spirit of anger and bitterness usually ends up harming the patient most of all. My own advice to friends and family is to settle claims early, rather than hold out for maximum gain.

Too often I have seen the physiological effect on people who became angry with their employer, or the driver of the other car, or the previous surgeon, or a spouse who lacked sympathy, or God. The anger must be dealt with, of course; it does not go away on its own. But if it is not dealt with, if it is allowed to fester in the mind and soul, the anger may release its poison in the body, affecting pain and healing. As Bernie Siegel says, "To hate is easy, but it is healthier to love."

Guilt

Fear shows up in laboratory tests and anger can contribute to a condition like RSD. I cannot point so precisely to a tangible proof of guilt's effect on pain. But after a career spent among leprosy patients, who are made to feel uniquely cursed by God, I know well that guilt compounds mental suffering. Counselors at chronic pain centers, too, report that their most challenging, "pain-prone" patients have deep-rooted feelings of guilt and may well interpret their pain as a form of punishment.

I have some personal experience with pain-as-punishment, for I studied under the English public school system when it still relied on caning to enforce discipline. Fresh from the Kolli hills of India, I had to go through a "civilizing" process in London that included several direct encounters with the cane. In retrospect, I recognize that the actual pain inflicted by a thin wooden rod striking the fatty tissue of the backside measures no more than six or maybe seven on a scale of ten. But at the time it felt like a nine or ten, especially if I sensed real anger in the one delivering the blows. I am sure that the aspect of punishment, especially the feeling of *unjust* punishment—Why did only I get caught?—intensified my perception of pain.

About this same time, I learned firsthand the devastating result of believing that human tragedies come about as a direct act of God. I was fifteen, and had just returned from a long hike in a meadow near London when my Aunt Eunice met me at the door. "Come into the dining room, Paul," she said, and I could tell from her pinched face and creased forehead that something dreadful had happened. When I followed her into the dark and heavy Victorian formal room, I concluded I must have done something terrible because Uncle Bertie was standing there, along with my Aunt Hope. My spinster aunts called upon Uncle Bertie, a huge man and father of thirteen, only when they thought I needed the gruff, stern influence of a masculine figure. My mind spun at a frantic pace: *What have I done?*

As I soon learned, I had done nothing. The three adults had gathered to break the news to me of the telegram from India announcing my father's death from blackwater fever. That day, and the next few days, my aunts made many attempts to explain and soften the blow of what had happened, using pietistic clichés they hoped would console me. But my adolescent mind found ways to turn their words of intended comfort into leering accusations. "Your father was a wonderful man, too good for this world." *But what about the rest of us—does that mean we're not good enough?* "God needed him in heaven more than we need him on earth." *No! I haven't seen Dad in six years. I need my dad!* "His work was finished here." *That can't be true! The church is barely beginning, and the medical work is growing. Who will care for the hill people now? And what about my mother?* "It's for the best." *How, tell me how, can it possibly be best?*

It took many years for my childhood faith to recover from my aunts' blows of kindness. Instinctively I felt that if God had decided to "take my father," as they kept saying, it must somehow be my fault. I should have needed him more, or at least worked harder to convince God that I loved my father. Meanwhile my mother, halfway around the world, was shouldering her own burden of guilt: *If only I had taken him for proper medical treatment right away and not delayed.** When I met her ship in England more than a year later, I could easily read the pain in her sagging posture and premature wrinkles.

This is not a book of theology, and I have no desire to wade into the deep subject of divine causation. Yet I have seen so much harm caused by guilt over this one issue that I would be remiss if I did not mention it as a pain intensifier. Hundreds of patients I have treated—Muslim, Hindu, Jewish, and Christian—have tormented themselves with questions of guilt and punishment. What have I done wrong? Why me? What is God trying to tell me? Why do I deserve this fate?

As a doctor and a committed Christian, I have one simple observation to make. If God is using human suffering as a form of punishment, he certainly has picked an obscure way to communicate his displeasure. The most basic fact about punishment is that it only works if the person knows the reason for it. It does absolute

*The phrase "if only" is a danger sign. Rabbi Harold Kushner tells of a January in Boston when he conducted funerals on two successive days, for two elderly women. He visited the grieving families of both women on the same afternoon. At the first home, the surviving son said, "If only I had sent my mother to Florida and gotten her out of this cold and snow, she would be alive today. It's my fault that she died." At the second home, the surviving son said, "If only I hadn't insisted on my mother's going to Florida, she would be alive today. That long airplane ride, the abrupt change of climate, was more than she could take. It's my fault that she's dead."

harm, not good, to punish a child unless the child understands why he or she is being punished. Yet most patients I have treated feel mainly confused, not chastened, by suffering. "Why me?" they say, not, "Oh, of course, I'm being punished for last week's lust."

In school I always knew why I was getting caned, even if I sometimes disagreed with the sentence. And in the Bible's accounts of punishment, the stories do not show individuals sitting around wondering what happened. Most of them understood exactly why they were being punished: Moses announced each of the Ten Plagues before the Egyptian Pharaoh; prophets warned corrupt nations years in advance. The classic story of suffering, in the book of Job, portrays a man who clearly was *not* being punished for evil deeds—God called Job "blameless and upright, a man who fears God and shuns evil."

These biblical examples have little in common with the pain and suffering most people undergo today. Millions of babies are born with birth defects every year. Whom is God punishing, and why? A drunk driver crosses a median strip and plows into a car. A man goes berserk and fires an automatic rifle into a crowded restaurant. What is the message? I see no close parallel between the suffering most of us experience today and the punishment presented in the Bible, which follows repeated warnings against specific behavior. (The Bible gives many other examples of suffering that, like Job's, had nothing to do with punishment. Jesus, in fact, went out of his way to refute the Pharisees' notion that blindness, lameness, and leprosy were signs of God's displeasure.)

When I was a child living in London, the elderly vicar of a neighborhood church slipped on a banana peel and fell on the sidewalk. We children joked about it: *Imagine, he fell on the way to church! A banana peel! Maybe he had his eyes closed, praying.* But then we learned he had broken his hip in the fall, and we stopped laughing. Weeks rolled by and the vicar was not released from the hospital. Infection set in, then pneumonia, and finally the vicar died. We felt ashamed of our laughter.

That experience stayed with me as I later tried to sort through the issues of guilt and punishment. Who was at fault? Obviously not the banana peel itself, which was perfectly designed to keep a banana fresh and clean until it is eaten, or drops to seed a new tree. And the incident could hardly be called an "act of God." God had not placed the banana peel on the pavement; it was left there by some thoughtless person who did not care about clean sidewalks or hazards to elderly people. Even at a young age I reasoned that though there had been a human agent, the litterer, the banana peel accident was just that, an accident, and implied no hidden message from God.

Eventually I concluded the same thing about my father's death. God did not steer a mosquito carrying malaria to my father and order it to bite him. By living in a region that harbored *Anopheles* mosquitoes, my parents assumed certain risks; I do not believe his infection came about as a direct act of God. Indeed, it seems safe to say that the vast majority of sicknesses and disasters have nothing to do with punishment.

I cannot always determine scientifically what has caused a given disease. And I cannot always answer "Why?" questions for my patients. Sometimes I ask them myself. But whenever I can, and whenever my patients seem open, I do my best to relieve them of oppressive, unnecessary guilt.

When my father died, my aunts quoted the text from Romans 8:28, "All things work together for good to them that love God." I felt relieved later on when I learned that the Greek original text is more properly translated, "In everything that happens, God works for good with those who love him." That promise, I have found to hold true in all the disasters and hardships I have known personally. Things happen, some of them good, some of them bad, many of them beyond our control. In all these things, I have felt the reliable constant of God's willingness to work with me and through me to produce some good.

Loneliness

Loneliness comes in the same package with pain since pain, perceived in the mind, belongs uniquely to me and cannot truly be shared. Tolstoy hinted at this truth in *The Death of Ivan Ilych:* "What tormented Ivan Ilych most was that no one pitied him as he wished to be pitied."

Yet, though no one else can perceive my physical pain, there is another, deeper sense in which pain can indeed be shared. Early in my career I heard a lecture from the anthropologist Margaret Mead. "What would you say is the earliest sign of civilization?" she asked, naming a few options. A clay pot? Tools made of iron? The first domesticated plants? "These are all early signs," she continued, "but here is what I believe to be evidence of the earliest true civilization." High above her head she held a human femur, the largest bone in the leg, and pointed to a grossly thickened area where the bone had been fractured, and then solidly healed. "Such signs of healing are never found among the remains of the earliest, fiercest societies. In their skeletons we find clues of violence: a rib pierced by an arrow, a skull crushed by a club. But this healed bone shows that someone must have cared for the injured person—hunted on his behalf, brought him food, served him at personal sacrifice."

With Margaret Mead, I believe that this quality of shared pain is central to what it means to be a human being. Nature has little mercy for animals weakened by age or disease: wildebeests scatter before a lioness, leaving the weak behind, and even a highly social wolf pack will not slow down to accommodate its injured member. Human beings, when they are acting *humanely* at least, do just the opposite. And the presence of a caring person can have an actual, measurable effect on pain and on healing. In one study of women with metastatic breast cancer, women who attended a mutual support group every week for one year felt better and lived almost two years longer than the women who did not attend the group, even though both groups received the same chemotherapy and radiation treatment.

I can hardly imagine facing severe pain without at least one friend or family member within reach. I remember the comfort my mother imparted to me as a child when I battled malaria and other tropical diseases. She held me consolingly as I shook with ague. When I felt the need to vomit, she helped me bend over to a certain position, placing one cool, firm hand on my forehead and supporting the back of my head with the other hand. I would relax, and my fear and consequently my pain would melt away. When I went to England for schooling, I could hardly bear the thought of illness. I wondered whether I would even be capable of vomiting without that reassuring hand on my forehead. Sickness inevitably came, and my aunts showed me the basin and left me alone. I felt like crying out, "Mother, I need you!"

My friend John Webb, who served as professor of pediatrics at Vellore, later took a position as head of pediatrics at a university in England. Having observed the effect of the family on children in India, he waged a battle in England to incorporate beds for mothers in the children's wards. Bureaucrats saw the proposal as a waste of money. Webb rightly saw it as an indispensable part of creating a healing environment for the child, by addressing the problems of fear and loneliness.

After seeing loneliness work its devastation on many suffering persons,* I have become an advocate of open wards for hospital care. Not many have joined my campaign; most patients prefer a private room to a semiprivate, and look upon open wards with horror. From the perspective of pain management, though, open wards offer many advantages.

During my medical training in London, I worked in a hospital divided into large wards of twenty to forty beds. Patients had little privacy and occasional difficulty sleeping. Yet I noticed that they tended not to complain about pain. Constant activity in the ward—someone was always telling a joke, singing a tune, or reading aloud—provided plenty of conscious distraction, one of the best techniques for pain relief. If the nursing supervisor arranged the patients with care, much as a hostess arranges guests at a dinner party, a spontaneous community would form.

In India I saw the ward concept taken to an extreme. Extended families practically moved in, squatting on the floor during the daytime to care for their sick relatives, and sometimes a large ward more closely resembled an Oriental bazaar than a place for convalescence. Some of the family members slept on a mat under the patients' beds at night. All these "intruders" startled me at first, until I realized what a remarkable service in pain management they performed. They helped control anxiety and offered a stroking touch when the patient needed one. Later, when I practiced medicine in the West, I looked back on that chaotic scene with nostalgia.

In modern hospitals, patients often lie in solitude with nothing to focus on except their pain. The only comparative study I know of was conducted in 1956: it found that in the same hospital complex, open ward patients received an average of 3.2 doses of

---

*Research suggests that loneliness may affect not merely the perception of pain but actual bodily health. Those who live alone have premature death rates at least double the national average. Among divorced people, the suicide rate is five times higher, and the fatal accident rate four times higher. Married cancer patients live longer than unmarried cancer patients. A study conducted by Johns Hopkins University determined the overall mortality rate to be 26 percent higher for widowers than for married men (the death of a spouse seems to have a much greater effect on the health of men than on that of women).

analgesic drugs after surgery, whereas a comparable group of patients in private rooms received an average of 13.4 doses. The modern tendency for very short hospital stays makes single rooms more sensible, but for long-term convalescence perhaps the St. Christopher's Hospice model offers the best compromise: the ward supervisor works out groupings of four or six compatible patients and reserves a few single rooms for those with acute symptoms or noisy behavior.

Ministering to the loneliness of a suffering person requires no professional expertise. When I have asked, "Who helped you most?" usually patients describe a quiet, unassuming person: someone who was there whenever needed, who listened more than talked, who didn't keep glancing down at a watch, who hugged and touched, and cried. One woman, a cancer patient, mentioned her grandmother, a rather shy lady who had nothing to offer but time. She simply sat in a chair and knitted while her granddaughter slept, and made herself available to talk, or fetch a glass of water, or make a phone call. "She was the only person there on my terms," said the granddaughter. "When I woke up frightened, it would reassure me just to see her there."

Sometimes as a physician I find that I have little to offer other than my personal presence. Even then, I am not powerless. My compassion can have a calming effect not only on the suffering person, but on the entire family.

I have never felt more helpless than the time in India when I treated a tiny baby named Anne. She was one of my first patients, brought to me by her young, idealistic missionary parents. Anne was their only child, and they were alarmed by a sudden onset of vomiting. By the time I saw the baby, after they had traveled a long distance to Vellore, she was terribly dehydrated. I examined her and reassured the parents that though Anne's intestines seemed to be completely blocked, I should be able to deal with it surgically. I operated immediately, removing the section of impacted and gangrenous bowel. It was a routine surgery, and a few days later baby Anne was delivered to the care of her relieved parents.

Within a week, however, the couple returned with their daughter. As I unwrapped the dressings around Anne's abdomen, I could smell the unmistakable odor of intestinal fluid seeping out of the surgical wound. I was perplexed and embarrassed. Back to the operating room Anne went, and I reopened the incision.

Strangely, the wound fell apart as soon as I cut the stitches, as if no healing had taken place. Inside the abdomen I found the intestine leaking and unhealed. This time I made a most meticulous closure using many fine stitches.

These were just the first two in a series of surgeries on Anne. It soon became clear that her body lacked some crucial element of the healing process. Could the problem be due to her earlier starvation and dehydration? I gave her protein and transfusions of fresh blood, but her tissues continued to behave as though they had no responsibility in healing. No alarms went off alerting one part of her body to another's need. We kept her nourished, and I tried every technique I could think of, even wrapping the intestinal junction with the filmy omentum the body uses to heal accidental wounds. But a surgeon is impotent without the cooperation of the body's cells. Skin flaps refused to adhere, muscles gaped apart, and sooner or later the intestinal juices trickled out.

I confess that I was unable to keep my "professional distance" around little Anne and her parents. Anne would lie with a sweet and trusting smile as I examined her, and her face would tug at my heart. She did not seem to feel much pain, but she grew thinner and thinner. I looked at her parents through tears, and just shook my head.

When Anne's tiny, wasted body was wrapped for burial, I cried in grief and helplessness. I cried during the funeral procession to the cemetery, almost as if it had been my own child. I felt like a miserable failure even though I suspected no doctor in the world could have kept little Anne alive for long.

For more than thirty years, in fact, I remembered Anne with a sense of failure. Then one day, long after I had moved to Louisiana, I got an invitation to speak at a church in Kentucky. Anne's father was pastor of the church, which was about to celebrate its centenary. I had not heard from him in several decades, and the letter came as a complete surprise. Out of obligation, and perhaps lingering guilt, I accepted his invitation.

When Otto Artopoeus introduced me from the pulpit, he said simply, "I don't need to introduce Dr. Paul Brand. I've told all of you about him. He is the doctor who cried at our Anne's funeral." The congregation nodded knowingly. Otto tried to say a few more words about his daughter and broke down.

That afternoon I went to the Artopoeus home for lunch, and around the table had gathered all of the children who came after

Anne, as well as the next generation of children whom they had produced. I was treated with great affection and yet also esteem, like a beloved dignitary who had stepped out of history into their lives. Clearly, I had become part of the family lore.

My first reaction on going to Kentucky had been a stab of guilt and embarrassment. After all, I had been the doctor who let the Artopoeus baby die. But when I got there, I found that the family had no memory of a surgeon who failed. The children seemed to treasure the oft-repeated story of a missionary surgeon who had cared for their sister Anne and who had wept with the family when she died.

Medically, I failed the entire family. But what I learned, some thirty years later, is that we in the health profession have more to offer than drugs and bandages. Standing side-by-side with patients and families in their suffering is a form of treatment in itself.

Helplessness

I have entered hospitals as a patient five different times, and each time the ability to manage pain deserted me when I walked through the front door. At home, where pain-relieving drugs are readily available, I rarely touch one. Because I like to stay fully aware of all my body is doing on my behalf, I try not to dull my perception. In the hospital, though, I found that such resolve went out the window. When the nurse rolled the pill cart to my room, I meekly swallowed the assigned pain relievers.

The main culprit, I now believe, was my sense of feeling helpless. Professionals brought me food on trays, bathed me, made my bed, and even tried to assist me in going to the bathroom. I also felt powerless in relationships: I could not easily express love to my wife, and most of my conversations with other people revolved around their concern and pity for me. Meanwhile, mail was piling up at home, my normal household and gardening tasks were going undone, and I was helpless to respond. My mind was foggy with drugs; my emotions drifted without a tether.

In an odd way, it seemed the world was now *rewarding* me for suffering. The mail brought cards and gifts from people I had not heard from in years. Others looked for ways to do my work for me. And, observing my neighbors, I noticed that the best way to get attention in the hospital was to groan and look miserable.

Recently, hospitals have begun to address the ways in which

they foster a sense of helplessness in patients like me. Some clinics that deal with chronic pain are attempting an "operant condition-ing" approach to pain. They do not deprive patients of pain med-ication, but they do concentrate on rewarding signs of progress. Staff members save their brightest smiles and warmest words of encouragement for patients who get up, move about the ward, and help others. This operant conditioning is so alien that doctors and nurses have to be specially trained to change their customary behavior.

Numerous studies have shown a clear relationship between a sense of control and the level of perceived pain. In laboratory experiments, rats that have some control over a mild electric shock—they can turn off the current by manipulating a lever—respond very differently than rats that have no access to such con-trol. The "helpless" rats experience actual harm: their immune system radically weakens and they become much more vulnerable to disease. Ronald Melzack says, "It is also possible to change the level of pain by giving people the *feeling* that they have control over it even though, in fact, they do not. When burn patients are allowed to participate in the debridement of their burned tissues, they claim that the process is more bearable."

I have treated patients with acute arthritis who have the same degree of degeneration but respond in opposite ways to the pain it produces. One woman stays in bed all day, clutching the affected hand in genuine agony, and will not even attempt to pick up a pencil. The other says to me, "Yes, my hand hurts. But I'd go crazy just lying around. I've got to work as best I can. After a while, I forget about the pain." Behind those two responses lies a great difference in personality, belief system, confidence, and expectations about health. The "pain-prone" person sees herself as a victim, unfairly cursed. The disorder defines her identity. The second sees herself as a regular human being somewhat slowed down by pain. I have had some arthritis patients who strike me as genuinely heroic about pain. In the morning they slowly force their stiff hands open; it hurts, yes, but the fact that they feel *in charge* gives them a measure of control that keeps pain from domi-nating.

I have mentioned that patients with terminal cancer tend to use less pain medication when given some control over the dosage. A recent invention called "patient-controlled analgesia" (PCA) goes a step further down the path pioneered by Dame Cicely

Saunders. PCA puts the patient in charge. A computerized pump containing a solution of morphine or another opioid is attached intravenously to the patient's arm, and the patient can administer a premeasured dose by pushing a button. The computer has built-in safety limits to prevent overdosing, but these usually prove unnecessary. Consistently, PCA patients experience less pain, use less analgesia, and have shorter hospital stays.

Squeezed by government and private insurers, hospitals have been forced to seek new ways to empower patients and thus speed up the recovery process. Doctors grumble about such clampdowns, but many admit in private that the pressure has indeed helped get patients on their feet faster. Until the late 1960s, for example, patients typically stayed in a hospital for three weeks after a heart attack, including a week or ten days completely immobile in bed. Now most coronary specialists would admit that that approach is unsound for the patient's psychological and physical health: it fosters a sense of helplessness and delays healing.

It has taken financial pressures for professionals in wealthy countries to recognize what other countries have never forgotten: our most important contribution is to equip the patient to regain control of his or her own body. In the words of the oncologist Paul K. Hamilton, "Materially, a doctor can only give medicine. The strength for coping with the disease rests within the patient; the task of the physician and health-care team is to help him or her discover and use that strength." In village India, I saw very little of the helplessness that can breed like bacteria in a modern hospital. People without access to much professional help knew they had to heal on their own, relying on the strength of family and community.

Some chronic pain clinics battle helplessness by negotiating "contracts" with their patients. First the staff encourages the patient to articulate a long-term goal: to play tennis, to walk a mile, to get a part-time job. Then, working as a team, they break the goal into smaller, weekly goals: holding a tennis racket, walking across the room with a cane, and then without a cane. Medical personnel chart the patient's weekly progress and praise each new step, thereby shifting the emphasis from helplessness to achievement.

We need not rely on paid professionals for such encouragement. Friends and relatives can accomplish the very same thing by forming a "contract" with the recovering person, and then rewarding any slight victory over helplessness. Far too often, however, well-intentioned helpers do just the opposite. I find when I am sick that everyone conspires to keep me from doing anything—"It's for your own good, of course," they say.

I have heard people with terminal diseases use the phrase "premortem dying" to describe what is in essence an enforced state of helplessness. The syndrome develops when relatives and friends try to make the dying person's last months more bearable. "Oh, you mustn't do that! I know you have always taken out the garbage, but *really*, not in your condition. Let me do it." "Don't burden yourself with balancing the checkbook. It would just create an unnecessary worry for you. I'll take care of it from now on." "I think you'd better stay home. Your resistance is so low." Suffering people, like all of us, want to cling to some assurance that they have a place, that life would not go on without a bump if they simply disappeared, that the checkbook would go unbalanced except for their expert attention. Wise helpers learn to seek out the delicate balance between offering help and offering too much help.

When I was in medical residency during World War II, I saw proof of the positive benefits that can result when patients feel useful. Britain was suffering heavy casualties on the European front and the military ordered a sudden call-up of nurses. Our hospital staff decimated, we had no choice but to ask patients to fill in. Patriotic feeling was running high, and most patients eagerly volunteered.

The nursing supervisor, a lively woman who would have made a fine drill instructor, assigned duties to every patient who could walk, and even a few in wheelchairs. They fetched bedpans, changed sheets, distributed food and water, and took temperature and blood pressure readings. The few remaining nurses concentrated on dealing with prescription drugs and IVs, and keeping records. The system worked well, and produced one rather extraordinary side benefit: patients got so caught up in caring for each other's suffering that they forgot about their own. I noticed a nearly 50 percent drop in demands for pain medication. On my night rounds, I found that patients who usually needed sleeping pills were peacefully asleep by the time I came around. After a few weeks of this emergency program, the hospital recruited more nurses and relieved the patients of their volunteer duties. Dosages almost immediately went back up, and the usual atmosphere of helplessness and lethargy wafted in.

Dr. Karl Menninger was once asked, "What would you advise a person to do if that person felt a nervous breakdown coming on?" His reply, "Lock up your house, go across the railway tracks, find someone in need and do something to help that person." In that spirit, if I had more years left on earth I might be tempted to franchise a new line of nursing care facilities designed to replace helplessness with a sense of meaning, somehow incorporating productive activities into the daily routine.

In England I visited one facility which combined a home for the elderly with a day-care program. The effect on the residents was amazing. It was difficult to tell who benefited more, the elderly babysitters who glowed with pride in feeling needed or the children who basked in all the attention. I did not check their medical charts, but I am confident the residents also required less pain medication.

Around the same time, I also visited a more traditional nursing home in a beautiful setting. The floor gleamed mica-white, and workers were scurrying about polishing handrails and furniture. The director, acting as my guide, pointed out the state-of-the-art medical equipment. He explained that this facility featured individual rooms to assure utmost privacy. When we went outdoors, I remarked with surprise that no patients were enjoying the spacious grounds, despite the warm spring weather. "Oh, we don't allow that," he replied. "We used to, but so many residents came down with colds and allergies that we decided just to keep them all indoors." In fact, he said, many patients were confined to bed: "These elderly are so fragile, you know—they're always in danger of falling and breaking a leg." As I strolled through the corridors, my heart sank. I saw well-tended patients living in immaculate rooms, with their spirits wasting away.

Fighting Back

I have a vivid memory of a fakir I treated in India. Although he came to me for treatment of a peptic ulcer, I was fascinated by his left hand, which he held up like a traffic cop perpetually signaling, Stop. He did not want me to work on the hand or arm, but he did tell me how it came about. Fifteen years before, he had taken a religious vow never to bring that hand down or use it again. The muscles atrophied, the joints fused, and the hand was now as fixed in its position as a tree limb.

That fakir with the rigid hand demonstrates the limits of medical care, for any possible corrective techniques were rendered useless by his resolve. The best hand surgeon and therapist in the world could not reverse the damage done to his hand because of a simple mental choice. It must have hurt him the first few days of his vow—I cannot hold my hand in that position for half an hour without feeling muscle cramps around my shoulder—but he shrugged it off when I asked about the pain. He had put both the arm and the pain out of his mind, literally.

To a very large extent, the course of healing in any individual patient depends on what takes place in the mind. The challenge of medicine is to find a way to harness the awesome powers of the mind in recovery.

The book *Anatomy of an Illness* tells the story of Norman Cousins's battle against ankylosing spondylitis, a crippling disease of the connective tissue of the spine. It includes this description of Cousins's stay in a hospital, a summary that perfectly captures what I have felt as a patient:

> There was first of all the feeling of helplessness—a serious disease in itself.
> There was the subconscious fear of never being able to function normally again. . . .
> There was the reluctance to be thought a complainer.
> There was the desire not to add to the already great burden of apprehension felt by one's family; this added to the isolation.
> There was the conflict between the terror of loneliness and the desire to be left alone.
> There was the lack of self-esteem, the subconscious feeling perhaps that our illness was a manifestation of our inadequacy.
> There was the fear that decisions were being made behind our backs, that not everything was made known that we wanted to know, yet dreaded knowing.
> There was the morbid fear of intrusive technology, fear of being metabolized by a data base, never to regain our faces again.
> There was resentment of strangers who came at us with needles and vials—some of which put supposedly magic substances in our veins, and others which took more of our blood than we thought we could afford to lose.
> There was the distress of being wheeled through white

corridors to laboratories for all sorts of strange encounters
with compact machines and blinking lights and whirling discs.

And there was the utter void created by the longing—
ineradicable, unremitting, pervasive—for warmth of human
contact. A warm smile and an outstretched hand were valued
even above the offerings of modern science, but the latter
were far more accessible than the former.

I have identified fear, anger, guilt, loneliness, and helplessness
as the responses most likely to intensify pain. As I read over
Norman Cousins's description, I see all five of these intensifiers at
work. They may seem intimidating adversaries to confront at a
time when suffering drains away energy. Yet there is good news. As
a French general supposedly said when informed that his army was
surrounded, "Wonderful! This means we can attack in any direction." We cannot always relieve pain successfully at stages one and
two, but all of us, regardless of physical condition, can do battle
with pain at level three, in the conscious mind.

Dr. Bernie Siegel says he sees three kinds of patients. About
15 to 20 percent have a kind of death wish. These have given up
on life, and may even welcome illness as a way of escape. A doctor
is severely handicapped in treating these patients because even as
the doctor struggles to get them well, they are resisting and trying
to die. About 60 to 70 percent of patients are in the middle. "They
perform to satisfy the physician," says Siegel. "They act the way
they think the doctor wants them to act, hoping that then the doctor will do all the work and the medicine won't taste bad. . . .
These are the people who, given a choice, would rather be operated on than actively work to get well."

The remaining 15 to 20 percent are what Siegel calls "exceptional patients." "They're not auditioning; they're being themselves. They refuse to play the victim." Siegel acknowledges that
this last group presents a challenge because they are often difficult
patients. In a hospital setting they do not meekly submit. They
demand their rights, get second opinions, question procedures.
But this group is also the most likely to get well.

Looking back on my own career, I must agree with Siegel's
categories. In the field of rehabilitation, my primary challenge has
been to get my patients to accept that they alone can determine
their fate. I can repair a hand; whether it works again is up to
them. I have not completed my job unless I somehow inspire them
to seek health so that they deeply *want* to get well. I have been

blessed to know many exceptional patients over the years, leprosy patients who overcame incredible odds to find a rich and fulfilling life for themselves.

One of the most "exceptional patients" I ever met, though, was Norman Cousins himself. I never treated Norman as a patient, but I knew him for almost thirty years and we corresponded occasionally during the period of his bout with ankylosing spondylitis and his later heart attack. I first met Cousins in the early 1960s, when he was in robust health and was editing *Saturday Review* magazine. Financier John D. Rockefeller III and Henry Luce of Time-Life had taken an interest in our leprosy work at Vellore, and they arranged for a meeting. I mainly remember Cousins's bright, active mind. He had boundless curiosity and seemed fascinated by every obscure detail of our research into pain.

The story of Norman Cousins's personal battle against suffering is well known, and there is no need to repeat many details here. He adopted a personal program of fighting back against "pain intensifiers," a program that has inspired patients around the world. For example, he battled the feeling of helplessness by posting a sign on his door limiting hospital personnel to one blood specimen every three days, which they had to share. (They had been taking as many as four blood samples in a day, mainly because it was more convenient for each hospital department to obtain its own samples.) He fought anger by borrowing a movie projector and watching movies by comedians like the Marx Brothers and Charlie Chaplin. He made the "joyous discovery that ten minutes of genuine belly laughter would give me at least two hours of painfree sleep."

Cousins's entire approach was based on his belief that, since negative emotions demonstrably produce chemical changes in the body, then positive emotions—hope, faith, love, joy, will to live, creativity, playfulness—should counteract them and help drive out the intensifiers of pain. In his last years, Cousins moved to the UCLA medical school and founded a research group to study the effect of positive attitudes on health.*

Cousins conducted a survey of 649 oncologists, asking them what psychological and emotional factors in their patients they

---

*The specifics of Norman Cousins's recovery plan are set forth in three of his books: *Anatomy of an Illness, Healing Heart,* and *Head First: The Biology of Hope.*

judged important. More than 90 percent replied that they attached the highest value to attitudes of hope and optimism. One of the most important gifts we in the health profession can offer our patients is hope, thereby inspiring in the patient a deep conviction that inner strength can make a difference in the struggle against pain and suffering.

In the early days of drug research, the new drugs being tested for pain would strongly outperform the standard treatments given as a control. The results were so striking that researchers began to question their techniques. They discovered a key factor: the doctors were unintentionally conveying confidence and hope to those patients who received the experimental drugs. By smile, voice, and attitude, the doctors were convincing patients of the probability of improvement. For this reason the "double-blind" method, which assures that neither doctor nor patient knows which drugs are being administered, became a standard testing procedure.

Near the end of his life, Norman Cousins wrote, "Nothing I have learned in the past decade at the medical school seems to me more striking than the need of patients for reassurance. . . . Illness is a terrifying experience. Something is happening that people don't know how to deal with. They are reaching out not just for medical help but for ways of thinking about catastrophic illness. They are reaching out for hope."

18
Pleasure and Pain

*In Italy for thirty years under the Borgias, they had warfare, terror,
murder, bloodshed—but they produced Michelangelo, Leonardo da Vinci,
and the Renaissance. In Switzerland, they have brotherly love, five
hundred years of democracy and peace, and what did that produce?
The cuckoo clock.*
Graham Greene, *The Third Man*

"Nature has placed mankind under the governance of two sovereign masters, pain and pleasure. It is for them alone to point out what we ought to do, as well as to determine what we shall do," said Jeremy Bentham, founder of University College in London. It seems only appropriate at the end of a book devoted to one of those masters to add a few words regarding the other, especially since the two are closely related. I have critiqued modern society for misunderstanding pain, for muffling it rather than listening to its message. I wonder whether we have also misunderstood pleasure.

By medical instinct I tend to consider first the body's point of view when I analyze a sensation. Freud stressed the "pleasure principle" as a prime motivator of human behavior; the anatomist sees that the body gives far more emphasis to pain. Each square inch of skin contains thousands of nerves for pain and cold and heat and touch, but not a single pleasure cell. Nature is not so profligate. Pleasure emerges as a by-product, a mutual effort by many different cells working together in what I call "the ecstasy of community."

In a diary entry after a concert, Samuel Pepys wrote that the sound of the wind instruments ravished him "and, indeed, in a word, did wrap up my soul so that it made me really sick, just as I have formerly been when in love with my wife." Pepys saw that, strictly from a physiological point of view, the ravishing sensation he got from beauty, or romantic love, bore an odd resemblance to nausea. He felt a kick in the stomach, a flutter, a muscular contraction—the same bodily reactions he might have to a twinge of illness.

Pleasure, like pain, takes place in the mind, and even more than pain is an interpretation only partly dependent on reports from the sense organs. Nothing ensures the same experience will prove pleasurable for two different people: sounds that enrapture a teenager at a rock concert may produce in her parents something akin to pain; the woodwind passage that transported Samuel Pepys may put that same teenager to sleep.

Unlikely Twins

The *Oxford English Dictionary* defines pleasure as a condition "induced by the enjoyment or anticipation of what is felt or viewed as good or desirable . . . the opposite of pain." Leonardo da Vinci saw things differently. He sketched in his notebooks a solitary male figure splitting into two, about belly height: two torsos, two bearded heads, and four arms, like Siamese twins joined at the waist. "Allegory of Pleasure and Pain," he entitled the study, commenting, "Pleasure and Pain are represented as twins, as though they were joined together, for there is never the one without the other. . . . They are made with their backs turned to each other because they are contrary the one to the other. They are made growing out of the same trunk because they have one and the same foundation, for the foundation of pleasure is labor with pain, and the foundations of pain are vain and lascivious pleasures."

For much of my life I would have, like the *Oxford English Dictionary*, classified pleasure as the opposite of pain. On a graph, I would have drawn a peak at each end and a trough in the middle: the peak at the left to represent the experience of pain or acute unhappiness, the peak at the right, pure happiness or ecstasy. Normal, quiet living occupied the ground in between. A healthy person, as I then saw it, faced resolutely away from pain and toward happiness.

Now, though, I agree more closely with da Vinci's depiction of pleasure and pain as Siamese twins. One reason, as I have made clear, is that I no longer see pain as an enemy to flee. From pain-deprived people I have learned that I cannot easily enjoy life without the protection provided by pain. There is another factor, too; increasingly I have become aware of the curious intertwining of pain and pleasure. I would redraw my graph of the range of human experience to show a single central peak with a surrounding plain. That peak would represent Life with a capital *L*, the point at which pain and pleasure meet, emerging from a flatland of sleep or death or indifference.

When I speak to church or medical groups I often tell stories from my childhood or my surgical career in India. "Oh, you poor thing," someone may respond, "growing up without plumbing or electricity or even radio. And the sacrifices you made working with such sad people in those harsh conditions!" I stare dumbfounded at the sympathizer, realizing how differently we must view pleasure and fulfillment. With the luxury of age I can look back on three-quarters of a century, and without a doubt the times that seemed to involve personal struggle now shine with a peculiar radiance. In my work with leprosy patients, our medical team faced hardship, yes, and many barriers, but the very process of working together to surmount those barriers yielded what I now remember as the most ecstatic moments of my life. And as I watch my grandchildren growing up in suburban America, I covet for them the richness of life that I enjoyed in the "primitive" conditions of the Kolli Malai range in India.

I have vivid childhood memories of strawberries. When Mother tried to grow strawberries in our garden, bugs, birds, cattle, and the unfriendly climate of the mountains conspired against them. If a few hardy fruits finally did manage to defeat their enemies, we would hold the ceremony of strawberries. With no refrigerator for storage, we had to eat them right away. My sister, Connie, and I shivered with anticipation. We gathered around the table with our parents and ogled, smelled, and savored the one or two bright, luscious strawberries. Then, under intense scrutiny from Connie and me, Mother divided the berries into four equal portions. We arranged the fruit on a plate, added milk or cream, and ate each portion slowly and delectably. Half the enjoyment came from the taste of the strawberry and half from the joy of sharing. Today, of course, I can go to a corner market near my home and buy a pint of strawberries, flown in from Chile or Australia, any month of the year. But the pleasure I get from eating those strawberries does not compare with my experience from childhood.

Perhaps the same principle helps account for a trend that seems almost universal in the reminiscences of older people: they tend to recall difficult times with nostalgia. The elderly swap stories about World War II and the Great Depression. They speak fondly of blizzards, the childhood outhouse, and the time in graduate school when they ate canned soup and stale bread three weeks in a row. Against a dim background of hardship and deprivation there came to light new resources of sharing and courage and interdependence that brought unexpected pleasure and even joy.

Currently, I sense an uneasiness in the United States and much of the West. The good life does not seem quite so good as promised. Critics worry that Americans are becoming soft and weak, a "culture of complaint" more likely to whine about a problem or file a lawsuit than strive to overcome it. Living in the United States for almost three decades, I have heard these concerns expressed by politicians, neighbors, and media commentators. To me, at the heart of the issue lies a basic confusion regarding pain and pleasure.

I may risk sounding like an old man reminiscing about "the good old days," but nonetheless I suspect that affluence has made the modern industrialized West a more difficult place in which to experience pleasure. This is a deep irony, because no society in history has succeeded so well in eliminating pain and exploiting leisure. Yet happiness tends to recede from those who pursue it. Ever elusive, it appears at unexpected moments, as a by-product rather than a product.

An encounter with two barbers, one in California and one in India, gave me an important insight into the nature of contentment, a state of deep-seated pleasure. I visited the first barber in Los Angeles just before embarking on an overseas trip in the 1960s. He worked in a shop of gleaming tile and stainless steel that featured the latest equipment, including four hydraulic chairs that went up and down at the press of a foot pedal. The owner was alone in his shop that morning and I was glad to learn he could accommodate me just before my flight.

A crusty man in his late fifties, this shop owner used the occasion to grouse about the miseries of modern barbering. "I can hardly make a living these days," he said. "I can't get responsible help. The barbers who work for me gripe about their tips and demand raises. They have no idea what a tough business this is. Everything I make I have to pay to the government in taxes." He went on with a bitter commentary on the laggardly state of the economy, the absurdities of work safety legislation, and the ingratitude of his customers. When I arose from his chair, I felt like asking for a therapist's fee. Instead, I had to pay him five dollars, an excessive sum for a haircut in those days.

A month passed, during which I made side trips to Australia and places in Asia before traveling to Vellore, India. Once again I needed a haircut. This time I visited a storefront barber shop across the street from the Vellore hospital. The barber motioned me toward his single chair, a rather crude contraption of rusty metal and cracked leather which lacked all upholstery stuffing. When I sat down he disappeared out the door and around the block, carrying a battered brass basin in which to fetch water. On his return he meticulously laid out an array of scissors, combs, a straight razor, and hand-operated clippers. I was struck by his air of quiet dignity. He was master of his craft, which he knew to be a worthy one. He took as much care arranging his instruments as did my nurses in the operating room across the street.

Just as the barber was noisily stropping the razor, preparing to cut my hair, his ten-year-old son showed up with a hot lunch from home. The barber looked at me apologetically and said, "Sir, you'll understand that this is my lunch time. Could I cut your hair when I'm finished?"

"Certainly," I replied, relieved that he was offering no special treatment to the foreigner wearing a doctor's coat. I watched as the boy spread the lunch on a banana leaf. Sitting on the floor, his bony legs crossed at the ankles, the father partook of rice, pickles, curry, and curds while the son stood beside him ready to replenish the food on the leaf. At the end, the barber let out a loud belch, a customary sign of satisfaction.

"I suppose your son will become a barber after you," I said, observing the reverent way the boy treated his father. "Oh, yes!" the barber beamed proudly. "I hope to have two chairs by then. We can work together until I retire. And then the shop will be his."

As the boy cleaned up, the father began work on my hair. Occasionally it felt as if his ancient clippers were pulling individual hairs out by the roots, but all in all I got a fine haircut. At the end he asked for the fee: one rupee, the equivalent of an American dime. I glanced in the mirror, favorably comparing this haircut with my last one, and as I did so I could not help comparing the two barbers as well. Somehow the one who earned one-fiftieth of the other's fee seemed to have the happier life.

I am grateful for my time in India. From people like the barber in Vellore I learned that contentment is an inner state, a truth that easily gets lost in the jangle of high-pressure advertising in the West. Here, we are constantly led to believe that contentment comes from the outside, and can only be maintained if we buy just one more product.

I found deep contentment in people who lived in conditions of poverty that we in the West would look upon with pity or horror. What is their secret? I often asked myself. Expectations account for some of the difference. The Hindu caste system, formally abolished in India just after I moved there, had heavily influenced the barber in Vellore by lowering his expectations about advancement. His father had been a barber, and his grandfather before him, and now he was rearing his own son to regard a barber's career as the peak of ambition. In the United States, a child grows up under the "log cabin to the White House" myth and feels ceaseless pressure to rise higher.

Although the barber in Los Angeles had attained a level of affluence far above anything the Vellore barber could dream of, he lived in a society of competition and upward mobility fueled by the engine of discontent. As his living standard rose, so did his expectations.* No doubt the Vellore barber lived in a mud-walled hut and owned a mere two or three pieces of furniture—but so did all his neighbors. As long as he had a mat to sleep on and a clean floor on which to spread his banana leaf, he felt content.

In a consumer society, expectations dare not plateau, because a growing economy depends on rising expectations. I appreciate the contributions made by consumer societies that strive for ever-improving products. In medicine I rely on such products every day. But I also believe that we in the West have something to learn from the East about the true nature of contentment. The more we let our level of contentment be determined by outside factors—a new car, fashionable clothes, a prestigious career, social status—the more we relinquish control over our own happiness.

---

*A recent poll asked Americans whether they thought they had achieved "the American dream." Ninety-five percent of those who made less than fifteen thousand dollars annually answered no; 94 percent of those who made more than fifty thousand dollars answered no.

Having lived in conditions of both poverty and affluence, I can compare the two. In the Kolli Malai of my childhood, we lived far more simply than do the poorest people in the United States today. The nearest village bazaar was five miles away (*walking* miles), the nearest railway forty miles. Although we had no electricity, oil lamps gave good light, and five gallons of oil per week sufficed for the entire family. Growing up, I had no running water, no television, few books, and only one manufactured toy that I can recall. Yet not for one moment did I feel deprived. On the contrary, the days went by far too fast for all I wanted to do. I made my own toys out of bits of wood or rock. I learned about the world not by watching nature specials on television, but by observing firsthand such wonders as the ant lion, the weaverbird, and the trap-door spider.

I contrast that environment with what I see too often now: children who rush around on Christmas Day from one electronic toy to another, bored with them all in a few hours. I do not mean to imply that one society is better than another; I have learned from both East and West. As a parent who has tried to rear children in both environments, though, I firmly believe that the modern world with all its affluence is indeed a more challenging place to find lasting pleasure.

The Greek king Tantalus, as punishment for the crime of stealing ambrosia from the gods, was condemned to an eternal torment of hunger and thirst. Water receded as he stooped to drink, and trees lifted their branches as he reached up to pluck their fruit. From this myth we get the word *tantalizing;* like most Greek myths, it offers a lesson worthy of contemplation. A double irony is at work: just as a society that conquers pain and suffering seems less able to cope with what suffering remains, so a society that pursues pleasure runs the risk of raising expectations ever higher, so that contentment lies tantalizingly out of reach.

Pleasure Redux

Modern technology, by mastering the art of controlling nature, has substituted a new reality for the "natural" reality known to the vast majority of people who have ever lived on this planet. Water flows from the tap at any hour; climate-control devices in cars and homes keep the temperature steady summer and winter; we buy shrink-wrapped steaks in cheerful supermarkets, far from the mess of a slaughterhouse; our bathroom shelves are lined with remedies for aches of stomach, head, and muscle. In contrast, those who live closer to nature tend to acquire a more balanced view of life that encompasses both pain and pleasure. In village India I grew up in stern conditions of heat and cold, hunger and good food, birth and death. Whereas now, living in a technologically advanced society, I am tempted to view all discomfort as a problem that should be solved.

"As the eagle was killed by the arrow winged with his own feather, so the hand of the world is wounded by its own skill," wrote Helen Keller. In subtle ways, technology allows us to isolate the pleasure phenomenon from its "natural" source and replicate it in a way that ultimately may prove harmful.

Taste illustrates the difference between "natural" and "artificial" pleasure. Taste buds distinguish only four categories—salty, bitter, sweet, and sour—which act as gauges to help us determine what foods are good for us. Remarkably, the body can adjust the level of perceived pleasure as an incentive to meet a particularly urgent need. In India I once experienced severe salt deprivation after perspiring all day in an operating room with no cooling system. I had painful abdominal cramps. Suspecting the cause, I forced myself to drink a tumbler of water into which I had stirred two teaspoonfuls of salt. To my amazement the drink tasted delicious, like nectar. My acute physiological need had altered my perception so that drinking brine truly gave me intense pleasure.

In a natural state, the body knows its needs and grades its responses to meet them. (For this reason, animals will travel miles in search of a salt lick.) However, as humans have gained the ability to extract and isolate the pleasurable aspects of food, we have introduced the possibility of upsetting the natural physiological balance. Now that we can efficiently mine, store, and then market salt, Western societies tend to consume too much. Some people have to go on low-sodium diets to counteract the bad effects.

The same principle applies to sweetness, a consistently pleasurable taste. We eat apples, grapes, and oranges to reward our taste buds, and simultaneously we obtain the benefit of their vitamins and nutrients. Refined sugar as such does not exist in nature, and the mastery of how to grow and process it in a concentrated form is a very recent achievement. In fact, the industrial world did not produce mass quantities until the nineteenth century, from which point sugar consumption increased exponentially—nearly

500 percent between 1860 and 1890 alone—opening a Pandora's box of medical problems.

Diabetes, obesity, and many other health problems stem from the overconsumption of sugar, a consequence of our modern ability to reproduce a pleasurable taste for purposes unrelated to nutrition. Modern corporations use sugar as a taste enhancer to increase sales of breakfast cereals, ketchup, and canned vegetables. Soft drinks are a ubiquitous source: the average American drinks more than 500 cans a year. Aggressive marketing has spread the sugar addiction to less developed societies who previously got sugar from beneficial fruit or from sugar cane (which is fibrous and makes the chewer work hard to derive sweetness).

As I look around me, I see many examples of the same pattern: society excels at the ability to isolate and repackage pleasure, thereby shortcutting its natural pathways. I hardly need mention the pleasure of sex, which marketers use to sell such products as beer, motorcycles, and tobacco. I cannot see any remote connection between sex and the addiction to tobacco, and yet advertisements would lead me to believe that smoking cigarettes will magically increase my sex appeal. The true end-product of cigarette smoking is damage to the heart and lungs; the true end of drinking beer is a potbelly; the true end of sugar-coated cereal is tooth decay. Why do we keep deceiving ourselves?

We moderns can even duplicate a sense of adventure—sweaty palms, a racing heartbeat, tensed muscles, an adrenaline high—in people who are slouched in plush theater seats watching a movie. Yet ersatz adventures ultimately do not satisfy. I may get some of the side effects, but not the full value I would gain from actually climbing a mountain or shooting rapids. I am living out someone else's adventure, not my own. Once an artificial environment has been created, though, it is easy for the young especially to confuse actual and vicarious pleasure—life as video game. They are tempted to experience life vicariously, sitting in front of a flickering television set, receiving sensory stimulation through the eyes and ears alone. They no longer see pleasure as something to reach for and attain after active struggle.

It is no accident that the worst epidemic of drug abuse takes place in technologically advanced societies, where expectations run high and reality often conflicts with the glamorous images dispensed by the media. Drug abuse shows the logical conclusion of a misdirected sense of pleasure, for illicit drugs grant direct access to the seat of pleasure in the brain. Not surprisingly, the short-term pleasure that comes from such direct access produces long-term misery. As the writer Dan Wakefield expressed it, "I used drugs the way I think most people really do, not primarily and habitually for 'kicks' or glamor but for blotting out pain, the pain of that interior or psychic void. . . . The irony is that the very substances—the drugs or alcohol—that one uses to numb the pain in this chemical, artificial way have the real effect of enlarging the very void they are seeking to fill, so that more and more booze and drugs are always needed in the never-ending quest to stuff the hole that is inevitably made larger by the increasing efforts to eliminate it."

Recently scientists have identified a "pleasure center" in the brain which can be stimulated directly. Researchers have implanted electrodes in the hypothalamuses of rats, who are then placed in a cage in front of three levers. Pressing the first releases a piece of food, the second lever yields a drink, and the third activates electrodes that give the rats an immediate but transient feeling of pleasure. Laboratory rats quickly figure out the three levers, and in these experiments the rats choose to press only the pleasure lever, day after day, until they starve to death. Why respond to hunger and thirst when they can enjoy the pleasures associated with eating and drinking in a more convenient way?

I would like to require every potential addict of crack cocaine to watch a video of the rats pushing levers, smiling on the way to their deaths. They demonstrate the seductive fallacy of pursuing pleasure artificially.

Listening to Pleasure

As with pain, I gain clues about pleasure from the body itself. All activities important for the body's survival and health provide physical pleasure when we do them right. The sex act, which ensures the survival of the species, gives pleasure. Eating food is not a chore but a pleasure. Even the body's maintenance task of excretion brings pleasure. I will refrain from describing the wonderful mechanisms involved in producing a good bowel movement—as well as the complications of constipation, which often results from ignoring the bowel's messages—but the astonishing fact is that the body amply rewards even this lowly function. Anyone who has pulled a car off a highway to a rest area just in time, or has dashed out at the intermission of a concert or football game, knows what I mean.

Perhaps because I have had to repair so many physical problems caused by overindulgence, I take a long-term view of pleasure. I recognize that gluttony may give short-term pleasure even as it sows the seed for future disease and pain. Hard work and exercise, which may seem like pain in the short term, paradoxically lead to pleasure in the longer term. I well remember the period of time when I was in prime physical shape. I was working in construction, several years before I went into medical school. After six months of physical labor I had shed all excess weight and built up muscles in my legs and upper body. Weekends, I took long walks through meadows and forests without tiring or having to stop and rest. On these walks, and sometimes even before sunrise as I was hurrying to catch the bus, I would suddenly become aware of the immense pleasure of a body working according to design. The Hebrew language has a wonderful word, *shalom*, which expresses an overall sense of peace and well-being, a positive state of wholeness and health. I felt shalom, as if my body's cells were calling out in unison, "All is well."

Back then I caught a tiny glimpse of what Olympic athletes must feel. I have consulted with a few such athletes for medical conditions, and it is a delight to examine a body tuned to the peak of performance. Olympians work as hard as anyone on earth, training six or eight hours a day in order to shave, say, a tenth of a second off a swimming mark. They know pain as a daily companion. Yet somehow the very process of physical struggle and mental discipline elevates them to a level of satisfaction that most of us will never know. Not once have I heard the winner of a marathon race say to the interviewer, "Yes, I'm proud to win the gold medal—but truthfully, it wasn't worth all the time and effort I spent training."

Pleasure and pain, da Vinci's Siamese twins, work together. Musicians, ballet dancers, athletes, and soldiers alike reach the pinnacle of self-fulfillment only through a regimen of effort and struggle. There are no shortcuts. When drug addicts enter recovery programs for help, they are sometimes assigned to a strenuous wilderness camp like Outward Bound, or to a term of work on a farm. The drugs had represented an escape from a way of life that lacked challenge. In the rigorous new environment, toil and sweat, fatigue and a good night's sleep, hunger and simple food combine to open new and appropriate pathways to happiness.

I have eaten many meals at fine restaurants. If you asked me to name the best meal I have eaten, however, without hesitation I would mention a dinner of rainbow trout grilled over a wood fire beside a river in India. The Brand family was vacationing with our friends the Webbs, twelve of us in all. It was a hot day, and John Webb and I fished in vain all morning and half the afternoon, wading upstream and downstream a mile in each direction to test various pools. Although the river was full of trout—we could see them clearly—in the still, unruffled water they could see us too, no matter how well we hid or tried to disguise ourselves. By midafternoon my muscles ached with the effort of casting. I was bruised from falling on the rocks as I scrambled between pools. My face burned from the sun. Our children were fast losing faith in us as providers of food; the younger ones were beginning to cry.

Then a cloud drifted over the sun and a breeze rippled the surface of the water. Fish after fish began to take our flies, and we reeled them in and flung them on the bank. When we had caught a dozen or so, we spread the fresh trout on chicken wire over the revived embers of a fire started long before. That meal was pure ecstasy. It consisted entirely of plain grilled trout laid on slices of bread, their natural oils serving as butter, yet I honestly cannot remember a taste to match it. I have ordered trout many times since, but no one has been able to duplicate the recipe. Apparently the hunger, the bruises and sunburn and mosquito bites, the near-failure and timely triumph were essential ingredients of my pleasure.

What I learned from trout fishing in the mountains of India has held true throughout my life. Nearly all my memories of acute happiness involve some element of pain or struggle: a massage after a long day in the garden, a scratching of an insect bite, a log fire after a hike in a snowstorm. Many include the element of fear or risk, such as my first time downhill skiing—I took up the sport at age 60—when by mistake I found myself flying down an expert run. The wind rushed past, my muscles tensed, my heart leapt, but when I made it to the bottom I felt for a moment like a champion.

Pain and pleasure come to us not as opposites but as twins, strangely joined. I love a hot bath at the end of a tiring day, especially if I feel pain in my back. The water must be truly hot. I balance on the edges of the tub, suspended just above the water, and carefully lower myself, back side first. When I have the temperature just right, I can only go in an inch at a time. The first sensation of water on skin, my nerve endings interpret as pain. Gradually they accept the environment as safe, and then finally report it as a tingling pleasure. Sometimes I cannot be sure whether I am feeling pleasure or pain. One degree hotter would bring certain pain; one degree cooler would diminish the pleasure.

I once read the philosopher Lin Yutang's summary of the ancient Chinese formula for happiness. As I went through his list of thirty supreme pleasures in life, I was startled to find pain and ecstasy inescapably mixed. "To be dry and thirsty in a hot and dusty land and to feel great drops of rain on my bare skin—ah, is this not happiness! To have an itch in a private part of my body and finally to escape from my friends and go to a hiding place where I can scratch—ah, is this not happiness!" Each of the supreme happinesses, without exception, included some element of pain.

Later I read the following passage in Saint Augustine's *Confessions:*

> What is it, therefore, that goes on within the soul, since it takes greater delight if things that it loves are found or restored to it than if it had always possessed them? Other things bear witness to this, and all are filled with proofs that cry aloud, "Thus it is!" The victorious general holds his triumph: yet unless he had fought, he would never have won the victory, and the greater was the danger in battle, the greater is the joy in the triumph. The storm tosses seafarers about, and threatens them with shipwreck: they all grow pale at their coming death. Then the sky and the sea become calm and they exult exceedingly, just as they had feared exceedingly. A dear friend is ill, and his pulse tells us of his bad case. All those who long to see him in good health are in mind sick along with him. He gets well again, and although he does not yet walk with his former vigor, there is joy such as did not obtain before when he walked well and strong.

"Everywhere a greater joy is preceded by a greater suffering," Augustine concludes. This insight into pleasure is one that we in the affluent West need to remember. We dare not allow our daily lives to become so comfortable that we are no longer challenged to grow, to seek adventure, to risk. An internal self-mastery builds when you run farther than you have run before, when you climb a mountain higher than any other, when you take a sauna bath and then roll in the snow. The adventures themselves bring exhilaration; meanwhile challenge, risk, and pain combine to bolster a confidence that may serve well in times of crisis.

In short, if I spend my life seeking pleasure through drugs, comfort, and luxury, it will probably elude me. Lasting pleasure is more apt to come as a surprising bonus from something I have invested myself in. Most likely that investment will include pain—it is hard to imagine pleasure without it.

Pain Transformed

When I return to India on hospital business, I like to drop in on some of my former patients, especially Namo, Sadan, Palani, and the others from the original New Life Center. They are middle-aged men now, with gray, thinning hair and wrinkles around the eyes. When they see me, they pull off their shoes and socks and proudly show me the feet they've managed to keep free of ulcers all these years. (Sadan is especially proud of his new shoes, which have Velcro strips instead of laces, making them more convenient for his damaged hands.) I examine their feet and their hands, congratulate them on their vigilance, and then we sit down together for a cup of tea.

We reminisce about old times and catch up on each other's lives. Sadan keeps records for a leprosy mission that oversees fifty-three mobile clinics. Namo has become a physiotherapist of national reputation. Palani heads up training in the physiotherapy unit of the Vellore hospital. I listen to their stories about work and family, and my mind goes back to the scarred, scared boys who first volunteered for experimental surgery.

I have never made much money in my lifetime of surgery, but I feel very rich because of patients like these. They bring me more joy than wealth ever could. And they bring me hope for other suffering people. In Namo, Sadan, and Palani I have indisputable proof that pain, even the cruelly stigmatizing pain of a disease like leprosy, need not destroy. "What does not destroy me makes me stronger," Dr. Martin Luther King, Jr., used to say, and I have seen that proverb come alive in many of my former patients.

Once, Sadan actually told me, "I am happy that I had the disease leprosy, Dr. Brand." I looked incredulous and he went on to explain, "Without leprosy I would have spent all my energy trying to rise in society. Because of it, I have learned to care about the little people." A statement from Helen Keller came to mind when I heard those words, "I am grateful for my handicap, for through it I found my world, my self, and my God." Although I would certainly never wish leprosy or Helen Keller's afflictions on anyone, I take comfort in the fact that somehow, in the mysterious resources of the human spirit, even pain can serve a higher end.

There is one last illustration of pain and pleasure working together that I must not overlook. Unlike my leprosy patients, who did not choose the battlefield on which they fought, some people voluntarily take on suffering as an act of service. These, too, find that pain can serve a higher end. I have met a few "living saints" in my time, men and women who at great personal sacrifice have devoted themselves to the care of others: Albert Schweitzer, Mother Teresa, disciples of Gandhi. As I have watched these rare individuals in action, though, any thought of personal sacrifice fades away. I find myself envying, not pitying them. In the process of giving away life they find it, and achieve a level of contentment and peace virtually unknown to the rest of the world.

M. Scott Peck writes, "Simply seek happiness, and you are not likely to find it. Seek to create and love without regard to your happiness, and you will likely be happy much of the time. Seeking joy in and of itself will not bring it to you. Do the work of creating community, and you will obtain it—although never exactly according to your schedule. Joy is an uncapturable yet utterly predictable side effect of genuine community."

I feel privileged to have served among the worldwide community of leprosy workers. Just as I learned most of what I know about pain from leprosy patients, I learned much of what I know about joy from the fine people who devoted themselves to their care. I have referred to some of them already—Bob Cochrane, Ruth Thomas, Ernest Fritschi—and as I think of the joy that arises spontaneously from service, others spring to mind. I mention them here at the end in tribute, not primarily because of their accomplishments, but because these are the ones who taught me about the highest level of happiness—life with a capital L.

I think of Dr. Ruth Pfau, a German medical doctor and nun who now works in Pakistan at a modern hospital. When I first visited her in the 1950s she had set up shop in an immense garbage dump by the sea. The air was humming with flies, and long before I reached her place a fetid smell burned my nostrils, a smell you could almost lean on. Dr. Pfau worked here because this was where leprosy patients, more than a hundred of them, had settled after being banned from Karachi. Coming closer, I could make out human figures, the patients, crawling over mountains of garbage in search of something of value. A single dripping tap in the center of the dump provided their only source of water. Nearby I found the neat wooden clinic where Dr. Pfau maintained an office. With Teutonic efficiency she had created an oasis of order in the midst of that squalor. She showed me meticulously kept records on each patient. The stark contrast between the horrible scene outside and the palpable love and concern inside her tiny clinic seared deep in my mind. Dr. Pfau was in the business of transforming pain.

I think of Abbé Pierre, son of a wealthy silk merchant in Lyon, France. Pierre had been a prominent politician before World War II. Afterward, devastated by the poverty he saw, he resigned his post and became a Catholic friar dedicated to helping the thousands of homeless beggars in France. He organized them in teams to scour the city for rags and bottles and scraps of metal. They built a warehouse from discarded bricks and started a business in which they sorted and recycled the enormous piles of junk they were collecting. Abbé Pierre obtained from the French government free land and some construction equipment (concrete mixers, shovels, wheelbarrows), which his workers then used to build their own dwellings. On the outskirts of nearly every large town in France, these "cities of Abbé Pierre" sprang up. Soon there were few homeless beggars left in France, and that explains how I happened to meet Abbé Pierre. He stopped by Vellore as part of a worldwide trip at a time when his organization, the Disciples of Emmaus, faced a crisis. As he explained to me, "I believe that every human being needs to be needed. My beggars must find someone worse off than they are, someone they can serve. Otherwise, we'll become a rich, powerful organization and the spiritual impact will be lost!" At Vellore, he found a suitable mission for his newly prosperous beggars: he agreed to have his followers donate a ward for the leprosy patients at the Vellore hospital. Only in service, said Abbé Pierre, could they find true happiness.

I think of a man we all called "Uncle Robbie," a New Zealander who turned up at Vellore one day, unannounced. He was a medium-size man, maybe sixty-five years old. "I have a little experience in shoemaking," he said. "I wonder if I could be of help to your leprosy patients. I'm retired now, and don't need money. Just a bench and a few tools." The facts of Uncle Robbie's life leaked out slowly. We were amazed to learn that he had been an orthopedic surgeon, had in fact been chief of orthopedics in all of New Zealand. He had given up surgery when his fingers began trembling. These details had to be pried out of Uncle Robbie; he was much more animated talking about shoes. He had learned how to work with leather, how to dip it and stretch it over a mold, then fill in all the hollow places with tiny scraps glued together. He would spend hours on a single pair of shoes, and keep making custom adjustments until the patient's foot showed no more stress points. Uncle Robbie (no one called him Dr. Robertson) lived alone in a guest room at the leprosarium—his wife had died some years before. He worked with us three or four years, training a whole platoon of Indian shoemakers, until he notified us one day, "You know, I think I've done my work here. I know of another large leprosarium in the north of India. And another on the coast." He departed, and over the next few years Uncle Robbie left a trail of service in the major leprosariums of India. Watching him labor so tenderly over the damaged feet of leprosy patients, I could hardly imagine him in the prestigious, high-pressure environment of orthopedic surgery back in New Zealand. He was an utterly unassuming man, and nearly everyone he met came to love him. No one ever felt sorry for Uncle Robbie—he was perhaps the most self-contented person I have ever known. He did his work for the glory of God alone.

I think of Sister Leela who, like Robbie, showed up at Vellore with no advance notice. She wore a plain sari in an odd style, rather like a nun's habit. She was indeed a Catholic nun, though not a member of any particular order. "I think I know how to heal ulcers on a leprosy patient's foot," she said to me, rather matter-of-factly. She needed only some felt, adhesive, and gentian violet (an antiseptic). I supplied these materials and assigned her some patients. Watching her at work was like watching a master sculptor. First she would skive, or shave, the felt into very fine layers. After treating the ulcer on a foot, she dabbed glue around the sore and then meticulously built up the felt in various thicknesses, depending on the contours of the foot. In effect she was creating a molded insole that would move with the foot rather than the shoe.

Sister Leela certainly did know how to heal ulcers, and she seemed quite happy to do just that all day long. Somehow, in this small but essential task, she had learned to find true joy through service. (Unless you have treated the ulcerous foot of a leprosy patient, you cannot imagine what a remarkable statement that is.) She stayed with us several years and then, like Uncle Robbie, felt the urge to move on. I lost track of Sister Leela for almost a decade, until I visited a leprosarium in Israel. There I saw a patient wearing an insole support formed of fine layers of felt. Sure enough, Sister Leela had stopped there. She had gone from Israel to Jordan, I was told. Several times later, in scattered parts of the world, I saw the same trademark felt treatment, and knew that Sister Leela had passed by.

I think too of Leonard Cheshire. In the earliest days of our project with leprosy patients, I was working in the mud storeroom we grandly called the "Hand Research Unit" when a distinguished-looking Englishman ducked in. "I have a special interest in the handicapped," he said, "and I hear you work with leprosy patients. Do you mind if I watch?" I welcomed him, and for the next three days this man sat in a corner, observing us. At the end of the third day he said to me, "I've noticed there are some people you have to turn away—those who are too old or too damaged to be helped by your surgeries. Those are the patients I'm interested in. I would like to help them." And Leonard Cheshire told me his story. During World War II he had served as group captain, an esteemed position in the Royal Air Force. He saw action in both Europe and Asia, earning the Victoria Cross and many other awards. At the very end of the war, President Harry Truman asked Winston Churchill to choose two British observers to accompany the *Enola Gay*, in order to demonstrate that the decision to drop the atomic bomb was an Allied, not a unilateral, decision. On that day, August 6, 1945, Leonard Cheshire looked out his cockpit window and saw an entire city of people vaporize. The experience profoundly changed him. After the war he began a new career devoted to the disabled, founding the Cheshire Homes for the Sick. Today, Cheshire's organization manages two hundred homes for the disabled in forty-seven countries (Cheshire himself died in early 1993). Among them is a home in Vellore, India, where about thirty leprosy patients live. Medically speaking, they are beyond help. But as Leonard Cheshire eloquently demonstrated to me, they are not beyond compassion and love.

I mention these five people because they have had a major part in forming my own beliefs about how pain and pleasure can sometimes work together. On the surface, they may seem uniquely unqualified: a garbage dump, a shelter for the homeless, a cobbler shop, a foot clinic, and a home for the disabled are unpromising settings in which to learn about pleasure. Nevertheless, these are some of the people I look back upon as happy in the deepest sense. They achieved a shalom of the spirit powerful enough to transform pain—their own pain as well as others'. "Happy are they who bear their share of the world's pain: In the long run they will know more happiness than those who avoid it," said Jesus (translation by J. B. Phillips).

A Mother's Bequest

What I learned from Dr. Pfau, Abbé Pierre, and the others reinforced one of the earliest lessons from my parents in the Kolli Malai range of India. My mother, especially, left me a strong legacy, one that it took me years to appreciate fully.

I have referred several times to my mother's life in the hills called "Mountains of Death," where I was born. I lived with my parents for nine happy years before going away to England for schooling. There I stayed with two aunts in a majestic house in a suburb of London, the estate home my mother had grown up in. The Harris family was a prosperous one, and the house contained numerous reminders of what life had been like for Evelyn, my mother, in her premissionary days. It was furnished in mahogany, its cabinets filled with priceless heirlooms.

My aunts told me that Mother used to dress with a certain flair, and showed me some of her silks and laces and long-plumed hats still hanging in the closet. She had studied at the London Conservatory of Art, and I saw the watercolors and oils she had painted years before. There were portraits of my mother as well; my aunts told me that the men students used to compete for the privilege of painting beautiful Evelyn. "She looks more like an actress than a missionary," someone had remarked at her farewell party before the voyage to India.

When my mother returned to England, though, after my father's death from blackwater fever, she was a broken woman, beaten down by pain and grief. *Could this bent, haggard woman possibly be my mother?* I remember thinking at the time. I made a foolish adolescent vow, so shocked was I at the change in her: *If this is what love does, I will never love another person so much.*

Against all advice, my mother returned to India, and there her soul was restored. She poured her life into the hill people, nursing the sick, teaching farming, lecturing about guinea worms, rearing orphans, clearing jungle land, pulling teeth, establishing schools, digging wells, preaching the Gospel. While I was staying in the manor house of her childhood, she was living in a portable hut, eight feet square, that could be taken down, moved, and reerected. She traveled constantly from village to village. On camping trips into the countryside she would sleep in a tiny mosquito net shelter that gave no protection from the elements (when storms came in the night, she wrapped herself in a raincoat and propped an umbrella over her head).

Mother was sixty-seven when I first went to India as a surgeon. We lived only a hundred miles apart, though it took a full twenty-four-hour journey to reach her place up in the hills. Her active years in the mountains had taken a toll. Her skin was weather-beaten, her body was infested with malaria, and she walked with a limp. She had broken an arm and cracked several vertebrae being thrown off a horse. I expected she would be retiring soon. How wrong I was.

At the age of seventy-five, still working in the Kolli hills, Mother fell and broke her hip. She lay all night on the floor in pain until a workman found her the next morning. Four men carried her on a string-and-wood cot down the mountain path to the plains and put her in a jeep for the agonizing hundred-mile ride over rutted roads. I was out of the country when the accident occurred, and as soon as I returned I scheduled a trip to the Kolli Malai with the express purpose of persuading Mother to retire.

I knew what had caused the accident. As a result of pressure on spinal nerve roots from the broken vertebrae, she had lost some control over the muscles below her knees. Limping, and with a tendency to drag her feet, she had tripped over a door sill while carrying a jug of milk and a kerosene lamp. "Mother, you're fortunate someone found you the next day," I began my rehearsed speech. "You could have lain there helpless for days. Shouldn't you think about retiring?"

She stayed silent, and I took the opportunity to pile on more arguments. "Your sense of balance is no longer so good, and your legs don't work well. It's not safe for you to live alone up here where there's no medical help within a day's journey. Think of it. Just in the last few years you've had fractures of your vertebrae and ribs, a concussion of the brain, and a bad infection on your hand. Surely you realize that even the best of people do sometimes retire before they reach eighty. Why don't you come to Vellore and live with us? We have plenty of good work for you to do, and you'll be much closer to medical help. We'll look after you, Mother."

My arguments were absolutely compelling—to me, anyway. Mother was unmoved. "Paul," she said at last, "you know these mountains. If I leave, who will help the village people? Who will treat their wounds and pull their teeth and teach them about Jesus? When someone comes to take my place, then and only then will I retire. In any case, why preserve this old body if it's not going to be used where God needs me?" That was her final answer.

For Mother, pain was a frequent companion, as was sacrifice. I say it kindly and in love, but in old age Mother had little of physical beauty left in her. The rugged conditions, combined with the crippling falls and her battles with typhoid, dysentery, and malaria, had made her a thin, hunched-over old woman. Years of exposure to wind and sun had toughened her facial skin into leather and furrowed it with wrinkles as deep and extensive as any I have seen on a human face. Evelyn Harris of the fancy clothes and the classic profile was a dim memory of the past. Mother knew that as well as anyone—for the last twenty years of her life she refused to keep a mirror in her house.

And yet with all the objectivity a son can muster, I can truly say that Evelyn Harris Brand was a beautiful woman, to the very end. One of my strongest visual memories of her is set in a village in the mountains, possibly the last time I saw her in her own environment. When she approached, the villagers had rushed out to take her crutches and carry her to a place of honor. In my memory, she is sitting on a low stone wall that circles the village, with people pressing in from all sides. Already they have listened to her praise them for protecting their water supplies and for the orchard that is flourishing on the outskirts. They are listening to what she has to say about God's love for them. Heads are nodding in encouragement, and deep, searching questions come from the crowd. Mother's own rheumy eyes are shining, and standing beside her I can see what she must be seeing with her failing vision: intent faces gaze with trust and affection on one they have grown to love.

No one else on earth, I realized then, commanded such devotion and love from those villagers. They were looking at a bony, wrinkled old face, but somehow her shrunken tissues had become transparent and she was all lambent spirit. To them, and to me, she was beautiful. Granny Brand had no need for a mirror made of glass and polished chromium; she could see her own reflection in the incandescent faces around her.

It was a few years later that my mother died, at the age of ninety-five. Following her instructions, villagers buried her in a simple cotton sheet so that her body would return to the soil and nourish new life. Her spirit, too, lives on, in a church, a clinic, several schools, and the faces of thousands of villagers across five mountain ranges of South India.

A co-worker once remarked that Granny Brand was more alive than any person he had ever met. By giving away life, she found it. Pain, she knew well. But pain need not destroy. It can be transformed—a lesson my mother taught me that I have never forgotten.

Afterword:
Leprosy and AIDS

———— ❖ ————

In the mid-1980s I began to notice a striking change when I spoke at conferences or church meetings. If I opened the floor to questions from the audience, the questions were increasingly less likely to relate to the subject of the address and more likely to center on the topic of acquired immunodeficiency syndrome (AIDS). Like no other health problem in recent times, the disease that results from human immunodeficiency virus (HIV) infection has stirred up fear and anxiety in the general population.

I also began hearing leprosy and AIDS mentioned in the same breath. "AIDS is the modern-day leprosy," said then–Surgeon General C. Everett Koop: "There are people who have the same attitude toward AIDS patients today that many people had toward leprosy patients one hundred years ago." Newspaper headlines were less polite: "AIDS victims are today's lepers!" blared one. Those headlines got the attention of my patients at Carville, Louisiana, who are now officially designated as suffering from Hansen's disease. Many of them remember the day when "leper" carried worse opprobrium than a curse word, and when infection constituted legal grounds for them to be torn from family and friends and locked away in isolation hundreds of miles from their homes.

My patients have mixed feelings about AIDS victims being called "the new lepers." Of course they hate the dreaded label that dredges up memories of harsher days. At the same time, they may have to stifle a self-satisfying sense that it's time some other group of people has a turn at knowing what true stigma feels like. They also know that even in the past their disease was never as bad as this new disease. None would want to exchange places with an AIDS patient.

As I write this, in 1993, the number of people in the world infected with leprosy, 10 to 12 million, roughly equals the number of those assumed to be infected with the human immunodeficiency virus. That is a temporary fluke of statistics: the figure for leprosy is now declining, while the figure for HIV infections is still increasing at a frightening rate. Of more significance, we have a proven cure for leprosy and to control the disease we need only apply resources on a global scale; far greater sums of money are going toward AIDS/HIV research than have ever been spent on leprosy, but to this point any solution eludes us.

At the end of a long career in leprosy work, I have a wonderful vantage point. The shroud of mystery that surrounded a terrible disease for centuries fell away in a very short period. It has been one of the great thrills of my life to see leprosy lose its fangs. In the county that includes Vellore, India, where I first started working with leprosy, the number of patients with active infection has declined from ten thousand to one hundred. The incidence of the disease has not changed much—about nine hundred new cases appear each year—but prompt treatment arrests the infection before the disease can work much damage. Less than 1 percent of all cases treated with multi-drug therapy have experienced relapse so far.*

The reconstructive surgeries I worked on so painstakingly— the tendon transfers, the nose replacements, the eyebrow transplants—are less frequently needed now. I can hardly believe the contrast as I walk through the grounds of certain former "leper colonies," once beehives of activity with hundreds of patients in all stages of deformity, and see a few old-timers living out their final days. With today's effective drugs, most patients are treated at home and the "leper colony" is a thing of the past. In places like Vellore, the terrible social stigma is slowly fading away as well. Family and fellow-villagers of new patients understand the disease and no longer ostracize one who reports an infection.

I long for the day that AIDS workers will have the effective tools to use in combating their disease that leprosy workers have

*Vellore represents the front lines of leprosy work. In other parts of the world the picture is not so rosy. Even though it takes less than two hundred dollars to cure a leprosy patient with a two-year course of multidrug therapy, fewer than half the leprosy sufferers in the world have access to such treatment.

now. In the meantime, as I look back over my medical career, I am struck both by parallels and by contrasts between the two diseases. The pathologies of leprosy and AIDS have little in common, but many similarities exist in the way the medical community and society have responded to them. Questions of public policy, such as quarantine and compulsory testing, keep surfacing in the discussion surrounding AIDS: these policies have a long history in the battle against leprosy, a history from which we can and should learn.

The Power of Stigma

In 1985, just as AIDS was beginning to loom large in public awareness, I made my first trip to mainland China. The visit provided at once a stark reminder of how leprosy had been treated for centuries and an ominous preview of what can happen when a disease like leprosy—or AIDS—becomes so stigmatized that even physicians are reluctant to treat it. Led by a remarkable man named Ma Heide,* Chinese public health officials had reduced the number of active leprosy patients from 500,000 to 70,000. But no attempt was being made to prevent injuries due to pain insensitivity or to repair hand and face deformities surgically.

Out of fear, most doctors would not dare to treat leprosy. On a trip to Nanjing we conducted our training program in a sparkling national center for dermatology, but no leprosy patient had ever been admitted to its modern operating room. Authorities had requested that we do demonstration surgeries on leprosy, and we asked the dermatologists whether we could use their operating rooms. After long consultations, the answer came back, "No." Leprosy surgery must be done at the leprosy hospital outside town, they said.

*An American of Lebanese descent, Ma Heide went to China as a young doctor in 1933. He found the conditions of poverty in Shanghai appalling: parents sold their sons into industry to work under slave labor conditions, and their daughters into prostitution (one out of fourteen houses was a brothel). Eventually, Heide joined Chairman Mao on his Long March. When the Communists succeeded in their takeover, he was the first foreigner to become a citizen of the new China. As adviser to the minister of public health, he waged an all-out campaign against venereal disease until it was eliminated as a problem in China, an accomplishment unprecedented in medical history. At that point Ma Heide shifted his attention to leprosy.

I have rarely seen anything as primitive as the "operating room" at the leprosy hospital. It had a table, but no proper sink to wash hands, and no instruments suitable for anything but amputations. It was, in essence, a chopping block. After amputating a patient's leg, the leprosy doctors would fit him with a wooden stump, fixed onto his leg by two metal pieces extending up the side. Of course, for these pain-insensitive patients, ulcers would quickly develop where the metal pieces rubbed against their skin. Less fortunate patients got no prostheses at all; these carried around a three-legged stool which they would place before them to rest the stump on before thrusting the good leg forward for the next step.

In another town near Nanjing there was a modern hospital devoted to hand surgery, but the same rules applied. No respectable hand surgeon would deign to treat a leprosy patient. My wife was scandalized by the leprosarium's "eye clinic," a bare room that no eye doctor had ever visited. Of the patients she examined that afternoon, 70 percent were blind. For many of them, blindness would have been prevented by a simple daily application of steroid drops.

I am afraid we made little lasting impact on Chinese attitudes toward leprosy patients. Stigma kept getting in the way of knowledge. We mentioned through our interpreter that one of our daughters had married a former patient. Later the interpreter came back and asked if he had mistranslated. Such a thing was impossible, he said—no doctor would let his daughter marry someone who had had leprosy. Once, I put my arm around a patient and stroked his hands as I examined them. The doctors around us sucked in their breath sharply. One of them later told me that single act impressed the doctors more than anything else we said or did in China.

I have often pondered the unique stigma that human society has long applied to leprosy, and now extends to AIDS. I have known of children shut up in a cave for years, or locked in a tiny upstairs room. I have known of villagers who burned down the hut of a leprosy patient and chased away the patient's family. I have seen firsthand the devastating impact of such rejection on my leprosy patients. And now, in the United States, I see haunting replays of that same rejection. Homes of AIDS patients are firebombed, and children banned from schools. HIV-positive homosexuals are disowned by their families; at a time when they most need emotional support, they get ostracism instead.

Where does such profound stigma come from? The origin of the word itself gives some clues. Derived from the Greek, it originally meant a mark on the skin. Sometimes, as in the case of a slave, the mark was applied by a branding iron and was called a "brand." Interestingly, the two words have gone in different directions. As slavery was abolished, mostly cattle and not humans were branded, and *brand* lost its negative connotation (for which I am indeed thankful!). Today, companies devote a great deal of money and attention to choosing brand names. Even as *brand* shed its negative aspects, though, *stigma* took them on.

The use of *stigma* has changed dramatically. In earlier times, pious followers of Jesus Christ would make scars on their palms to identify with the scars of the crucifixion; they wore these *stigmata* with pride, not shame. In my own lifetime, medical textbooks taught us to look for the *stigmata*, or visible signs, of various diseases. Now, of course, the word is almost always used in a negative sense. Minorities and suffering people rightly fear being *stigmatized*.

It might be helpful, in considering leprosy and AIDS, to rethink our modern use of the word *stigma*. From a doctor's perspective, there is both "good" and "bad" stigma. In our work with leprosy, we did not regret that the disease made itself known visibly, for we relied on these visible stigmata to identify which people needed further examination and treatment. The wonderful advances in leprosy control would never have happened had there been no marks to help us recognize the afflicted.

For thousands of years societies have relied on visible stigmata to protect against epidemics. The Old Testament gives explicit instructions about people with skin diseases; they were identified by the priest and segregated outside the camp to prevent the disease from spreading. Most societies also quarantined people with leprosy, for fear of contagion.

The problem with stigma is that it easily progresses from good to bad, and then becomes difficult to reverse. Human history contains many examples of "bad stigma" expressed in cruel and unwarranted ways. Medieval princes collected midgets, monsters, and hunchbacks for personal entertainment. Ancient Greeks sometimes tossed disabled people from mountains, the Japanese drove them into snowdrifts, Eskimos set them adrift on ice floes. We may be more sophisticated and subtle in modern times, but each of us still carries around an unconscious ranking of illnesses and deformities that affects our attitudes toward suffering people. Today we reserve for sufferers of leprosy, AIDS, and a few other diseases a special stratum of fear and rejection.

Overreactions

Often in medicine, what begins as a reasonable and sensible fear grows into an unreasonable and harmful overreaction that is difficult to overturn. Leprosy offers a telling example. As effective treatment became available, and as the facts about leprosy's low rate of contagion became known, those of us involved in leprosy work lost our fears. In places like China, though, the medical community still lags far behind. And it will likely take generations for overall society to catch up with the advances in our knowledge about leprosy. "Bad stigma" tends to linger long after the reasons for it have disappeared.

In India, when I first sent cured leprosy patients back to the villages, they returned to the hospital, asking for cosmetic surgeries on their eyebrows and noses. Villagers stigmatized them as long as visible signs of the disease remained, even though they posed no actual danger. The same problem explains why patients in the United States are so adamant about being classified as Hansen's disease patients: the word *leprosy* has too much bad stigma associated with it. Despite all we know about controlling leprosy, it remains—along with AIDS—on a very short list of diseases that make a person ineligible to enter the United States.

HIV infection, unlike leprosy, has no visible marks to betray its presence, at least in early stages. It has no "good stigma" to warn potential sexual partners, or to help authorities with control and treatment. That very absence heightens the irrational fears of society, contributing to the "bad stigma." Anyone— neighbor, lover, relative—could be a carrier of this deadly virus. HIV-infected patients themselves hesitate to come for testing or treatment, afraid they will suffer discrimination if the news leaks out.

The parallels between leprosy and AIDS are most evident when comparing the "bad stigma" attached to each. I have tried to identify the source of the extreme stigma that surrounds these diseases. In both cases, I believe, the stigma comes from (1) the peculiar horror of the disease symptoms, (2) fear of contagion, and (3) belief that the disease is a curse of God.

Peculiar horror of the disease

I have written at length about the horrors of leprosy, some-times called the "creeping death." A disease that affects the hands and face cannot easily be hidden. In the early days, before sulfone drugs, leprosy often led to fatal complications as well. Leproma nodules grew inside the cool lining of the nasal passages, blocking the nose and forcing patients to breathe through the mouth. Bacilli next infiltrated the gums, causing teeth to loosen, and then spread into the pharynx and larynx. First the voice became hoarse, then the patients had difficulty breathing, and in the final stage a tracheostomy was the only way to keep air flowing in (some of my early patients at Chingleput and Carville still bore the scars from these operations).

AIDS may lead to visible manifestations—Kaposi's sarcoma, thrush, malnutrition—and usually proves fatal, but somehow I think the peculiar horror of the disease lies elsewhere. It repre-sents a kind of bodily disloyalty, wherein the body loses the ability to deal with the most ordinary problems. Danger lurks every-where: diarrhea, a common cold. The body has surrendered its vital function of protecting itself against outside invaders.

At this point, I cannot hold out tangible hope for sufferers of AIDS. Some of the best minds in the scientific world are attempt-ing to unlock the secrets of HIV, but so far the virus has proved elusive. What I can do is recall the days when leprosy was viewed with the same fear and revulsion. The laborious research of people like Bob Cochrane and the drug researchers at Carville finally paid off. Leprosy can now be cured, its horrors prevented. I pray for the day when we can say the same for AIDS.

Fear of contagion

In both diseases the fear of widespread contagion is based on myth. Neither disease is highly infectious, except to specific at-risk groups.

Leprosy can only be contracted by the small percentage of people (around 5 percent) who lack natural immunities. I am heartened to see that in places like Vellore, where good training and access to leprosy health care are available, the stigma based on exaggerated fears of contagion goes away. The children of my for-mer patients are now marrying nonpatients, something unthinkable just a generation ago. It disturbs me, though, that hysteria does not so easily abate in the most educated countries; here, the "bad stigma" persists. I find more ignorance and fear of leprosy in countries like Japan and the United States than in India. As recently as 1987, government plans to treat leprosy patients at a general outpatient clinic—in San Francisco, center of AIDS rights activism!—had to be abandoned because of public protest.

As most people now know, HIV infection only spreads as a result of certain well-defined activities that involve the exchange of bodily fluids. Compared to other viruses, in fact, HIV is rather difficult to spread. Thus the main groups who need fear contagion are those who engage in unsafe, promiscuous sex or who otherwise (through sharing needles, for example) come in intimate contact with another person's bodily fluids.

With respect to AIDS, I am frankly mystified by the way politics has taken precedence over sound medical policy—on both sides. The subject has become so polarized that it is hard to discuss AIDS without putting oneself into one or the other advocacy group. Both sides retrench into hardened positions and little helpful dialogue takes place.

On the one hand, many in the general public live with an exaggerated fear of their own risk. We already have a "vaccine," in a manner of speaking, that will go a long way toward preventing the spread of AIDS for most people. It does not require abstinence from sex, merely faithfulness to one partner. Never has there been such a fearful epidemic with such a simple solution. The medical profession knows this fact, but many hesitate to speak up for fear of a backlash against "interfering with behavior and life-style."

Promiscuity, not sexual orientation, is the central issue from a medical perspective. For this reason, I find hypocritical those heterosexuals who use the AIDS epidemic as an opportunity for "gay-bashing" while continuing to engage in promiscuous sex themselves. In Africa and parts of Asia, AIDS spreads primarily through heterosexual contact.

On the other hand, I am astonished at the AIDS activists who go to any length to protect the rights of the person infected with HIV. Having lived with the effect of "bad stigma" on leprosy patients, I readily understand an individual's right to privacy and the resistance to compulsory testing. But there are other rights to consider as well. The HIV-positive person can pass on a lethal virus if he or she continues to share unclean needles or practice promiscuous sex. In the name of protecting personal freedoms, lobbying groups insisted that San Francisco bathhouses remain open even after the initial facts about the AIDS epidemic had become known; as a result, thousands more patrons were exposed. For a time, these same groups also opposed screening procedures for blood banks.

The AIDS issue has become so politicized that, while it is standard medical procedure to require testing and contact tracing for other sexually transmitted diseases, the rules do not apply to HIV, a much more dangerous threat. In some states, an orthopedic surgeon has no legal right to test a patient for HIV infection before performing surgery. Thus a surgeon who will put himself or herself at grave risk cannot identify that risk in advance. I cannot help wondering whether such fierce insistence on the infected person's personal rights is not contributing to the "bad stigma" that surrounds AIDS.

Curse of God

In Europe, much stigma directed against leprosy stemmed from an unfortunate translation of a word in the Hebrew Bible. In truth, the symptoms described in Leviticus bore little relation to the disease we now call leprosy, but over time *leper* took on a moral taint, a sign of supernatural judgment. In the Middle Ages a priest, not a doctor, examined a person suspected of having leprosy. If the disease was confirmed, the afflicted person was taken to the church, where the priest read a "Leper Mass" and scattered ceremonial dust over his head, signifying the death before death. Thus condemned, the victim was led to the cemetery to witness the filling of an open grave, a symbol of his burial.

"Remember that you are dead to the world; that you have no home, no family . . . nothing," the priest intoned at the graveside. The priest then read a list of harsh rules that would govern the leprosy sufferer's life from that moment on. He must renounce all property and inheritance. He could never again enter a church, marketplace, tavern, house, or public meeting place. He could not walk on narrow streets or speak to children, or speak to anyone downwind. He was given a distinctive uniform—in France the robe had a red *L* sewn onto it—and a bell or rattle to sound whenever anyone approached. He was allowed one possession: a wooden bucket on a long pole which he could hold out to beg for food.

Leprosy has always carried the stigma of divine curse. "Flee the leper as you would flee the lion," said Mohammed. All over the world, and most markedly in countries like Japan which never had exposure to the Bible, the disease was taken as a sign of supernatural judgment. Hindus in India, who traditionally viewed leprosy as punishment for some crime in a former life, implemented repressive measures similar to those in Christian Europe. A good Hindu would not touch anyone suffering from leprosy, enter a victim's house, or, in some cases, even look on the sight of leprosy. The official Leper's Act in India, which remained on the statute book until 1984, sanctioned mandatory incarceration for anyone infected with the disease.

Apart from some misguided efforts to associate leprosy with the final stage of venereal disease, there was no attempt to identify a cause-and-effect relationship between behavior and disease. The existence of a disease with such "creeping death" manifestations was assumed to be prima facie evidence of God's condemnation. In the same way, the terrible bubonic plague in Europe called forth many wild-eyed prophets who pointed to the buboes as proofs of God's judgment.

Like no other disease in modern times, AIDS shares with leprosy the stigma of divine curse. Furthermore, it offers a more direct cause-and-effect tie to behavior, and many self-proclaimed prophets have seized on that fact. For some Christians, AIDS appears to manifest a direct relationship between behavior and suffering-as-punishment. One question often comes up: Did God send AIDS as a specific, targeted punishment?

As a Christian I disapprove of sexual promiscuity and drug abuse, behavior patterns that are responsible for the majority of cases of HIV infection. I believe society has wisely honored the Ten Commandments and other such codes as expressing lasting moral truth. Yet, as I have also made clear in this book, I stand against the notion that God is in the business of dispensing specific illnesses. I view the Ten Commandments as a kind of "owner's manual" for healthy life on this planet, not unlike the owner's manual I receive when I buy a Ford automobile. I am free to disobey flagrantly the manual's recommendations that I change the oil periodically, and if I do I will bear the consequence. But this is hardly a judgment or "curse" from Ford. It is the consequence of my behavior.

Many people resent a moral code like the Ten Commandments, and regard it as an arbitrary list of rules—God's way of keeping us from having too much fun. I see it as exactly the opposite: a prescription for the most joy-filled and healthy life, a life of shalom. I happen to believe that a society works best when a day is set aside to honor God; when children respect parents; when stealing, murder, and adultery are forbidden; when people do not lie to each other and covet each other's possessions.

I am a doctor, not a theologian, but after living in several cultures I am ready to diagnose *promiscuity* as the disease of our modern age. To me, the word covers far more than a sexual connotation; it implies a kind of irresponsibility or hedonism, a spirit of "Have fun today; tomorrow will take care of itself." We approach politics that way, accumulating a massive debt that our children and grandchildren will have to pay off. We are irresponsible toward the environment, clear-cutting forests, wasting topsoil, burning hydrocarbons, and failing to deal with population growth. These policies may one day lead to global catastrophe, but I hardly see this as a direct "curse" of God. If such catastrophe happens, it will be the outcome of promiscuous behavior, of disregarding the owner's manual.

Indisputably, behavior choices affect health: obesity increases the risk of heart disease, drinking increases the risk of liver ailments, and sexual promiscuity increases the risk of venereal disease. I think back to Dr. Luther Terry, the Surgeon General who had the courage to declare that a popular habit, smoking, was harmful to health and should be abandoned. The reason his pronouncement took courage is that people do not like to be told how to behave. They would rather hear that if you want to smoke you should take a vaccine to prevent any possible harm, or that if you get lung cancer a doctor can fix it.

In the twenty-five years since Luther Terry's pronouncement against smoking, other behavior-related sicknesses have moved in, even as smoking has begun to move out. AIDS is the latest and probably the worst of such illnesses. Many protest vigorously against the notion that AIDS is behavior-related, but in plain fact AIDS would never have become the epidemic it is apart from such behavior as intravenous drug abuse and sexual promiscuity. The response of the public to the AIDS epidemic has been predictable: "Fix it. Find a vaccine."

Today, few have the courage to say that the problem with AIDS is mostly behavioral and the only solution available right now is a behavioral solution. The sexual revolution of recent decades was an experiment. It may have had some good points; it certainly had some negative effects, notably the rise in sexually transmitted diseases (which now afflict one in five Americans) and the acute secondary effect on children of broken homes. Now we know that an overwhelmingly dangerous sickness, AIDS, has been added to the negative side of the ledger.

People don't like doctors, politicians, or even preachers meddling in their behavior, and I will add only this to the current discussion: the "owner's manual" of morality was written for our benefit, not to restrict our freedoms. As I enter my sixth decade of marriage I can say without a flicker of hesitation that the basic human virtue of faithfulness to one sexual partner is the most joyful way of life. I have always lived free of any fear of sexually transmitted diseases. I have always trusted my wife completely, and she me. We have each been able to channel love and commitment and intimacy to one person—a lifelong investment that is now, in old age, paying rich dividends.

Ex-smokers have discovered a great bonus: not only do they run a reduced chance of lung cancer and heart disease, but they also find that life without smoking is more enjoyable. They can run upstairs or sprint for a bus without gasping or coughing. That positive message should be our approach to the debate about sexual promiscuity as well: faithfulness is better for everyone, and is foundational for happy family life.

As a Christian physician, I must quickly add that no matter how we feel about the harm of abandoning moral law, we must always be in the vanguard of those who would bring comfort and help to the suffering person. I serve on the board of an organization called World Concern, which directs a large AIDS program in Thailand. There, the majority of prostitutes, sold into the trade as teenagers, now carry HIV and endanger their customers. How should we respond to such victims? To me, the answer is clear. When I address Christian physicians on the subject of AIDS, I challenge them to act with compassion, as Jesus would have, and minister to the suffering person in his or her need. Jesus set the pattern by reaching out and *touching*—an act of unimaginable courage in those days—people afflicted with leprosy. When confronted with a woman caught in the very act of adultery, he responded by saying, "If any of you is without sin, let him be the first to throw a stone at her." And then he, the only one without sin in that story, proceeded to show her mercy.

Medical Lessons

I well remember the fear I felt in my earliest days of experimental surgery on leprosy patients. We did not know about the low contagion rate of leprosy back then, and all health workers lived in dread of catching the disease. I have read the account of one early doctor in Hawaii who stuffed cotton in his nose, wore rubber gloves day and night, and held his breath while bandaging leprosy patients. Others became addicted to the morphine they took to quell their fears. My field of orthopedic surgery introduced special risks, because we were often working with splinters of bone. In the first few years of surgery I recorded thirteen pricks by needle or bone. I later realized that these accidents, having no ill effects, proved my natural immunity to leprosy.

If I had been working with AIDS patients, though, I would have exposed myself to far greater danger, since a single prick from a needle or sharp splinter of bone can transfer a virus that may be 100 percent fatal. Not long ago at a meeting of the Southern Orthopaedic Association I heard a stirring address by Dr. Ollie Edmunds of the Tulane Medical College. Dr. Edmunds treats hemophiliac children who have contracted AIDS through blood transfusions. "These children are very special people and we develop a special relationship," he said. "I just couldn't give them up as patients, despite the risk to me."

Dr. Edmunds led a discussion on how the surgeon can try to guard against infection. One surgeon in the room described wearing thimbles on the tips of his fingers to prevent needle pricks. Another mentioned the need to wear two pairs of gloves, one of them perhaps being cotton, but he admitted that a sharp object will penetrate fabric as well as rubber.

During the course of this discussion I had flashbacks to my days in medical school fifty years ago. Then, too, we had lengthy discussions on how to prevent infection in the operating room, but for the opposite reason. In those preantibiotic days, the patient was in mortal danger from infection that the surgeon might introduce. Now the tables have reversed: the patient endangers the surgeon.

In my day, staphylococcal osteomyelitis posed the greatest danger. In operations on bone, despite all aseptic precautions a staphylococcus germ sometimes would get into the wound and establish itself in bone. Surgeons identified a commmon source: If a splinter of bone or a needle point slightly pricked or tore a rubber glove, a drop of the surgeon's sweat (which often carries staphylococcus) might pass through the hole and contaminate the bone. To prevent such a danger, we were drilled in the "no-touch technique" of orthopedic surgery.

As a general principle, nothing that might come in contact with the wound could be handled by the hands of a surgeon or nurse, even though those hands were encased in sterile gloves. The instrument nurse never touched the instruments at all. She picked up the instrument with two large pairs of sterile forceps and handed them to the surgeon. The surgeon took the handle end, which never touched the wound, and used the business end as his only contact inside the wound. We also practiced rigorously the art of sewing up wounds without our hands being in the wound. We held the needles in needle holders, grasped the point of the needle with a different forceps, and drew it through the tissue. Even today I can tie knots as fast with forceps as I can with my hands. After much practice, the operation became a beautifully smooth drill, and at the end of the operation we would all show each other our gloved hands to demonstrate there was no blood on them.*

*India did not know the word *disposable* and for the sake of economy we used the same gloves over and over, resterilizing them between each use. At the end of a day's surgery the operating room nurses would collect all the gloves and inflate them, blowing them up like balloons and holding the ends closed while they checked for needle holes or tears, which would bubble when the gloves were held under water. The nurse patched such holes with fragments of rubber taken from discarded gloves. As I watched this ritual over the years, I saw that we surgeons prick our gloves far more frequently than most of us realize. Today in the West all gloves are discarded at the end of each surgery, and the surgeon rarely knows whether the gloves used remained intact or not. Out of habit, I still inflate my own gloves when I take them off, in order to check whether I have violated the aseptic technique.

This disciplined technique gradually fell into disuse once penicillin came on the scene and health workers realized that even if staphylococcus entered the bone, penicillin could destroy it. I continued to use the technique sometimes in India, however, and trained my assistants in it. In conditions indoors and outdoors, we rarely had any problems with infection introduced into the surgical wounds.

As I heard the discussion at the meeting of the Southern Orthopaedic Association, it occurred to me that this "no-touch" technique, a relic of surgery from fifty years ago, might be exactly appropriate for today's surgeons who operate on AIDS patients. In our day we were taking such elaborate measures to ensure that no germs from our hands got into the wound of the patient. Today, the same technique might prevent the patient's germs from penetrating the gloves of the surgeon. I discussed the technique with Ollie Edmunds after the meeting. Having been trained much later than I, he was unaware of the old style, and agreed it might be a good idea to practice while operating on AIDS patients. Since then, I have learned that some medical schools have revived variations of the "no-touch" technique for this reason, an instance of the wisdom of the past serving urgent new needs of the present.

The long history of leprosy work offers other lessons that can inform current medical policy toward AIDS. For example, when fear of an AIDS epidemic first began to enter public consciousness, loud cries for "quarantine" went up. I do not hear much discussion of quarantine these days—although the nation of Cuba has apparently imposed a strict quarantine on their HIV-infected patients—but some may wonder why the medical profession did not endorse such a policy. Human rights issues aside, isn't the most effective way to stop the spread of an epidemic to separate out all carriers of the disease?

Leprosy treatment provides an important insight. In Hawaii, for example, the Act to Prevent the Spread of Leprosy (1865) authorized the "arrest" of leprosy "suspects," and anyone found with leprosy was subject to lifetime banishment to the colony at Kalaupapa on the island of Molokai. Between 1865 and 1965, when the policy was finally abandoned, some eight thousand leprosy sufferers were sent to Kalaupapa; nearly one hundred survivors remain there today. This is how one native Hawaiian, a composer and hula master, remembers his banishment:

Again the militia took over.
Soldiers escorted us to the wharf for farewell.
Prisoners, we were marched aboard,
  victims of leprosy, branded for exile.
Abandoned, cut off from family and dear ones,
  we were left alone with our grief, with our love.
Rain of tears streamed from leper eyes.
Leper cheeks glistened with raindrops in the sun.
Never again would we look upon this land of ours,
  this lovely harbor town.

In Hawaii, as in most places, medical authorities abandoned
quarantine not because they believed the danger from disease had
lessened, but because quarantine proved counterproductive. I
heard many stories illustrating this fact from the old-timers at the
leprosy hospital in Carville. People who noticed symptoms of leprosy would hide out and not report to a doctor for fear of being
shipped to a colony. Or, they would wait until their children were
grown before reporting in. As an ironic result of quarantine, then,
some cases of leprosy always went undetected, keeping alive the
potential for contagion.

The history of leprosy in Spain clearly demonstrates the
unintended consequences of quarantine. Under the Franco
regime, Spain had a rigid policy of compulsory notification. All
leprosy patients had to register their condition with the authorities, and were then assigned to live in colonies. After Franco died,
the government lifted these regulations. The very next year the
number of reported cases doubled. The following year, the
reported cases doubled again. Public health officials concluded
that three-fourths of the leprosy cases in Spain had been in hiding.
Half of them sought treatment the first year the law changed; half
of them waited another year to see whether the government had
been setting a trap.

In India I participated in widespread campaigns against leprosy and also against other infectious diseases and epidemics. I too
found that attempts to segregate patients usually failed because of
the patients' strong resistance to enforced isolation. Some always
found ways to escape the authorities and hide their disease. I concluded that in most cases quarantine simply does not work.

On the other hand, I absolutely support the epidemiological
necessity of *identifying every possible case* of an infectious disease.
This becomes a challenge when, as in leprosy (and AIDS), the

patient's desire for secrecy conflicts with the sound medical need to control the disease. At first in India we conducted leprosy clinics separately from other hospital outpatient clinics. We found that only those patients who had obvious marks of the disease showed up. Early cases who were still unmarked, or who could hide their marks under clothing, would not expose themselves and be identified as "lepers." Thus they remained a source of infection to others, even as the disease continued to progress untreated in them.

Leprosy missions began to open free "skin clinics" in strategic towns and in hospitals, where skin diseases of all kinds could be seen and treated. Leprosy patients soon learned that the doctors and nurses at these clinics could be trusted to observe confidentiality, and so they went to them voluntarily as soon as they had any suspicion of the disease. For similar reasons, I support the need for "anonymous" HIV testing centers. Concerned individuals must be able to trust that the results will be confidential; otherwise we create a disincentive that works against our goal of identifying active infections.

The Church's Response

One of the major differences between leprosy and AIDS, and the one that grieves me most, is the response of the Christian church. Although the church surely added to the misery of leprosy sufferers with its "curse of God" message, at the same time individuals rose up from within the church to lead the way in treatment. In the Middle Ages, religious orders devoted themselves to the care of leprosy. And even in recent times scientific leadership in the disease has tended to come from missionary doctors, because they were the only ones willing to work with leprosy patients.

I remember a comment made by Mother Teresa. She was running a clinic for leprosy patients in Calcutta, and invited me to help train her sisters. "We have drugs for people with diseases like leprosy," she said. "But these drugs do not treat the main problem, the disease of being *unwanted*. That's what my sisters hope to provide."

Much of my work in India was funded by the Leprosy Mission in England, parent organization to the American Leprosy Missions. Why is it, I have sometimes wondered, that we have Christian missions devoted exclusively to leprosy? I know of no arthritis mission or diabetes mission. The answer, I think, relates to the incredible stigma that has surrounded leprosy for so many centuries. To work with leprosy required more than a natural instinct of compassion; it required a kind of supernatural calling. People such as Father Damien, who ministered to leprosy patients in Hawaii and then contracted the disease himself, believed that human beings, no matter what their affliction, should never be cast aside. It was up to the church to care for the sick, the unwanted, the unloved.

When I moved to Carville in 1965 I learned that the history of that institution was all too typical of leprosy work worldwide. The first seven patients, chased out of New Orleans, were smuggled by authorities up the Mississippi on a coal barge. (In 1894 U.S. laws forbade people with leprosy from traveling on any form of public transportation.) They landed at an abandoned, rundown plantation that the State of Louisiana had procured under the pretense of starting an ostrich farm, not wanting to alarm neighbors. A few slave cabins were still standing, populated mainly by rats, bats, and snakes. The seven patients moved into the "Louisiana Leper Home," but the state had difficulty recruiting workers for the leprosarium. Finally the Daughters of Charity, an order of Catholic nuns, volunteered. These saintly women, nicknamed "The White Caps," did much of the initial labor. Getting up two hours before daylight to pray, wearing starched white uniforms in bayou heat, the nuns drained swamps, leveled roads, and repaired buildings for the new leprosarium. Their successors were still serving at Carville when I worked there a few years ago.

I hope and pray that in a hundred years or so, when the definitive history of the AIDS epidemic is written, the Christian church will play an equally noble role. So far, I see few signs. Government and publicly funded research is now providing the kind of scientific expertise on AIDS that mission hospitals provided for leprosy, and I see no need for the church to try to duplicate those efforts. But I do see an urgent need for the church to help break through the stigma surrounding AIDS and to respond with compassion and dignity. Because of my experience with leprosy patients, I know the difference such a response can make.

Once while living in Louisiana I saw a beautiful illustration of the church combating "bad stigma." The owner of a furniture store in Columbia, Mississippi, came with his family to Carville full of tears and questions. He had just been diagnosed with leprosy, and it felt to him like a death sentence. Who would ever shop at his store again? Would he become ugly and deformed? Would he live? How could he tell his extended family, his neighbors, his church that he had leprosy? I sat with him and told him the facts about leprosy, and in the process I learned he was an elder of his church. He asked me to help break the news to the congregation, and to allay their fears about contagion. I agreed to return with him to Columbia, and together we held several meetings with church groups. In a remarkable way, the entire church rallied around the family. The man's furniture business did not fall off. His church became a center of information on leprosy.

My favorite memory of a church's embracing a leprosy patient revolves around a patient in India named John Karmegan. He came to us in such an advanced state that we could do little for him surgically. We did, however, offer him a place to stay and employment in the New Life Center. John was a troublemaker from the beginning. Dark in complexion, he had borne the brunt of racism before contracting leprosy. Now, because of paralysis, his attempts to smile produced something more like a leer, and because people often responded with a gasp or a gesture of fear he simply learned not to smile. My wife, Margaret, stitched one of his eyelids partly closed to protect his sight, and this made his appearance even more unusual.

Several times we caught John stealing from other boys in the village. He treated fellow-patients cruelly and defied all authority, going so far as to organize hunger strikes against us. By almost anyone's reckoning, he was beyond rehabilitation.

Not by Granny Brand's reckoning. Perhaps attracted by John's very irredeemability, she adopted him as a special target of her evangelism. She took to John and spent time with him, and eventually he became a Christian. We baptized him in the cement tank used for construction materials.

Neither conversion nor baptism had much immediate effect on John's personality. He made friends with a few patients, but years of rejection had poisoned him against all nonpatients. "You're paid to do this work," he would say to me and the other health workers. "It's not because you're Christians, or because you care about me. It's because you're paid. Nobody likes an ugly face, and nobody wants a leper."

One day John made the same accusation at our church on the leprosarium grounds. "You're paid to take communion with me. It's your job. What would happen if I went to town? Do you think those people would let me in their church?" I had no answer for him.

Not long afterward I went to the leaders of the Tamil church in Vellore and talked to them about John. "Everyone can tell he has leprosy," I said. "He has a deformed face, his eyes are poor, and his hands are very clawed. But I can assure you his disease has been arrested. He poses no danger to others. Would you let him visit?" The elders agreed he could visit.

"Can he take communion?" I asked, knowing that the church used a common cup. The elders looked at each other hesitantly, and discussed the matter at length, but in the end they decided he could also take communion.

A few days later I accompanied John to the church, which met in a plain, whitewashed brick building with a corrugated iron roof. It was a tense moment for both of us. I could hardly imagine the trauma and paranoia a leprosy patient must feel attempting for the first time to enter that kind of public setting. We stood together at the back of the church. John's paralyzed face showed no reaction, but his trembling gave away his inner turmoil. I prayed silently that no church member would show him rejection.

As the congregation stood to sing the first hymn, an Indian man seated toward the back half-turned and saw us. We must have made an odd couple: a white foreigner standing next to a leprosy patient with patches of his skin in garish disarray. I held my breath.

And then it happened. The man put down his hymnal, smiled broadly, and patted the bench next to him, inviting John to join him. John could not have been more startled. Haltingly, he made shuffling half-steps to the row and took his seat. I breathed a prayer of thanks.

That one incident proved to be the turning point of John's life. Medical treatments, compassionate care, rehabilitation—each step had helped, but it was a stranger's inviting a deformed Christian brother to break bread with him that truly changed John. He emerged from that service shining with joy.

Years later, after I had moved to America, I visited Vellore and made a side trip to a factory set up to employ the disabled. The manager wanted to show me a new machine that produced tiny screws for typewriter parts. As we walked through the noisy plant, which reeked of diesel fuel, he shouted at me that he wanted to introduce me to his prize employee. This man had just won the Swedish typewriter company's All-India prize for producing the most parts with the fewest errors.

When we arrived at the prize employee's work station, he turned to greet us and I found myself looking at the unmistakable crooked face of John Karmegan. He wiped the grease off his stumpy hand, shook mine, and grinned with the ugliest, loveliest, most radiant smile I had ever seen. Then he held out for my inspection a handful of the small precision screws that had won him the prize.

A simple gesture of acceptance may not seem like much. For John Karmegan, however, it proved decisive. Because of the love shown in a tiny church in Vellore, John's old wounds healed. Perhaps for the first time, he felt free of the oppressive burden of shame and rejection. He felt like a human being again. The marks of his disease—the stigmata—had not changed. But as a verse in the New Testament puts it, "Perfect love drives out fear." It drives out stigma as well.

Acknowledgments

Dr. Paul Brand and Philip Yancey have coauthored two previous books, *Fearfully and Wonderfully Made* and *In His Image*, both published by Zondervan Publishing House, a division of HarperCollins. Recently Dr. Brand has also written *The Forever Feast*, published by Servant Publications. Some of the stories in this book of memoirs appear in different form in these other books, and the authors wish to thank the publishers for their cooperation. Also, Dorothy Clarke Wilson's *Ten Fingers for God* proved to be an invaluable resource.

The authors are deeply grateful to those who gave wise and needed guidance in improving the manuscript, especially Judith Markham, Tim Stafford, Harold Fickett, Pauline Brand, David and Kathy Neely, and the book's editors, Karen Rinaldi and John Sloan.

Bibliography

Ackerman, Diane. *A Natural History of the Senses*. New York: Random House, 1990.

Berna, Steven. *Pain and Religion: A Psychophysiological Study*. Springfield, Ill.: Charles C. Thomas, Publisher, 1972.

Brand, Paul. *Clinical Mechanics of the Hand*. Saint Louis: C. V. Mosby Company, 1985.

Brand, Paul, and Philip Yancey. *Fearfully and Wonderfully Made*. Grand Rapids, Mich.: Zondervan Publishing House, 1980.

————. *In His Image*. Grand Rapids, Mich.: Zondervan Publishing House, 1984.

Brody, Saul Nathaniel. *The Disease of the Soul: Leprosy in Medieval Literature*. Ithaca, N.Y.: Cornell University Press, 1974.

Callahan, Daniel. *What Kind of Life: The Limits of Medical Progress*. New York: Simon and Schuster, 1990.

Cannon, Walter B. *The Wisdom of the Body*. New York: W. W. Norton and Company, 1939.

Cassell, Eric J., M.D. "The Nature of Suffering and the Goals of Medicine." *New England Journal of Medicine* 306, no. 11 (1982): 639–45.

Castillo, Stephani J. "Viewer's Discussion Guide for *Simple Courage*, a One-Hour Television Documentary." Honolulu: Olena Productions, 1992.

Christman, R. J. *Sensory Experience*. Scranton, Penn.: Intext Educational Publishers, 1971.

Cousins, Norman. *Anatomy of an Illness as Perceived by the Patient*. New York: W. W. Norton and Company, 1979.

————. *Human Options*. New York: W.W. Norton and Company, 1981.

————. *The Healing Heart: Antidotes to Panic and Helplessness*. New York: Avon Books, 1983.

————. *Head First: The Biology of Hope*. New York: E. P. Dutton, 1989.

Dougherty, Flavian, ed. *The Deprived, the Disabled, and the Fullness of Life*. Wilmington, Del.: Michael Glazier, 1984.

Eccles, John C., *The Human Mystery*. New York: Springer-Verlag, 1979.

———. *The Human Psyche*. New York: Springer-Verlag, 1980.

Eccles, Sir John, and Daniel N. Robinson. *The Wonder of Being Human: Our Brain and Our Mind*. New York: Free Press/Macmillan, 1984.

Feeny, Patrick. *The Fight against Leprosy*. New York: American Leprosy Missions, 1964.

Frank, Jerome D. *Persuasion and Healing*. Baltimore: Johns Hopkins University Press, 1973.

Frankl, Viktor E. *The Doctor and the Soul*. New York: Alfred A. Knopf, 1965.

Grass, Günther, *Show Your Tongue*. New York: Harcourt Brace Jovanovich, 1988.

Greene, Graham. *Ways of Escape*. New York: Simon and Schuster, 1982.

Gregory, R. L., ed. *Illusion in Nature and Art*. New York: Charles Scribner's Sons, 1973.

Gregory, R. L. *Eye and Brain: The Psychology of Seeing*. New York: McGraw-Hill Book Company, 1978.

Hansel, Tim. *You Gotta Keep Dancin'*. Elgin, Ill.: David C. Cook Publishing Company, 1985.

Hardy, James D., Harold G. Wolff, and Helen Goodell. *Pain Sensations and Reactions*. New York: Hafner Publishing Company, 1967.

Harth, Eric. *Windows on the Mind*. New York: William Morrow and Company, 1982.

Hunt, Morton. *The Universe Within: A New Science Explores the Human Mind*. New York: Simon and Schuster, 1982.

Illich, Ivan. *Medical Nemesis: The Expropriation of Health*. New York: Pantheon Books, 1976.

Jagadisan, T. N. *Fulfillment through Leprosy*. Tamil Nadu, India: Kasturba Kusta Nivaran Nilayam, 1988.

Kline, David. "The Power of the Placebo." *Hippocrates* (May/June 1988):24–26.

Komp, Diane M. *A Window to Heaven: When Children See Life in Death*. Grand Rapids, Mich.: Zondervan Publishing House, 1992.

Lankford, L. Lee. "Reflex Sympathetic Dystrophy." *Rehabilitation of the Hand: Surgery and Therapy*, ed. by Hunter, Schneider, Mackin, and Callahan. St. Louis: C. V. Mosby Company, 1990, 763–75.

Lapierre, Dominique. *The City of Joy*. New York: Warner, 1985.

Lewis, Thomas, M.D. *Pain*. New York: Macmillan Company, 1942.

Lipton, Sampson. *Conquering Pain*. New York: Arco Publishing, 1984.

Loeser, John D. "Phantom Limb Pain." *Current Concepts in Pain* 2. no. 2 (1984): 3–8.

Lynch, James J. *The Broken Heart: The Medical Consequences of Loneliness*. New York: Basic Books, 1977.

Macfarlane, Gwyn. *Alexander Fleming: The Man and the Myth*. Cambridge, Mass.: Harvard University Press, 1984.

Melzack, Ronald. "The Perception of Pain." *Scientific American* 233 (February 1961): 1–13.

———. *The Puzzle of Pain*. New York: Basic Books, 1973.

———. "The Tragedy of Needless Pain." *Scientific American* 262 (February 1990): 27–33.

———. "Phantom Limbs." *Scientific American* 264 (April 1992): 120–26.

Malzack, Ronald, and Patrick D. Wall. *The Challenge of Pain*, rev. ed. London: Penguin Books, 1988.

Menninger, Karl. M.D. *The Vital Balance: The Life Process in Mental Health and Illness*. New York: Viking Press, 1963.

Miller, Jonathan. *The Body in Question*. New York: Random House, 1978.

Moore, Henry Thomas. *Pain and Pleasure*. New York: Moffat, Yard and Company, 1917.

Mooris, David B. *The Culture of Pain*. Berkeley: University of California Press, 1991.

Muller, Robert. *Most of All, They Taught Me Happiness*. New York: Doubleday and Company, 1978.

Naipul, V. S. *India: A Wounded Civilization*. New York: Alfred A. Knopf, 1977.

———. *India: A Million Mutinies Now*. New York: Viking Press, 1990.

Oatley, Keith. *Brain Mechanisms*. New York: E. P. Dutton, 1972.

Olshan, Neal H. *Power over Your Pain—Without Drugs*. New York: Beaufort Books, 1983.

Pace, J. Blair. *Pain: A Personal Experience*. Chicago: Nelson-Hall, 1976.

Peck, M. Scott. *The Road Less Traveled.* New York: Simon and Schuster, 1978.

Penfield, Wilder, *The Cerebral Cortex of Man: A Critical Study of Localization of Function.* New York: Macmillan Company, 1950.

———. *The Mystery of the Mind: A Critical Study of Consciousness and the Human Brian.* Princeton, N.J.: Princeton University Press, 1975.

Penn, Jack. *The Right to Look Human: An Autobiography.* Johannesburg: Hugh Keartland Publishers, 1976.

Penrose, Roger. *The Emperor's New Mind: Concerning Computers, Minds, and the Laws of Physics.* New York: Oxford University Press, 1989.

Register, Cheri. *Living with Chronic Illness.* New York: Free Press, 1987.

Russell, Wilfrid. *New Lives for Old: The Story of the Cheshire Homes.* London: Victor Gollancz, Ltd., 1980.

Ryle, Gilbert. *The Concept of Mind.* Chicago: University of Chicago Press, 1949.

Sacks, Oliver. *A Leg to Stand On.* New York: Harper and Row, 1984.

———. *The Man Who Mistook His Wife for a Hat and Other Clinical Tales.* New York: Simon and Schuster, 1985.

———. "Neurology and the Soul." *The New York Review of Books* (November 22, 1990), pp. 44–50.

Scarry, Elaine. *The Body in Pain: The Making and Unmaking of the World.* New York: Oxford University Press, 1985.

Selye, Hans. *From Dream to Discovery: On Being a Scientist.* New York: McGraw-Hill Book Company, 1964.

———. *The Stress of Life,* rev. ed. New York: McGraw-Hill Book Company, 1976.

Selzer, Richard. *Mortal Lessons: Notes on the Art of Surgery.* New York: Simon and Schuster, 1976.

———*Confessions of a Knife.* New York: Simon and Schuster, 1979.

Shenson, Douglas. "When Fear Conquers: A Doctor Learns abouts AIDS from Leprosy." *New York Times Magazine* (February 28, 1988), pp. 35–48.

Siegel, Bernie S. *Love, Medicine & Miracles.* New York: Harper and Row, 1986.

Snyder, Solomon. "Matter over Mind: The Big Issues Raised by Newly Discovered Brain Chemicals." *Psychology Today* (June 1980), pp. 66–76.

Soelle, Dorothy. *Suffering*. Philadelphia: Fortress Press, 1945.

Somervell, T. Howard. *Knife and Life in India*. London: Livingstone Press, 1955.

Sontag, Susan. *Illness as Metaphor*. New York: Farrar, Straus and Giroux, 1978.

———. *AIDS and Its Metaphors*. New York: Farrar, Straus and Giroux, 1989.

Stacy, Charles B., Andrew S. Kaplan, and Gray Williams, Jr., and the Editors of Consumer Reports Books. *The Fight against Pain*. Yonkers, N.Y.: Consumer Reports Books, 1992.

Stein, Stanley, with Lawrence G. Blochman. *Alone No Longer*. Carville, La.: The Star, 1974.

Szasz, Thomas S., M.D. *Pain and Pleasure: A Study of Bodily Feelings*. New York: Basic Books, 1957.

This Spreading Tree: The Story of the Leprosy Mission from 1918 to 1970. London: Leprosy Mission, 1974.

Thomas, Lewis. *Late Night Thoughts on Listening to Mahler's Ninth Symphony*. New York: Viking Press, 1983.

———. *The Youngest Science: Notes of a Medicine-Watcher*. New York: Viking Press, 1983.

Tiger, Lionel. *The Pursuit of Pleasure*. Boston: Little, Brown and Company, 1992.

Tournier, Paul. *Creative Suffering*. San Francisco: Harper and Row, 1982.

Valenstein, Elliot S. *Great and Desparate Cures: The Rise and Decline of Psychosurgery and Other Radical Treatments for Mental Illness*. New York: Basic Books, 1986.

Vaux, Kenneth L. *This Mortal Coil: The Meaning of Health and Disease*. New York: Harper and Row, 1978.

Veninga, Robert L. *A Gift of Hope: How We Survive Our Tragedies*. Boston: Little, Brown and Company, 1985.

Wakefield, Dan. *Returning: A Spiritual Journey*. New York: Penguin Books, 1988.

Wall, Patrick D. "'My Foot Hurts Me': An Analysis of a Sentence." *Essays on the Nervous System; a Festschrift for Professor J. Z. Young*. Oxford: Clarendon Press, 1984.

Wall, Patrick D., and Ronald Melzack, ed. *Textbook of Pain*. London: Churchill Livingston, 1984.

Waylett-Rendall, Janet. "Therapist's Management of Reflex Sympathetic Dystrophy." *Rehabilitation of the Hand: Surgery and Therapy*, ed. James M. Hunter, M.D., Lawrence H. Schneider, M.D., Evelyn J.

MacKin, P.T., and Anne D. Callahan, M.S., O.T.R. St. Louis: C. V. Mosby Company, 1990, pp. 787–89.

Weisenberg, Matisyohu, ed. *Pain: Clinical and Experimental Perspectives*. St. Louis: C. V. Mosby Company, 1975.

Whitfield, Philip, and D. M. Stoddart. *Hearing, Taste, and Smell: Pathways of Perception*. New York: Torstar Books, 1984.

Wilson, Dorothy Clarke. *Granny Brand: Her Story*. Chappaqua, N.Y.: Christian Herald Books, 1976.

————. *Ten Fingers for God: The Life and Work of Dr. Paul Brand*. Grand Rapids, Mich.: Zondervan Publishing House, 1989.

Wolf, Barbara. *Living with Pain*. New York: Seabury Press, 1977.

Yancey, Philip. *Where Is God When It Hurts?* Grand Rapids, Mich.: Zondervan Publishing House, 1990.

Zinsser, Hans. *As I Remember Him: The Biography of R. S.* Boston: Little, Brown and Company, 1940.